A COMPREHENSIVE P[

MEDICAL
GENETICS

A COMPREHENSIVE PRIMER ON

MEDICAL GENETICS

Theodore F. Thurmon, MD

Professor of Pediatrics
Director of Medical Genetics
Louisiana State University
School of Medicine
Shreveport, LA

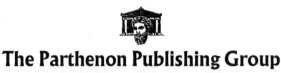

The Parthenon Publishing Group
International Publishers in Medicine, Science & Technology

NEW YORK   LONDON

Published in the USA by
The Parthenon Publishing Group Inc.
One Blue Hill Plaza, PO Box 1564
Pearl River, New York 10965, USA

Published in the UK and Europe by
The Parthenon Publishing Group Limited
Casterton Hall, Carnforth
Lancs. LA6 2LA, UK

Library of Congress Cataloging-in-Publication Data
Thurmon, Theodore F., 1937–
   A comprehensive primer on medical genetics /
Theodore F. Thurmon.
       p. cm.
   Includes bibliographical references and index.
   ISBN 1-85070-066-4
   1. Medical genetics--Programmed instruction. I. Title.
   [DNLM: 1. Genetics, Medical outlines. QZ 18.2 T539c 1999]
   RB155.T537   1999
   616'042--dc21
   DNLM/DLC
   for Library of Congress   99-10581
                                               CIP

British Library Cataloging in Publication Data
Thurmon, T.F.
   A comprehensive primer on medical genetics
   1. Medical genetics
   I. Title
   6.6'.042

ISBN 1-85070-066-4

Printed and bound in the USA

Contents

Acknowledgments: This book resulted from recurrent revisions to a manuscript for the still unpublished second edition of another (*Thurmon TF. Rare Genetic Diseases*. Cleveland: CRC Press, 1974). It would not have reached this stage without help. Dr. Victor A. McKusick provided massive initial and maintenance infusions of knowledge. Dr. Samuel H. Boyer taught me concise thinking. Dr. Marie Louise Buyse shared the vision that order can be found in information chaos. Dr. Susonne A. Ursin gathered much of the data for the original version. Suzanne Greenwood Thurmon shouldered the massive burden of organizing and indexing the text. Numerous other mentors, colleagues, and students contributed in many ways. The personnel of the Medical Libraries at the Louisiana State University Schools of Medicine in Shreveport and in New Orleans were immensely and incessantly helpful.

Illustrations were produced individually by the author at Cameo Studio. Original ink drawings were either scanned into computer files and edited, or rendered directly into computer files with graphics software. The pixel size was 0.26 mm (~ 96 dpi) because of the intended use in teaching materials. Higher resolution drawings do not reproduce well on some display devices. Also in the interest of reproduction, bit-mapped graphics were used instead of vector graphics. In some cases, illustrations in the literature were used as models. Illustrations modeled from the literature are identified by notation within the illustrations and are used by permission.

PREFACE

The primary use of this *Primer* has been that of a set of notes for a course in medical school. It has grown in pace with the breadth of the subject and has become a textbook which characterizes the specialty of Medical Genetics. The "notes" format seems to aid in comprehension and memory so it has been preserved. No other textbook of Medical Genetics explains all of the pivotal themes of this subject or the actual management of the clinical problems. Other textbooks cover many points well but all of them leave deep unbridged gaps of knowledge that tantalize the reader who meets genetic diseases face-to-face.

To document all of the concepts in this *Primer*, it was necessary to bring in material from many sources and assimilate it into an understandable form. General references are listed after this Preface. The main purpose of that list is documentation; however, so many tried and true concepts of Medical Genetics are so diametrically opposed to popular notions that these references may help in the re-learning process. More specific references are listed after each chapter. The "notes" format may suffice for persons who already have an elementary understanding of Genetics but supplemental reading can aid comprehension at all levels.

Methods of programmed instruction were used to construct the chapters so the *Primer* can be used for self-instruction. It also supports a problem-based-learning approach. It is intended to introduce Medical Genetics to medical students or to graduates who have not yet had a course in this subject but may also serve to bring others up to speed in Medical Genetics. "Up to speed" can be loosely interpreted to mean what a knowledgeable person might wish to know about this field. Health professionals who provide services to persons with genetic problems, and well-educated patients and their family members have found parts of this volume interesting and helpful in understanding the genetic problems that confront them. It has been used by candidates for degrees other than the MD and has proven to be a worthwhile general introduction to the field of human genetics. It contains basic knowledge of Medical Genetics needed by primary-care physicians.

Each item in the *Primer* represents a concept that is important to either the understanding or the practice of medical genetics. The items are presented as core concepts with little exposition. Each concept has been extensively checked against current references and represents accepted dogma (either patently correct or, at least, majority opinion). In rare instances, such as the semantics of the terms, polygenic and multifactorial, the concepts stem from the author's personal experience and investigations; however, their accuracy has also been documented. In addition to the core concepts, numbers of lists and tables that are useful in study and in clinical practice are included. The material in the Appendices is of special interest.

Chapters after the first build upon the concepts in previous chapters so that a logical order of thought is established. Molecular Genetics is covered before Mendelian Genetics since the aim is comprehension rather than historical correctness. Mathematical aspects are covered in enough detail that the reader is not required to make conceptual leaps, i.e., all of the steps are there (a characteristic that may be unique to this volume). It is the view of the author that the mathematical aspects are crucial to the understanding of the meaning of genetics in modern life. Abominations of public policy and squandering of public funds have arisen directly from failure to comprehend these aspects of the science.

The science of Medical Genetics is composed of a mixture of two disciplines, Genetics and Medicine. Basic genetics occurs almost exclusively at the microscopic or molecular level. In even the most overt of genetic events, no part of the genetic mechanism is perceived by the senses. This aspect is reviewed in Chapter 1, Tenets of Genetics. It is a vast area of science which is mostly the purview of scholars other than physicians. Emphasis is placed on the principles that are important to the understanding of observable genetic events. These principles have changed relatively little during the current rapid pace of research in this field. Persons with a background in Genetics may find little new in this chapter.

The next three chapters describe Genetic Animism. In the primal state, Genetics is an efficient plan for how to live on the planet Earth. Left alone, it would remain, for the most part, unperceived. Our departures from the primal state fan this smoldering phenomenon into flame and give it life. The term for imbuing an otherwise inanimate object with life is animism. Another way of looking at this phenomenon is that the object already has life and that there are things which we do that allow us or force us to perceive it. The perception of most interest to us is genetic disease. These chapters concern what we do to the genetic mechanism to make it produce countable numbers of cases of genetic diseases, and about the epidemiology of this process.

Chapter 5 is the first of four chapters about the tools of the trade, techniques of diagnosis in the clinic and in the laboratory. These subjects are prone either to omission from medical education, or to misconception. The physician needs to know what to look for, how to find it, which tests to order, why the tests cost so much and how to evaluate the test results.

Chapter 9 concerns our genetic uniqueness. Many of the concepts have legal meaning in tracing derivation. Disease can arise due to molecular confusion between self and non-self. Success in transfusion and other forms of transplantation requires detailed knowledge of genetic characteristics so that there can be as close a match as possible between the recipient and the donor. Twinning is a natural phenomenon that tests the rules of self and non-self and often results in disease.

Chapter 10 begins a discussion of common clinical problems by reviewing the principles and problems of developmental genetics. It leads into a chapter on congenital anomalies which is supplemented by a monograph on syndrome identification in Appendix 3. The index of that monograph is of topical interest in that it dispels notions of the diagnostic value of specific features. With few exceptions, most features and combinations of features are shared by several disorders. The same is true of disorders of later onset (Ball MJ [1980]).

The next four chapters treat of the more frequent genetic diseases, and thereby provide a working answer to the perennial question as to which genetic diseases are the "significant" ones. To a patient or a patient's relative, the significant disease is the one afflicting that patient but frequency has to loom large as a measure of significance to the physician since the more frequent diseases are more likely to be seen by the physician. The more frequent diseases also account for the most human suffering and the greatest expenditure of medical care resources.

Chapter 16 departs into more unusual disorders. The first page lists all genetic diseases for which we have reliable incidence data. In this chapter on Genetic Erudita, we discuss the rarest of them. These diseases have been imbued with significance by various authorities but a primary physician may never have a patient with any of them. However, their etiologies run the gamut of mechanisms of causation of genetic diseases so it is of value to use them as vehicles of study. Their frequency is disproportionately high in Medical Genetics clinics.

Chapter 17 concerns Pharmacogenetics and Genetic Therapeutics. It contains concepts important to the first rule of our profession, *primere non nocere* (first, do not harm). Genetic variations not related to any disease can result in disease if drugs are used indiscriminately. Those concepts are extended into areas of popular interest along the lines of "first, do not misunderstand." Naturally occurring genetic variation can appear to be the result of xenobiotics if not analyzed properly. Successful treatment of a genetic disease requires careful study of each case. One finds that most diagnoses are really categories, but it is the details of each case that determine results.

Chapter 18 begins a section about Applied Genetics. Medical practice treats mostly of diseases with a genetic basis but most of what is practiced is medicine. There is also a practice of genetics. It concerns the identification of patients who merit Medical Genetics services, the assessment of the amount of genetic risk in diverse situations, and the mechanisms of management of that risk. In chapter 19, ethical guidelines are also discussed.

Though there were some well-meaning persons involved, the old concept of eugenics as the science of achieving some imagined ideal human was mostly the product of sick and ignorant minds. Through Applied Genetics, there are things that we can do to assist individuals to realize the fullest potential of their genetic characteristics. This is the new eugenics.

A chapter on Public Health Aspects outlines practical considerations of the epidemiology of genetic diseases. The discussion is mostly heuristic but there is a sufficiently broad set of topics as to impart to the reader some of the principles that are important to this sector of Medical Genetics. An added attraction is a discussion of some diseases for which the actions of special interest groups have placed specific responsibilities on the physician. The table, Indications for Proband Services, serves as a worthwhile guide to what Medical Geneticists do.

Theodore F. Thurmon
LSU School of Medicine
Shreveport, LA
July 1, 1998

BIBLIOGRAPHY

Ball M J. Features of Creutzfeld-Jacob disease in brains of patients with familial dementia of Alzheimer type. Canad J Neurol Sci 1980;7:51-51.

Behrman RE (editor). *Nelson Textbook of Pediatrics*, 14th edition. Philadelphia: Saunders, 1992.

Benson PF, Fensom AH. *Genetic Biochemical Disorders*. Oxford Monographs on Medical Genetics No. 12. New York: Oxford, 1985.

Berini RY, Kahn E. *Clinical Genetics Handbook*. Oradell, NJ: Medical Economics Books, 1987.

Bernstam VA. *Pocket Guide to Gene Level Diagnostics in Clinical Practice*. Boca Raton: CRC Press, 1993.

Bodmer WF (editor). *Inheritance of Susceptibility to Cancer in Man*. New York: Oxford, 1982.

Connor JM, Ferguson-Smith MA. *Essential Medical Genetics*. Oxford: Blackwell, 1991.

Darnell J, Lodish H, Baltimore D. *Molecular Cell Biology*, 2nd edition. Scientific American Books. New York: WH Freeman, 1990.

DeGrouchy J, Turleau C. *Clinical Atlas of Human Chromosomes*, 2nd edition. New York: Wiley, 1984.

Edlin G. *Human Genetics*. Boston: Jones & Bartlett, 1990.

Emery AEH, Rimoin DL. *Principles and Practice of Medical Genetics*, 2nd edition. New York: Churchill Livingstone, 1990.

Evans MI. *Reproductive Risks and Prenatal Diagnosis*. Norwalk, CT: Appleton & Lange, 1992.

Filkins K, Russo JF. *Human Prenatal Diagnosis*, 2nd edition. New York: Marcel Dekker, 1990.

Fuhrmann W, Vogel F. *Genetic Counseling*, 2nd edition. Heidelberg Science Library. New York: Springer-Verlag, 1976.

Gardner EJ, Simmons MJ, Snustad DP. *Principles of Genetics*, 8th edition. New York: Wiley, 1991.

Gelehrter TD, Collins FS. *Principles of Medical Genetics*. Baltimore: Williams and Wilkins, 1990.

Gershon ES. Genetics of the affective disorders. Hospital Practice, 1979;March Issue, 117-122.

Goedde HW, Agarwal DP (editors). *Alcoholism. Biomedical and Genetic Aspects*. New York: Pergamon Press, 1989.

Harper P. *Practical Genetic Counseling*, 3rd edition. Boston: Wright, 1988.

Hollingsworth DR, Resnik R (editors). *Medical Counseling Before Pregnancy*. New York; Churchill Livingstone, 1988.

Holmes GL. Diagnosis and Mangement of Seizures in Children. Philadelphia: Saunders, 1987.

Holton JB. The Inherited Metabolic Disease. New York: Churchill Livingstone, 1987.

Hommes FA (editor). *Techniques in Diagnostic Human Biochemical Genetics. A Laboratory Manual.* New York: Wiley-Liss, 1990.

Jones KL. Smith's Recognizable Patterns of Human Malformation. 4th edition. Philadelphia: Saunders, 1988.
- The basic "picture book", illustrating 292 disorders diagnosable by inspection.
- Introduction and Chapters 2 through 7 comprise a brief textbook of basic Medical Genetics and Dysmorphology.

Levitan M. Textbook of Human Genetics. New York: Oxford, 1988.

Lynch HT, Hirayama T (editors). Genetic Epidemiology of Cancer. Boca Raton: CRC Press, 1989.

Mange AP, Mange EJ. *Genetics: Human Aspects*, 2nd edition. Sunderland, MA:Sinauer, 1990.

McKusick VA. *Mendelian Inheritance in Man. Catalogues of Autosomal Dominant, Autosomal Recessive, and X-linked Phenotypes*, 10th edition. Baltimore: The Johns Hopkins Press, 1992.
- An annotated bibliography of 4937 genetic disease phenotypes.
- An ethical and legal essential to the practice of medicine.
- Pages ix to clxxiv comprise a brief textbook of advanced Medical Genetics.

Moore KL. *The Developing Human. Clinically Oriented Embryology*, 3rd edition. Philadelphia: Saunders, 1982.

Muench KH. *Genetic Medicine*. New York: Elsevier, 1988.

Murphy EA, Chase GA. *Principles of Genetic Counseling*. Chicago: Year Book Medical Publishers, 1975.

Nora JJ, Fraser FC. *Medical Genetics. Principles and Practice*, 3rd edition. Philadelphia: Lea & Febiger, 1989.

Patten BM. *Human Embryology*. New York: McGraw-Hill, 1968.

Pierpont MEM, Moller JH. *Genetics of Cardiovascular Diseases*. Boston: Martinus Nijhoff Publishing, 1987.

Romero R, Pilu G, Jeanty P, et al. *Prenatal Diagnosis of Congenital Anomalies*. Norwalk CT: Appleton & Lange, 1988.

Sadler TW. *Langman's Medical Embryology*. Baltimore: Williams & Wilkins, 1990.

Scriver CR, Beaudet AL, Sly WS, et al (editors). *The Metabolic and Molecular Bases of Inherited Disease. 7th Edition*. New York: McGraw-Hill, 1995.
- The first nine chapters are an important supplementary textbook.
- The remainder is useful for management of individual metabolic diseases.

Shepard TH. *Catalog of Teratogenic Agents*, 6th edition. Baltimore: The Johns Hopkins Press, 1989.
- An annotated bibliography of 1353 teratogenic agents.
- Includes data on man and experimental animals, mostly the latter.

Stine GJ. The New Human Genetics. Dubuque: Wm.C.Brown, 1989.

Suzuki DT, Griffiths AJF, Miller JH, et al. *An Introduction to Genetic Analysis*, 4th edition. New York: WH Freeman, 1989.

Thompson, MW, McInnes RR, Willard HF. *Thompson & Thompson Genetics in Medicine*. Philadelphia: Saunders, 1991.

Tsaung MT, Faraone SV. *The Genetics of Mood Disorders*. Baltimore: The Johns Hopkins Press, 1990.

Vandenberg SG, Singer SM, Pauls DL. *The Heredity of Behavior Disorders in Adults and Children*. New York: Plenum Medical Book Company, 1986.

Vogel F, Motulsky AG. *Human Genetics. Problems and Approaches*, 2nd edition. New York: Springer-Verlag, 1986.

Watson JD, Tooze J, Kurtz DT. *Recombinant DNA. A Short Course*. Scientific American Books. New York: W.H.Freeman, 1983.

Weaver DD (1989): *Catalogue of Prenatally Diagnosed Conditions*. Baltimore: The Johns Hopkins Press, 1989.

Wyngaarden JB, Smith LH, Bennett JC. *Cecil Textbook of Medicine*, 19th edition. Philadelphia: Saunders, 1992.

1. A eukaryote has its DNA in a nuclear membrane;
    - a prokaryote does not. Most knowledge of molecular genetics was
    - discovered in prokaryotes and later extended to eukaryotes.

- DNA is:
    - 10% non-coding highly repetitive sequences,
    - 30% moderately repetitive sequences and
    - 60% non-coding unique sequences.

- The rare DNA sequences that code for amino acid chains are
    - structural genes and are interspersed
    - in moderately repetitive DNA with much more frequent non-coding sequences.

- Ultracentrifugation of DNA yields one main band and
    - several small satellite bands which contain highly repetitive sequences, including
        - microsatellite simple sequence length polymorphisms (SSLP), 1 to 4 nucleotides long, mostly 2, throughout the genome, and
        - minisatellite variable number tandem repeats (VNTR), 11 to 60 nucleotides long, in heritable patterns mostly toward the telomeres.

    Polymorphism, from Gr. πολν μορφη: multiple forms (of a gene). Originally the occurrence of alleles too frequently to be due to recurrent mutation (Ford), but subsequently defined in usage by frequency: idiomorph < 0.01, polymorph between 0.01 and 0.99, monomorph > 0.99.

- Each of the two strands in the DNA double helix has a backbone of deoxyribose
    - attached to nucleotides that are paired through hydrogen bonds, with
        - adenine (A) complementary to thymine (T) and
        - cytosine (C) complementary to guanine (G).

- Two results of DNA nucleotide pairing are:
    - precise repair and precise replication.

- Eukaryotes have B-DNA which has
    - 10 nucleotides per right-handed turn
        - due to the amount of hydration,
    - but segments may form left-handed Z-DNA when methylated,
        - which renders the DNA genetically inactive.

- At a gene locus, the strand of DNA that is the functional gene is called the
    - coding or sense strand,

    while the opposite strand at that locus is called the
    - antisense strand.

- The RNA molecule differs from DNA in that it has
    - ribose in place of deoxyribose and
    - uracil (U) in place of thymine (T).

DNA is placed into a tube which contains layers of sucrose in graded concentrations. The tube is then centrifuged. The bottom of the tube is punctured and the contents pumped through a meter that reads absorption of UV light at 260 nm.

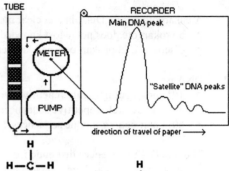

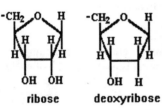

ribose   deoxyribose

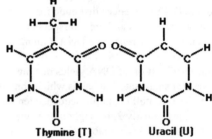

Thymine (T)   Uracil (U)

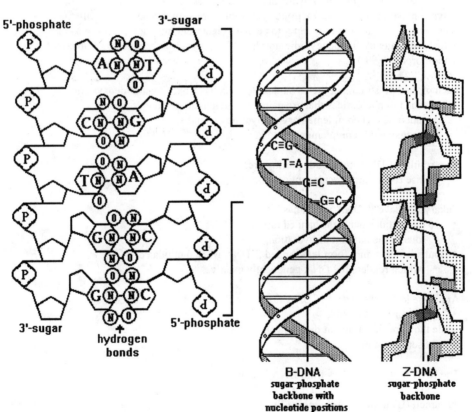

5'-phosphate   3'-sugar

3'-sugar   hydrogen bonds   5'-phosphate

B-DNA
sugar-phosphate backbone with nucleotide positions

Z-DNA
sugar-phosphate backbone

2.   DNA in the chromosome is wound twice around each
   •   nucleosome which are globular structures composed of
      •   two units each of 4 major histones and 1 linker histone.

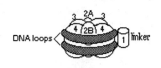

NUCLEOSOME
with histones numbered

Arrangement of nucleosomes
in the solenoid with linker histones internal

   •   Nucleosomes with complexed DNA are twisted into a
      •   helical structure called a solenoid.

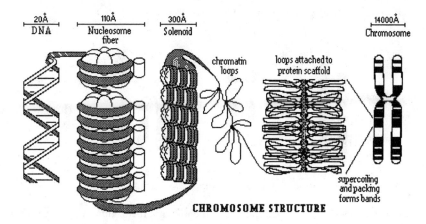

CHROMOSOME STRUCTURE

   •   Solenoids loop into 50-200 kb domains attached to the protein scaffold of the chromosome
      at scaffold attachment regions (SAR) between expressed genes,
      •   the scaffold is composed mainly of topoisomerase II,
      •   with lesser amounts of Sc 1 and Sc 2,
      •   as well as trace amounts of several regulatory DNA-binding proteins.

   •   Supercoiling and packing of solenoid loops forms chromosome bands which are constant
      identifiers but of unknown functional significance.

   •   Chromosome 1 contains about
      •   15 centimeters of DNA which at metaphase is compacted into
      •   3 micrometers.

   •   Euchromatin stains lightly and contains the expressed genes. It is termed
      •   facultative heterochromatin when it becomes inactivated.

- Constituitive heterochromatin stains deeply and is made up mostly of
  - highly repetitive sequences of DNA.

- Chromosomes are grouped by the position of the centromere:
  - Acrocentric: near one end. Submetacentric: off-center. Metacentric: near the middle.

- Major parts of a chromosome include:
  - the short arm, p,
  - the long arm, q,
  - the primary constriction or centromere, and
  - telomeres, which are tandem repeats of TTAGGG, an average of 10 kb in length.
    - Telomeres decrease by 40-90 bases per year of age.

- Acrocentric chromosomes have satellites, which are
  - separated from the tips of the short arms by secondary constrictions.

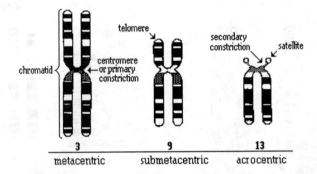

- The centromere contains a specific type of heterochromatin that forms a distinctive alpha satellite DNA made up of alphoid repeat DNA units of 170 base pairs, each of which is bound to a set of proteins that make up the kinetochore to which the spindle fibers attach.

- Humans have 2 sex chromosomes (X and Y), and 22 autosomes (1 through 22):

Group	Characteristic	Group	Characteristic
A (1 - 3)	metacentric	E (16 - 18)	metacentric or submetacentric
B (4 - 5)	submetacentric	F (19 - 20)	metacentric
C (6 - 12, X)	metacentric or submetacentric	G (21, 22, Y)	acrocentric with satellites
D (13 - 15)	acrocentric with satellites		(Y has no satellites)

- RNA from the secondary constrictions of the acrocentric chromosomes is
  - used in the nucleolus for synthesis of ribosomes.

- Chromosome bands are named by numbering them in a
  - sequential hierarchy outward from the centromere, i.e.,
  - 21q22 indicates sub-band 2 of major band 2 of the long arm of chromosome 21.

- A karyotype is the chromosome constitution with respect to number and morphology,
  - the term also being used for a photograph or print of the metaphase chromosomes of a single cell ordered by size, shape and banding pattern.

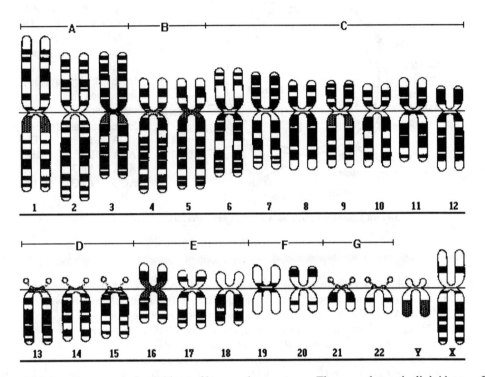

Note: This is a diagram of a haploid set of human chromosomes. The normal state is diploid, two of each chromosome. One is of maternal origin and one of paternal origin but each is genetically somewhat different from parental chromosomes because of crossovers during meiosis. However, there are few if any differences visible in the microscope.

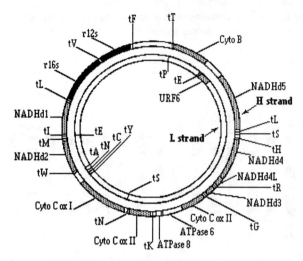

The mitochondrial chromosome is transcribed in toto and then cleaved into separate mRNAs. The tRNAs and rRNAs are used for mitochondrial protein synthesis.

Mitochondrial genes follow a genetic code different from nuclear genes:

Codon	Nucleus	Mitochondrion
UGA	ter	TRP
AUA	ILE	MET
AGA	ARG	ter
AGG	ARG	ter

t = transfer RNA (followed by 1 letter amino acid code)   r = ribosomal RNA

Chromosome M or 25

- The mitochondrial chromosome is a circular double helix of DNA of 16,539 base pairs,
  - containing 13 polypeptide subunits of oxidative phosphorylation enzymes, with
  - 2 rRNA genes, and 22 tRNA genes, necessary for their expression.
  - There are several alleles for each gene, some of which function poorly.
    - These disease-causing alleles accumulate with age.
  - Each mitochondrion contains about 10 of these chromosomes.
  - A typical somatic cell contains about 1,700 mitochondria.

- When mitochondria divide, segregation of the mitochondrial chromosomes is quantitative,
  - so subpopulations of cells tend to drift toward homoplasmy,
    - a condition in which all mitochondria have the same allele at a particular locus.
  - However, total homoplasmy is seldom realized,
    - so the normal state is some degree of heteroplasmy.

- Nearly all mitochondria of the zygote are contributed by the ovum, so
  - transmission of mitochondrial diseases is through the maternal line.
  - During oogenesis, mitochondria accumulate, so the ovum contains
    - about 10,000 mitochondria, or about 100,000 mitochondrial chromosomes.
  - However, a "bottleneck" of unknown nature results in only between 1 and 6 types of
    - mitochondrial chromosomes being represented in the zygote.

3. Two functions of DNA are:
  - exact transmission of genetic information, and
  - specification of sequences of amino acids in peptides.

- DNA replication is
  - semiconservative, each strand generating a new daughter strand
  - bidirectionally from a point of origin called a replicon which is
    - single in prokaryotes and
    - multiple in eukaryotes, each separated by 50 - 100 kb.

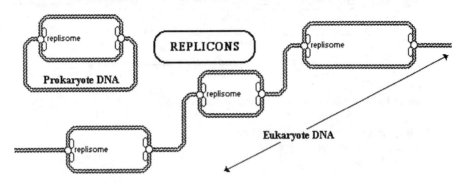

- DNA replication creates a daughter strand in a 5'→3' direction, so is
  - continuous for the leading strand but
  - discontinuous for the lagging strand.

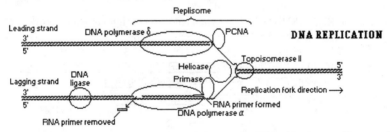

A protein similar to DNAa of *E. coli* activates the replisome. Helicase unwinds DNA and Topoisomerase II separates the strands. The Primase-DNA polymerase α complex attaches to the lagging strand. A 10 nucleotide RNA primer is formed where the strand meets Primase. DNA polymerase α elongates the strand in a 5' to 3' direction to form an Okizaki fragment of about 1000 nucleotides complementary to the lagging strand and then removes the RNA primer. DNA ligase fuses the fragment with the growing daughter strand, resulting in 3' to 5' elongation of the lagging chain. An accessory protein, Proliferating Cell Nuclear Antigen is required for leading strand synthesis and coordination of synthesis of both strands.

- Primase synthesizes the
  - RNA primer on the DNA template in the initial steps of DNA synthesis.

- At the replication fork,
  - short Okazaki fragments are synthesized and
  - linked by DNA ligase to form the lagging strand.

- In the process of transcription
  - triplet DNA codons produce primary RNA
  - which has nucleotides complementary to the sense strand of DNA.

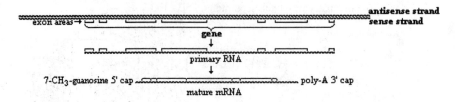

- Primary RNA is processed into messenger RNA (mRNA)
  - by excision of introns,
  - splicing of exons, and addition of a
  - 7-methyl guanosine 5' cap and a
  - poly-A 3' tail.

- The 5' cap facilitates binding of mRNA to ribosomes.

- One of the functions of introns is to promote splicing of exons.

- Ribosomes are formed of three types of
  - ribosomal RNA (rRNA) which are encoded by a contiguous segment of
  - nucleolar-associated DNA.

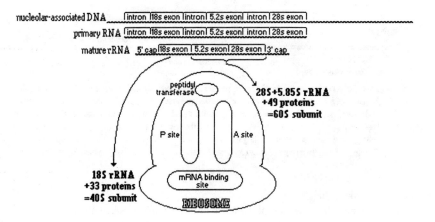

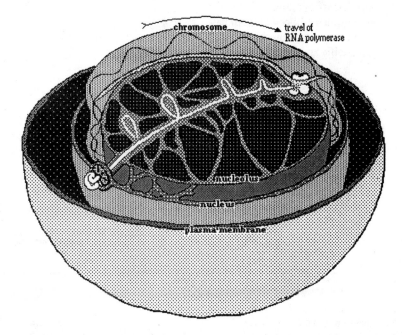

Physical Relationships During Processing of Pre-rRNA to Ribosomal Subunits

RNA polymerase I unwinds the sense strand of DNA from the chromosome and forms pre-rRNA. It is bound by proteins into the nucleolar fibrous network which intensifies around it and assembles spliceosomes that loop out the introns and splice the exons. The resulting rRNA molecule is transmitted along the nuclear fibrous network through a nuclear pore into the cytoplasm. Ribosomal and nucleolar proteins and, for the 60S subunit, the 5.85S rRNA, associate with the pre-rRNA as it is being processed, completing virtually all parts of the ribosomal subunit in the nucleolus. The 5.85S rRNA is synthesized outside of the nucleolus.

- Transfer RNA (tRNA) is distinguished from other forms of RNA
  - by its loops,
  - one of which (anticodon loop) has
    - 3 bases complementary to an mRNA codon that codes for a
    - specific amino acid according to the genetic code.

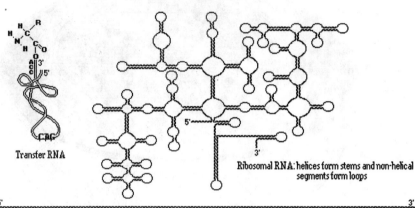

Transfer RNA

Ribosomal RNA: helices form stems and non-helical segments form loops

Messenger RNA: single-stranded

- Ribosomes translate
  - triplet nucleotide codons of messenger RNA into amino acids and produce
  - linear chains of amino acids called polypeptides.

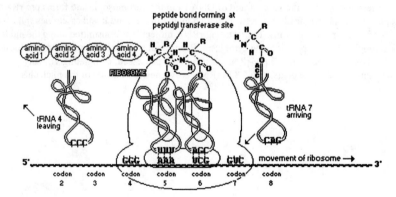

- Polypeptide synthesis is
  - initiated by the mRNA codon AUG and is
  - terminated by either UAA, UAG or UGA.

- Polypeptide chains become proteins by:
    - intra-chain folding and bonding,
    - combination with other amino acids, and
    - chemical removal of segments.

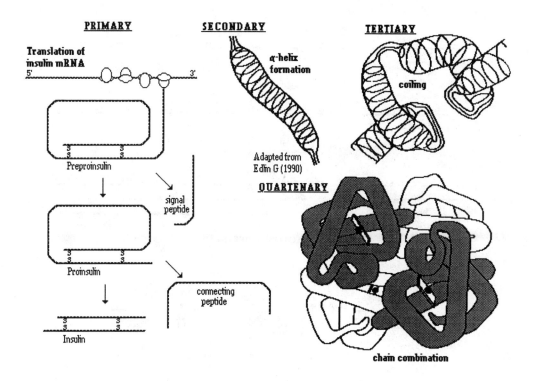

- Gene regulation in eukaryotes involves processes similar to the
  - operon of prokaryotes, important to which are
  - consensus sequences of DNA upstream from the transcriptional unit.

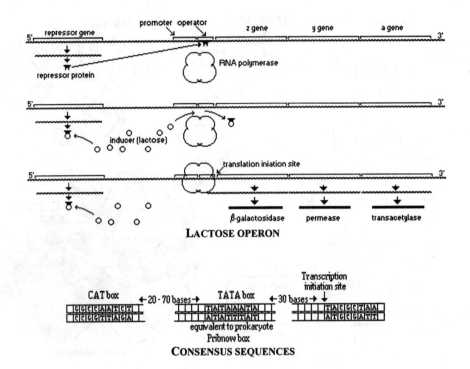

LACTOSE OPERON

CONSENSUS SEQUENCES

- Flanking regions on either side of a structural gene often function to
  - regulate gene expression and
    - their malfunction can produce a genetic disease in the
    - presence of a normal gene.

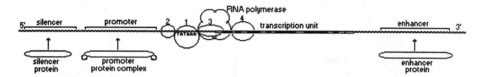

Eukaryotic gene regulation is mediated primarily by protein products of other genes, although numbers of other types of molecules may be required to complex with specific proteins to permit their regulatory functions. Enhancers or silencers may be located at distant sites on either side of a gene and may function bidirectionally, e.g., a silencer may decrease transcription when its protein product is present but may act to allow enhancers to work when it is inactive. More specific promoter regions are located upstream from the transcription unit and near to it. Transcription factors act directly to initiate transcription when the balance of other factors allows their activation. In the illustration, transcription factor 1 interacts with the TATA box, allowing factor 2 to attach to DNA and complex with factor 1. They then complex with factor 3 which attaches to DNA and protects it from digestion. RNA polymerase then attaches to the complex and factor 4 anchors it to DNA. Transcription then begins.

EUKARYOTIC GENE REGULATION

4.   Differentiated cell fuction occupies the G1 phase or Gap I.
  • Non-dividing, resting cells enter a "G0" state and do not proceed to the S phase.
  • Chromosome number is diploid 2N.

•   Late in G1 in dividing cells, DNA synthesis inducer appears, centrioles separate.

G1 (gap 1) 50%	S (synthesis) 28%	G2 (gap 2) 17%	M mitosis
differentiated cell function	DNA synthesis	synthesis of RNA followed by synthesis of chromosomal proteins	
DNA synthesis inducer appears at end of phase			5%
2N	2N	2N 4N	2N

TIME —→

PHASES OF THE CELL CYCLE. Intervals for cells growing in culture. G1 may be much longer in somatic cells.

•   The S phase or DNA synthesis: centrioles replicate, DNA unravels, each helix
  • acting as template for synthesis of a complementary copy or daughter strand
  • not formed into a chromosome so chromosome number remains 2N.

•   G2 phase or Gap II: synthesis of RNA that codes proteins that form chromosomes.
  • Centrosomes, each containing 2 centrioles, separate.
  • Chromosome number is 2N at the beginning of G2 and 4N at the end.

•   The M phase: mitosis.
  • No organized synapsis.
  • Crossing over is rare.

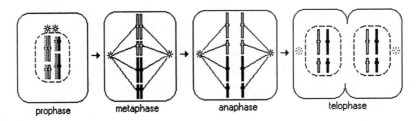

| prophase | metaphase | anaphase | telophase |

•   Prophase (chromosome number is 4N):
  • nucleolus breaks down, nuclear membrane breaks down,
  • centrosomes migrate and form the poles of the mitotic spindle.
  • chromosomes condense around the duplicated DNA,
  • centromeres duplicate,
  • each chromosome becomes visible as a pair of sister chromatids
    • close to the other chromosome but not in tetrad association.

- Metaphase: a spindle fiber from each centriole attaches to each
  - chromatid at the centromere.
  - Chromosome number is 4N.

- Anaphase: Chromatids separate, each going to a different pole.
  - Chromosome number is 4N.

- Telophase: Nuclear membranes form around chromosomes at each pole,
  - centrioles fade, chromosomes thin and elongate,
  - cytoplasm divides (cytokinesis).
  - Nucleoli reform and daughter cells enters G1.
  - Chromosome number at beginning is 4N and at end is 2N.

- Meiosis requires 2 divisions.

- Prophase I: differs from mitotic prophase in that
  - chromosomes appear to be long single threads when they become visible in spite of the fact that DNA has already duplicated.
  - Chromosome number is 4N.
  - There are several definable stages:

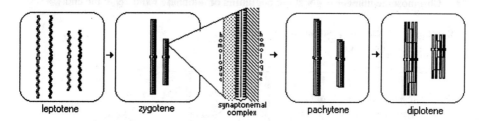

leptotene   zygotene   synaptonemal   pachytene   diplotene
                                     complex

- Leptotene: thready chromosomes with visible chromomeres.

- Zygotene: formation of the synaptonemal complex, a proteinaceous structure
  - associated with pairing (synapsis). Homologs appear to fuse into bivalents.
  - A brief burst of DNA synthesis associated with crossing-over.

- Pachytene: crossing over occurs but chiasmata are not visible.
  - Bivalents become tetrads as chromatids form on new DNA and become visible.

- Diplotene: bivalents loosen leaving chiasmata. Fetal oocytes begin to
  - reach this stage by week 12 of gestation then chromosomes thin and smudge
  - (dictyotene) in the primary oocytes until they are ovulated.

- Metaphase I: chromosomes migrate to the equatorial plane,
  - A spindle fiber from one centriole attaches to a centromere of one chromosome of a pair while a spindle fiber from the opposite centriole attaches to other.
  - This type of attachment leads to a reduction division.
  - In oogenesis, metaphase I occurs at the time of ovulation.
  - Chromosome number is 4N.

- Anaphase I: spindle fibers draw chromosomes toward centrioles.
  - Chromosome pairs segregate, one member of the pair going to one pole and one going to the opposite pole.
  - Chromosome number is 4N.

- Telophase I: Nuclear membranes form around chromosomes at poles,
  - chromosomes thin and elongate,
  - cytoplasm divides (cytokinesis).
  - The 46 chromatids in each daughter cell represent only 23 chromosomes so this was a reduction division.
  - In oogenesis, one daughter cell receives very little cytoplasm, and becomes a polar body.
  - The other becomes a secondary oocyte.
  - Chromosome number is 4N at the beginning of telophase I and 2N at the end.

- Interphase I: Brief chromosomal condensation.
  - Polar body enters G1.

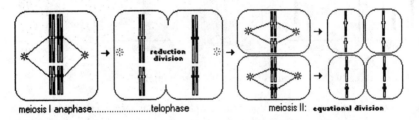

meiosis I anaphase.......................telophase   meiosis II: **equational division**

- Prophase II: Secondary oocyte and both secondary spermatocytes enter a stage similar to mitotic prophase.
  - In oogenesis, meiosis stops here unless there is fertilization.

- Metaphase II, Anaphase II: Similar to mitosis except that the chromatids are sisters;
  - a spindle fiber from one of the centrioles attaches to only one of the chromatids causing an equational division.

- Telophase II: Since Anaphase I resulted in 23 paired chromatids,
  - Telophase II leaves 23 single chromatids in each daughter cell (gamete).
  - Chromosome number is N (haploid).
  - In oogenesis, one daughter cell becomes the second polar body and enters G1
  - while the other becomes an ovum.
  - Since it must have already been fertilized to reach this gamete stage, the ovum's nucleus immediately becomes the female pronucleus which has motility and moves toward the male pronucleus.
  - Telophase in the first polar body usually does not proceed to cytokinesis.

- Interphase II: spermatid enters G1, matures into sperm.
  - Upon entry into the ovum, it matures further into the male pronucleus.

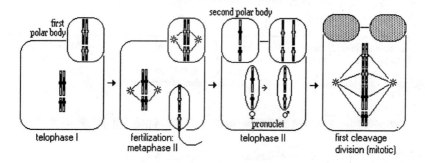

- Formation of the zygote occurs when female and male pronuclei approximate and loose their membranes.
  - Each haploid set of chromosomes replicates and the first cleavage division,
  - a mitotic division, ensues, initiating embryonic development.

- Cross-overs between members of a chromosome pair during mitosis is
  - called somatic recombination and,
  - in heterozygous individuals, can produce clones of homozygous cells.

- Cross-overs between chromatids of one chromosome during mitosis is
  - called sister chromatid exchange.

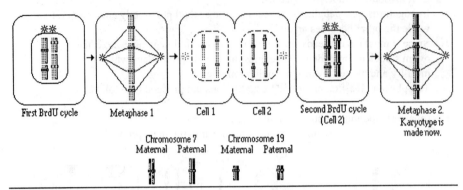

First BrdU cycle   Metaphase 1   Cell 1   Cell 2   Second BrdU cycle (Cell 2)   Metaphase 2. Karyotype is made now.

Chromosome 7   Chromosome 19
Maternal Paternal   Maternal Paternal

Visualization of sister chromatids. BrdU replaces thymidine in the cell culture medium. It is incorporated into the replicating DNA strand. In the next cycle of cell division, that strand is a template and the DNA replicated from it has BrdU in both strands. Special staining techniques are used to stain the unifiliary differently from the bifiliary BrdU DNA. In the illustration, two sister chromatid exchanges are seen on the maternal 7q, one on maternal 7p, and one on paternal chromosome 19q.

- Primary oocytes whose chromosomes remain exposed in suspended prophase for years until ovulated are predisposed to chromosomal mutations.

- Spermatogonia develop in great numbers from self-renewing stem cells requiring numerous DNA replications which produces a large probability of single gene mutations with age.

5.   Restriction enzymes protect bacteria from invasion by foreign DNA;
  - modification enzymes protect their own DNA through methylation of newly replicated strands.

- Type II restriction enzymes act as homodimers with reverse orientation so they
  - cleave DNA at palindromic sites, symmetric inverted repeats,
  - comprising 4 to 8 nucleotides, averaging 1 site per 1000-6000 nucleotides,
  - producing fragments with sticky ends when the sequence is offset, or
  - blunt ends when the sequence is the same in both DNA strands.

- Reverse transcriptase is an
  - enzyme from RNA tumor viruses that can be used to produce a
  - complementary DNA (cDNA) probe by
  - reverse transcription of a messenger RNA if there is
  - some mechanism to capture and stabilize the ordinarily evanescent mRNA.

Enzyme	Source	Recognition Site	Cleavage Results
EcoRI	Escherechia coli	✂ GAATTC / CTTAAG ✂	GAATTC G / G CTTAAG
TaqI	Thermus aquaticus	✂ TCGA / AGCT ✂	TCGA T / T AGCT
SmaI	Serratia marcescens	✂ CCCGGG / GGGCCC ✂	CCC GGG / GGG CCC

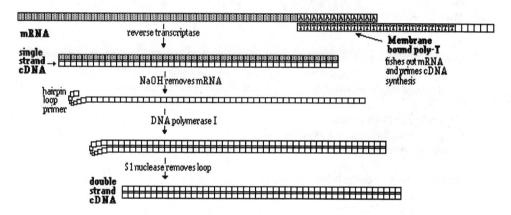

- Restriction enzyme fragments of cDNA with sticky ends can be recombined
    - with a vector that has been cleaved to produce similar sticky ends, then
    - cloned in large quantities by allowing the vector to reproduce in a host.

- Vectors include:
    - Plasmids which carry up to 10 kilobase lengths of DNA
    - Bacteriophages λ which carry up to 15
    - Cosmids which carry up to 49
    - Bacteriophages P1 which carry up to 100
        - P1 artificial chromosomes (PAC) extend this to 150
    - Bacterial artificial chromosomes (BAC) which carry up to 300
    - Yeast artificial chromosomes (YAC) which carry up to 2 megabases.

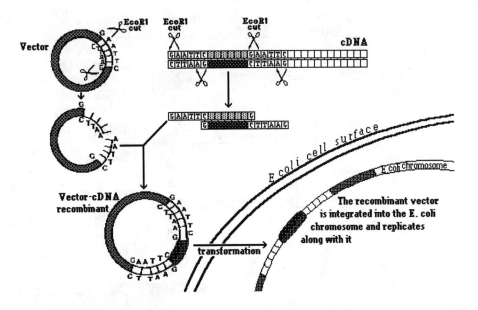

- A genomic library is prepared by cloning all of the
  - DNA fragments produced by a restriction nuclease while a
  - cDNA library is prepared by cloning all fragments of a cDNA probe.

- Sequencing of DNA fragments
  - determines the structure of genes and
  - allows construction of genes and use of them to obtain gene products.

- Somatic cell genetics deals with post-meiotic genetic changes;
  - it began with the use of cultured cells of somatic origin in the study of
    - genetic organization,
    - expression and
    - regulation

- John Littlefield isolated
  - human/mouse cell hybrids cells by co-culturing
    - human cells lacking hypoxanthine-guanine phosphoribosyl transferase and
    - mouse cells lacking thymidine kinase
  - by exposing the co-culture to hypoxanthine-aminopterin-thymidine (HAT) medium that killed all cells except for spontaneous hybrids.

- Harry Harris used
  - inactivated Sendai virus to greatly increase the rate of
  - cell fusion in co-cultures resulting in synkaryons which have
    - nuclei with chromosomes from more than one cell.

- Human/mouse fused cells are called heterokaryons because the
  - chromosomes are from different species; they
    - spontaneously lose human chromosomes
    - allowing localization (mapping) of genes to chromosomes
    - by determining the phenotypes associated with remaining chromosomes.

- Deletion mapping is done by hybridizing mouse cells with
  - cells from persons with chromosome deletions
    - and determining which functions are absent,
  - allowing localization of genes for those functions to the deleted regions of the chromsomes.

- Complementation analysis is done by co-cultivation of cells from
  - two persons who have a similar metabolic disease which
    - corrects the metabolic abnormality if the diseases are due to mutant genes from different loci or
    - fails to correct if the diseases are caused by different abnormal alleles at the same locus.

- Other direct gene mapping techniques include
  - in-situ hybridization
  - restriction site mapping and
  - chromosome walking.

 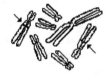 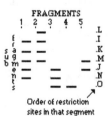 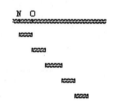

CELL HYBRIDIZATION	**IN-SITU HYBRIDIZATION**	**RESTRICTION SITE MAPPING**	**CHROMOSOME WALKING**
The arrow points to a human chromosome in a mouse cell nucleus	The arrows point to genes localized by cDNA hybridization	A segment of DNA is digested into large fragments which are separated by size. Each fragment is further digested into subfragments which are also separated by size. Sites are mapped by overlaps.	CDNA is prepared from a DNA segment between 2 restriction sites. It is sequenced and a small part of the sequence is used to prepare a primer which is used to initiate cDNA for the next segment. The next segment is sequenced, and the process is repeated.

6.   Mutagens identified in experimental animals include
- radiation,
- chemicals affecting replicating DNA: nucleotide base analogues
- chemicals affecting non-replicating DNA: alkylating agents, acridine orange

- Human data support belief in the same mutagens; however,
  - only radiation has been proven to increase the human mutation rate.

- The doubling dose of a mutagen is
  - the amount that increases the mutation rate to twice the spontaneous rate,
    - for X-ray determined to be 40 rem in mice and
    - estimated to be 156 rem in man.

- Mutagens are not known to be responsible for human genetic disorders;
  - all cases are thought to stem from spontaneous mutations,
    - errors inherent in replication of DNA or chromosomes.

TYPE	SITE	EFFECTS	RESULTS
Point	Single nucleotide	Substitution Insertion Deletion	Neutral Nonsense Missense Frame shift Aberrant mRNA splicing
DNA segment	Multiple contiguous nucleotides	Insertion Deletion	"Nonsense" Frame shift
Point (?)	"Mutation generator"	Unequal crossover Gene conversion Replication slippage	Meiotic instability of microsatellite DNA
Point (?)	Abnormal DNA ligation (?)	Chromosome breaks Sister chromatid exchange	Mitotic instability of chromosomes
Chromosome	Parts of chromosomes	Translocation Pericentric inversion Complex Uniparental disomy	Partial or total deletion Partial or total duplication Deletion plus duplication
	Whole chromosomes	Nondisjunction Nonconjunction Uniparental disomy	Deletion Duplication
Genome	Total	Maturation division failure during gamete formation	Triploidy Tetraploidy

CLINICALLY IMPORTANT MUTATION

- Single nucleotide "point" mutations have been studied most extensively; however,
  - other types are more frequent causes of human genetic disorders.

- A point mutation that changes an mRNA codon to UAA, UAG or UGA is called a
  - nonsense mutation; no amino acid is incorporated, polypeptide synthesis stops;
    - hence, these are called terminator codons.

Early students of human mutation raised antibodies to a protein in a laboratory animal and used them to test patients for the presence or absence of the protein, usually an enzyme. In most studies, it was found that, though the enzyme activity had been lost, the protein was still present. This was termed cross-reacting material positive or CRM+, in comparison to the rare instances in which the protein was absent (CRM-). After-dinner discussions often considered the point that most mutations in bacteria were CRM-, the opposite of findings in humans. This is now thought to be due to the bias of ascertainment of human enzyme defects which are more likely to be discovered if they are mild enough to allow reproduction.

There is a loose connection between CRM- and nonsense mutants: If the terminator codon occurs in the gene prior to the sequences that produce the antigenic portion of the protein, a CRM- state results. However, a mutation in a regulator site distant from the gene can result in no gene product with no mutation in the gene itself. This would also be CRM-.

The CRM is often colloquialized into "crim." Hurried references to "crim-positive" or "crim-negative" states have helped confuse a generation of students who can find nothing similar in a dictionary, and is a factor in the arcane reputation of genetics.

- Neutral mutations result in incorporation of the same amino acid;
  - both UUU and UUC code for phenylalanine.

5' base	Middle base				3' base
	U	C	A	G	
U	UUU phe	UCU ser	UAU tyr	UGU cys	U
U	UUC phe	UCC ser	UAC tyr	UGC cys	C
U	UUA leu	UCA ser	UAA**ter	UGA**ter	A
U	UUG leu	UCG ser	UAG**ter	UGG trp	G
C	CUU leu	CCU pro	CAU his	CGU arg	U
C	CUC leu	CCC pro	CAC his	CGC arg	C
C	CUA leu	CCA pro	CAA gln	CGA arg	A
C	CUG leu	CCG pro	CAG gln	CGG arg	G
A	AUU ile	ACU thr	AAU asn	AGU ser	U
A	AUC ile	ACC thr	AAC asn	AGC ser	C
A	AUA ile	ACA thr	AAA lys	AGA arg	A
A	AUG*met	ACG thr	AAG lys	AGG arg	G
G	GUU val	GCU ala	GAU asp	GGU gly	U
G	GUC val	GCC ala	GAC asp	GGC gly	C
G	GUA val	GCA ala	GAA glu	GGA gly	A
G	GUG val	GCG ala	GAG glu	GGG gly	G

*iniator   **terminator

THE GENETIC CODE
(mRNA assignments)

- Missense mutations result in incorporation of the wrong amino acid
  - GUU codes for valine; a change to GCU would put alanine there.

- Frame-shift mutations are due to either insertion or deletion of a nucleotide
  - changing the reading of all subsequent nucleotides
    - because they are read as codons (sets of 3 nucleotides).

THE RED ODO GRA NAL LDA YTO

↑ insertion

Examples of frame-shifts of a three-letter code: THE RED DOG RAN ALL DAY TOO

↓ deletion

THE RED OGR ANA LLD AYT OO

- Point mutation near mRNA splice junctions causes aberrant splicing resulting in
  - exon skipping in most cases but can lead to
  - cryptic splice site utilization.

- Mutations causing thymine dimers have been used to study
  - DNA repair mechanisms which include:
    - photoreactivation
    - excision or dark repair
    - postreplication or recombination repair
    - SOS repair.

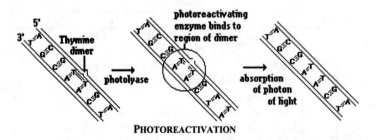

PHOTOREACTIVATION

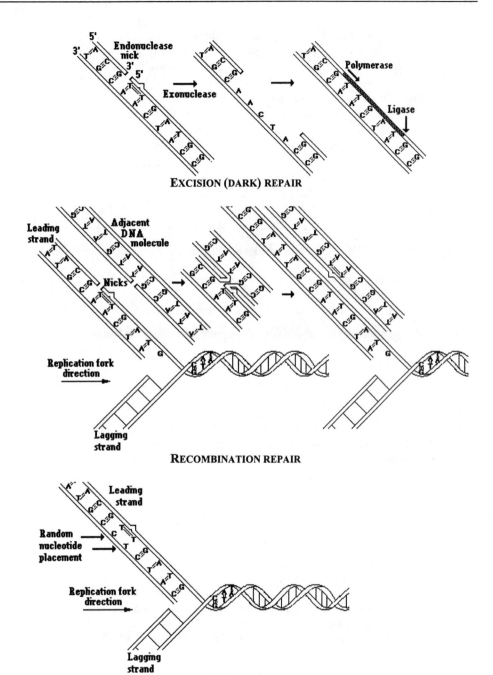

EXCISION (DARK) REPAIR

RECOMBINATION REPAIR

SOS REPAIR

- A point mutation that is not repaired becomes an allele, from Gr. αλληλ: one another, or an
  - alternate form of a gene that may occupy a locus, and, if it persists, forms a
    - genetic equilibrium with the original gene in the population.

- The Hardy-Weinberg law states that, at equilibrium,
  - if there are two alleles A and a with frequencies p and q in a population,
  - the frequencies of homozygotes (AA or aa) and heterozygote (Aa) is the binomial expansion of $(p + q)^2$:

	Alleles	A		a
	Allele (gene) frequencies	p		q
	Genotypes	AA	Aa	aa
	Genotype frequencies	p^2	2pq	q^2
X-linked recessive	Genotype (male)	A		a
	Genotype frequencies (male)	p		q

- With appropriate corrections for bias of ascertainment,
  - p is calculated as 1-q, since $(p + q)^2 = 1$,
  - q^2 can be defined as the incidence of autosomal recessive disorders,
  - $2pq + q^2$ is the incidence of autosomal dominant disorders,
    - essentially 2q since q^2 is near 0 and p is near 1.

- For X-linked recessive genes in males, the hemizygous state results in
  - the gene frequency and the genotype frequency being identical
  - hence the ratio of affected males to affected females is q/q^2 or $1/q$.

- The mutation rate, μ, can be estimated from the rate of genetic lethals, m,
  - point mutation disorders that do not allow reproduction
  - so result in losses of genes which must be replaced by mutation
  - to maintain genetic equilibrium.

- For autosomal dominant genetic lethals, the mutant is a heterozygote, Aa
  - with frequency ≈ 2pq; essentially 2q since p is near 1, so
  - μ = m/2

- Rates of autosomal recessive genetic lethals do not readily allow estimation of μ.
  - Both alleles have usually been transmitted from carriers (frequency = 2pq x 2pq).
  - Very rarely, one could be transmitted, and one a new mutation (frequency = 2pq x μ).
  - It would be exceedingly unusual for both to be new mutations (frequency = $μ^2$).
  - Hence, the likelihood of any case resulting from new mutation is vanishingly small.
    - For cystic fibrosis, $μ^2$ ≈ 0.0000000001, (2pq x μ) ≈ 0.0000004, (2pq x 2pq) ≈ 0.002.

- 2/3 of x-linked recessive genetic lethal mutations are in females so are not evident.
  - The 1/3 that are in males = m;
  - hence $\mu = m/3$.

- The rate of spontaneous single nucleotide mutations
  - is 1:100,000 loci per gamete per generation.

- Single nucleotide mutation rate estimates higher than 1:100,000 suggest either
  - a high rate of non-penetrance or
  - genetic heterogeneity, usually the latter:
    - over 70 mutations cause Duchenne muscular dystrophy,
    - over 100 mutations cause β-thalassemia.
    - over 400 mutations cause cystic fibrosis,

- Each individual is estimated to be heterozygous for 4 lethal equivalents,
  - mutant recessive genes that would be lethal if homozygous.

- Rates of mutations of types other than point mutation are not well characterized;
  - about 1% of cultured normal human cells have mitotic instability;
  - some human length polymorphisms due to meiotic instability have a rate of 5%;
  - some chromosome duplications have a rate of 10% in human conceptuses.

- Mutations that cause meiotic instability appear to be point mutations which change the copy number of short tandem repeats (STR) of microsatellite DNA by causing
  - replication slippage (skipping of several codons by the replication site)
    - which deletes a segment from the daughter strand,
  - gene conversion (non-reciprocal recombination)
    - which replaces part or all of a gene with all or part of another gene, and
  - misalignment during crossover ("Lepore" mutation)
    - which deletes a segment from one strand and duplicates it in the other,
  - these mechanisms leading to visible chromosome aberrations in some cases.
  - Gene conversion and crossover misalignment also repair mutations.

- Mitotic instability is characterized by the same phenomena in somatic cells,
  - also probably instigated by point mutations, and
  - more often accompanied by visible chromosome aberrations.

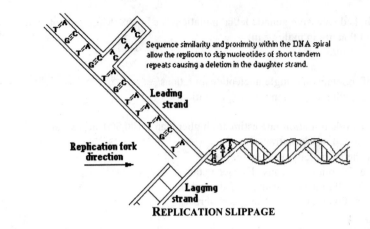

Sequence similarity and proximity within the DNA spiral allow the replicon to skip nucleotides of short tandem repeats causing a deletion in the daughter strand.

Leading strand

Replication fork direction →

Lagging strand

REPLICATION SLIPPAGE

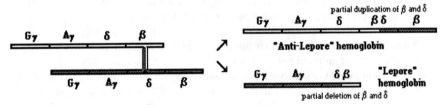

partial duplication of β and δ

"Anti-Lepore" hemoglobin

"Lepore" hemoglobin

partial deletion of β and δ

CROSSOVER MISALIGNMENT

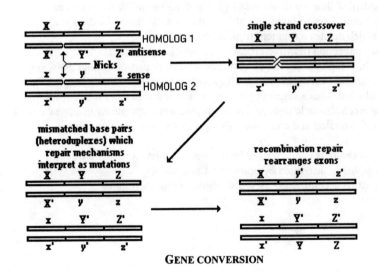

HOMOLOG 1

antisense

Nicks

sense

HOMOLOG 2

single strand crossover

mismatched base pairs (heteroduplexes) which repair mechanisms interpret as mutations

recombination repair rearranges exons

GENE CONVERSION

- Nondisjunction may
  - duplicate or delete
    - whole chromosomes.

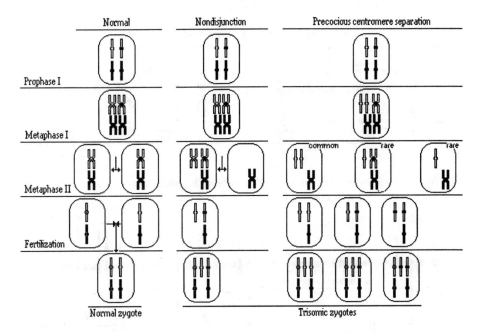

Meiotic nondisjunction has been thought to be the most frequent cause of Down syndrome; however, recent studies indicate that nonconjunction is more frequent, as long known in other species. Failure of orienting mechanisms at the equator allow a bivalent to undergo precocious centromere separation during meiosis I rather than during meiosis II, rendering the chromosome 21 homologs as unpaired univalents that are randomly distributed to the poles. When both arrive at the same pole, fertilization of the resulting gamete produces trisomy. Maternal age is the major known factor leading to nonconjunction.

Down Syndrome Data

Parent	Total	Error in Meiosis I	Error in Meiosis II
Mother	95%	77%	23%
Father	5%	22%	78%
Nonconjunction	68%	50%	18%

- Persons with normal phenotypes may harbor chromosome translocations or
  - inversions and gametogenesis in these persons may result in
    - transmission of the translocation or inversion with
    - no phenotypic abnormalities in offspring.

- Segregation during gametogenesis in persons with chromosome translocations or
  - inversions may also cause an abnormal phenotype in offspring due to
    - duplication or deletion of parts of chromosomes.

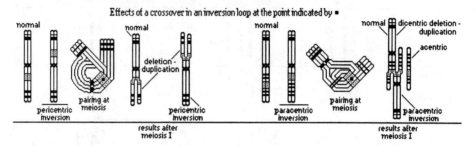

Effects of a crossover in an inversion loop at the point indicated by ■

- Exchange of parts of nonhomologous chromosomes is called
  - reciprocal translocation.

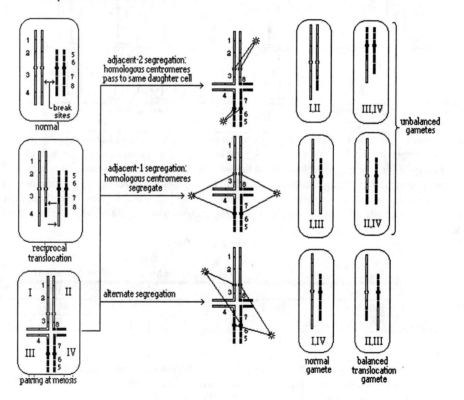

- Transverse fission of the centromeres and fusion of nonhomologous centromeres is
    - Robertsonian translocation, the "balanced" state accompanied by
        - loss of the smaller derivative chromosome but causing
        - no discernable phenotype although there are only 45 chromosomes.

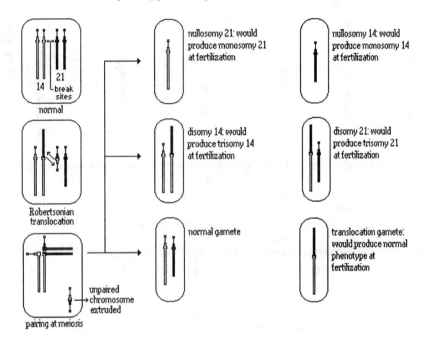

- The classic (Darlington) concept of isochromosome formation involves
    - abnormal horizontal centromere fission during cell division,
        - resulting in short arms in one daughter cell and long arms in the other,
    - however, recent studies indicate that it is usually due to unequal crossover,
        - resulting in an isodicentric chromosome that looks like an isochromosome.

- Ring chromosomes result from
    - terminal deletions of the tips of p and q with
    - fusion at the deletion points.

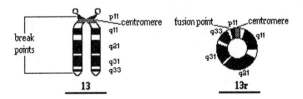

- Complex events involving chromosomal breaks during gametogenesis in persons with normal chromosomes may result in either
  - deletion or
  - duplication of parts of chromosomes.

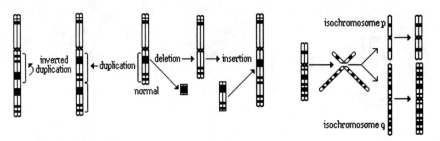

- The same mechanisms may cause chromosome heteromorphisms which are
  - heritable variations in chromosome structure not associated with any phenotypic abnormality at the current level of perception:
    - pericentric inversion of 9,
    - variable size of centromeric heterochromatin of 1, 9, & 16,
    - size and shape of satellites of 14, 15, 21, & 22,
      - involving both repetitive DNA and ribosomal genes,
    - fragile sites on 2q13, 6p23, 9q32, 12q13, 20p11 and Xq27.

- After fertilization, chromosome aberrations may occur in the early embryo, i.e.,
  - mitotic non-disjunction leading to a trisomic cell line in a euploid embryo, or
  - reversion leading to a normal cell line in a trisomic embryo
    - and, if both resulting cell lines are viable, this is called mosaicism.

- Triploidy may result from:
  - duplication of female pronucleus (usually produces intact fetus):
    - tetraploid oogonium (99%)
    - polar body fusion (?%)
  - duplication of male pronucleus (usually produces poorly differentiated fetus):
    - dispermy (70%)
    - tetraploid spermatogonium (30%)

- Tetraploidy and higher counts may result from
  - multispermic fertilization,
  - post-fertilization failure of cytokinesis.

Additional references:

Arnstein N. Mitochondrial DNA mutations and aging. Am J Hum Biol 1995;7:117.

Brocolli D, Cooke H. Aging, healing and the metabolism of telomeres. Am J Hum Genet 1991;52:657-660.

Choo KH, Earle E, Shaffer L, et al. Molecular characterization of human t(14q21q) Robertsonian translocation. Proceedings of the 8th International Congress of Human Genetics. Abstract 1647. Am J Hum Genet 1991;49 (Suppl):296.

Comings DE. Mechanisms of chromosome banding and implications for chromosome structure. Ann Rev Genet 1978;12:25-46.

Ford EB. Polymorphism. Biol Rev 1945;20:73-88.

Fraser-Roberts JA, Pembrey ME. *An Introduction to Medical Genetics*. New York: Oxford, 1985.

Harnden DG, Klinger HP (editors). *ISCN 1985. An International System for Human Cytogenetic Nomenclature (1985)*. New York: S. Karger, 1985.

Jeffreys AJ, Royle NJ, Wilson V, et al. Spontaneous mutation rates to new length alleles at tandem-repetitive hypervariable loci in human DNA. 1988;Nature 332:278-281.

Krawczak M, Reiss J, Cooper DN. The mutational spectrum of single base-pair substitutions in mRNA splice junctions of human genes: causes and consequences. Hum Genet 1992;90:41-54.

Kuhn EM, Therman E. No increased breakage in three Bloom syndrome heterozygotes. J Med Genet 1979;16:219-222.

Marchington DR, Hartshorne GM, Barlow D, et al. Homopolymeric tract heteroplasmy in mtDNA from tissues and single oocytes: Support for a genetic bottleneck. Am J Hum Genet 1997;60:408-416.

Peterson MB, Frantzen M, Antonarakis SE, et al. Comparative study of microsatellite and cytogenetic markers for detecting the origin of the nondisjoined chromosome 21 in Down syndrome. Am J Hum Genet 1992;51:516-525.

Poulton J. Transmission of mtDNA: Cracks in the bottleneck. Am J Hum Genet 1995;57:224-26.

Russell PJ. *Lecture Notes on Genetics*. Boston: Blackwell Scientific, 1980.

Schull WJ, Masonari O, Neel JV. Genetic effects of the atomic bombs: A reappraisal. Science 1981;213:1220-1227 and 1205.

Waggoner DD, Magenis RE. Origin and phenotype of mosaic trisomy 21. Proceedings of the 8th International Congress of Human Genetics. Am J Hum Genet 1991;49 (Suppl):288.

Wallace DC. Mitochondrial genetics: A paradigm for aging and degenerative diseases? Science 1992;256:628-32.

Wilson GG. *Restriction enzymes: A brief overview*. The NEB Transcript (New England Biolabs, Beverly, MA 01915) 1993;5:1-5.

1. Factors that alter Hardy-Weinberg proportions govern the occurrence of genetic disorders:
   * new mutations
   * selection
   * non-random mating: (assortative mating and inbreeding)
   * migration.

* For most genes, mutation results in many alleles that persist within a population, so the Hardy-Weinberg proportions are represented as:

$$(p+q+r \ .... \ n)^2=1$$

   EXAMPLE: For 5 alleles, the equation would be $(p+q+r+s+t)^2=1$ which expands to:
   $$t^2+2st+s^2+2rt+2rs+r^2+2qt+2qs+2qr+q^2+2pt+2ps+2pr+2pq+p^2=1$$
   and this means that individual genotypes are quite rare.

* Fitness (f) is the proportion of mutated genes transmitted to the next generation (paralleling number of offsprings), while the
   * selection coefficient (s) is the proportion not transmitted; hence,
   selection is equivalent to prevention of reproduction.

* Selection against an autosomal dominant phenotype can lower its incidence to the mutation rate within one generation while
   * selection against an autosomal recessive phenotype would require 10 to 20 generations to decrease its incidence half the distance to the mutation rate;
   relaxing selection results in equivalent rates of increase.

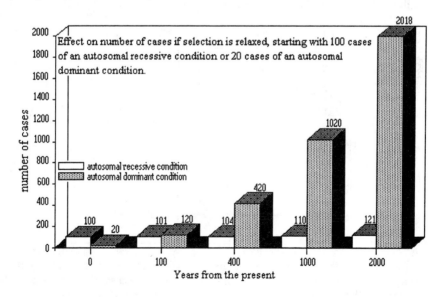

- A heterozygote advantage exists when
  - the heterozygote (Aa) is fitter than either homozygote (AA and aa)
  - and results in a balanced polymorphism that holds the frequency of the mutant gene above the mutation rate since 2pq is a much larger number than q^2.

- Stabilizing selection (equivalent to heterozygote advantage)
  - favors the intermediate phenotype (Aa) over phenodeviants (AA and aa)
  - directional selection favors the intermediate and one of the phenodeviants, and
  - disruptive selection favors both phenodeviants.

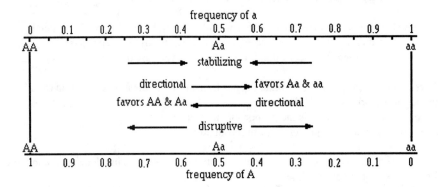

- Assortative mating is reproduction between persons who have similar genetic traits.
  - It affects gene frequency like directional selection if unidirectional,
  - or like disruptive selection if bidirectional.

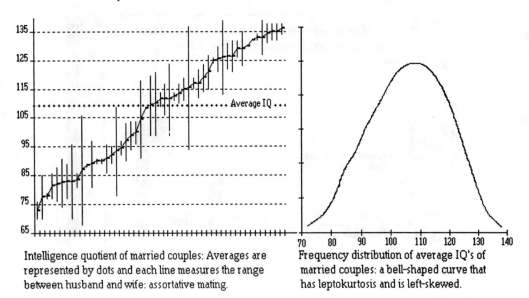

Intelligence quotient of married couples: Averages are represented by dots and each line measures the range between husband and wife: assortative mating.

Frequency distribution of average IQ's of married couples: a bell-shaped curve that has leptokurtosis and is left-skewed.

- Inbreeding is reproduction between relatives.
  - It affects gene frequency like disruptive selection.

Generation	AA	Aa	aa
0	0	100	0
1	25	50	25
2	37.5	25	37.5
3	43.75	12.5	43.75
4	46.9	6.25	46.9
∞	50	0	50

EFFECT OF CLOSE INBREEDING

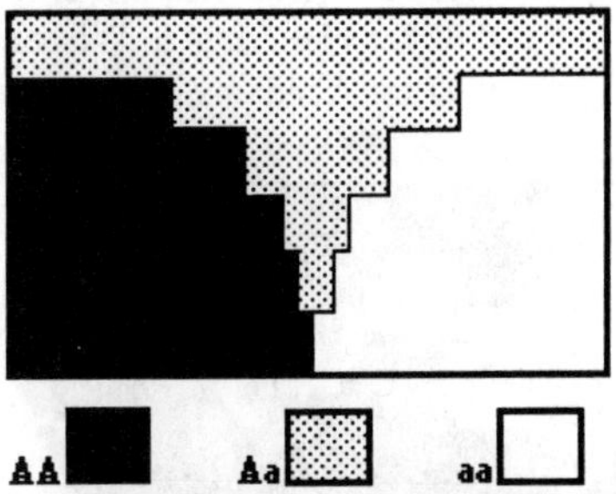

Adapted from Suzuki DT, Griffiths AJF, Lewontin RC (1989)

  - Inbreeding causes high frequency of autosomal recessive disorders in small population isolates.

- The coefficient of inbreeding (F) is
  - the probability that an individual is homozygous at a locus
    - having received both alleles from an identical ancestral source and is calculated as:

$$F = \frac{(0.5)^n}{2}$$

  - where n is the degrees of relationship separating the individual's parents.

- The coefficient of inbreeding of a population (K) is
  - the average consanguinity within a population and is calculated as:

$$K = \sum\left[\frac{F_i - M_i}{N-1}\right]$$

  - where F is the coefficient of inbreeding for i degrees of relationship.
  - M is the number of marriages between relatives of i degrees of relationship and
  - N is the population size.

- Outbred U.S. populations have K estimates around 0.0008 while
  - estimates in small genetic isolates range from
    - 0.001 for Redbones in Vernon Parish to
    - 0.02 for Hutterites in Wisconsin to
    - 0.07 for Acadians in St. Martin Parish.

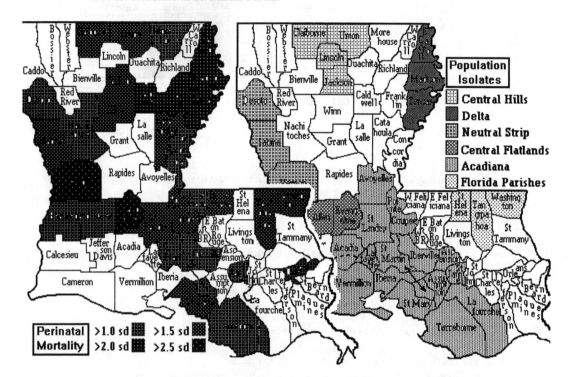

- Socio-cultural characteristics of isolates with high K contribute to elevated frequencies of genetic disorders that are not autosomal recessive traits:
  - low mobility: keeps all cases in one place.
  - altruism: decreases reproductive competition.
  - large family sizes: increases numbers of cases.

2.   Genetic drift is
   • gradual genetic change
      • due to chance fluctuation in gene frequency in small populations.
Within each population, it affects gene frequency like directional selection.

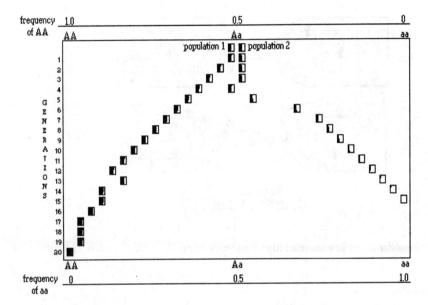

Random genetic drift. Each initial population was all heterozygotes (orange). Within 20 generations, 41% of the populations had drifted into homozygosity, i.e., had become fixed, as either AA homozygotes (scarlet) or aa homozygotes (white). The course of two of the populations to fixation is illustrated [Buri P (1956): Gene frequency in small populations of mutant Drosophila. Evolution 10:367-402.]

   • The neutralist theory of polymorphism holds that
      • genetic drift accounts for current allelic frequencies.

   • The selectionist theory holds that
      • selection accounts for current allelic frequencies.

   • Most striking degrees of blood group polymorphism appear to represent drift but
      • disease associations with blood groups and
      • hemolytic disease of the newborn may be mechanisms of selection;
      • also, Fy(a-b-) protects against malaria.

- The founder effect, a form of rapid genetic drift, is
  - the shrinkage of the breadth of genetic variation that occurs when a new
    - population is formed by a few migrants from a larger parent population.

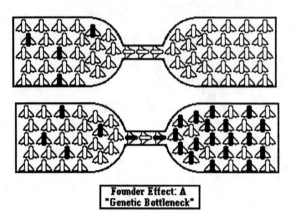

Founder Effect: A "Genetic Bottleneck"

- Founder effect is a cause of high frequency of rare genetic disorders in small population isolates.

3. Gene flow is
   - gradual change in gene frequency due to admixing of ethnic groups
     - after one group migrates into the environment of the other.
   - It affects gene frequency like stabilizing selection
   - and may also introduce new genetic disorders into an ethnic group.

4. Mendel's first law is that of unit inheritance which means that
   - the characteristics that are inherited are conferred by single entities
     - later named "genes."

- Mendel's second law is that of segregation which means that
  - during gametogenesis, gene pairs separate, each gamete containing only one.

- Mendel's third law is that of independent assortment which means that
  - members of different gene pairs enter gametes independently of one another.

- A homozygote is a person who has the same allele at both loci of a gene but
  - a heterozygote has a different allele at each locus.

- Males are hemizygous for genes of the X chromosome.

- Phenotype expression of a recessive allele can be detected only when it is
  - homozygous or hemizygous but
  - a dominant allele is expressed whenever present.

- Analysis at a level of phenotype close to the gene may detect expression of recessive alleles in heterozygotes.

- In a compound heterozygote, each of the two alleles is a different mutant gene:
  - a frequent explanation of non-typical diseases.

- Autosomal genes are on chromosomes other than the sex chromosomes.

- Autosomal phenotypes may be sex-limited or sex-influenced:

SEX LIMITED	
Expression only in males:	Precocious puberty
	Hypogonadism (recognition easier)
Expression only in females:	Hydrometrocolpos

SEX INFLUENCED	
More common in males:	Baldness
	Hemachromatosis
More common in females:	Congenital adrenal hyperplasia
	(recognition earlier)

- Pleiotropy exists when
  - one gene produces several apparently unrelated abnormalities.

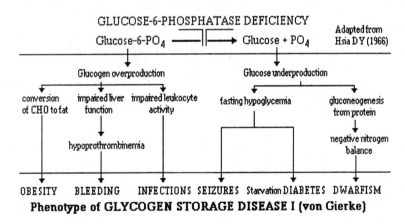

Phenotype of GLYCOGEN STORAGE DISEASE I (von Gierke)

Pleiotropy illustrated by the multifaceted phenotype of GSD I, a disease in which the connections between the genetic defect and the observed abnormalities have been dissected biochemically. The biochemical basis of most other genetic diseases is not known so there is usually no obvious basis for the abnormalities caused in differing systems by one gene.

- Genetic heterogeneity exists when
  - several different genes seem to produce the same abnormality.

Clinical Heterogeneity of Charcot-Marie-Tooth (CMT) Disease

The different forms are distinguished clinically by age of onset and rate of progression.

Genetic type	Age of onset	Rate of progression
Autosomal recessive	first decade	rapid
X-linked recessive	second decade	intermediate
Autosomal dominant	third decade	slow

Order of appearance of findings:
1. leg muscle wasting, especially peroneus; foot drop
2. pes cavus, hammer toes
3. indifference to pain in toes
4. equinovarus, scoliosis
5. hand muscle wasting, claw hand

Molecular Heterogeneity of Charcot-Marie-Tooth (CMT) Disease

form [McKusick number]	features	locus	type	defect
1A [118220, 601097] *myelin defect*	nerve conduction velocity <40 m/s, hypertrophic nerves, Schwann cell "onion bulbs"	17p11.2	AD	PMP22 duplications or missense mutations
1B [118200, 159440]		1q22	AD	MPZ missense mutations
1C [601098]			AD	?
2A [118210] *axon defect*	nerve conduction velocity >40 m/s, axon loss	1p36	AD	?
2B [600882]		3q13	AD	?
4A [214400]	like CMT1A but earlier onset and more severe	8q13	AR	?
4B [601382]			AR	?
5 [600361]	nerve conduction velocity ~40 m/s, extensor plantar reflex		AD	?
X1 [302800]	like CMT1A but earlier onset	Xq13.1	XD	Cx3 missense mutations
X2 [302801]		Xp22.2	XR	?
X3 [302802]		Xp24	XR	?

Differential Diagnosis of Charcot-Marie-Tooth (CMT) Disease

disease [McKusick number]	disease [McKusick number]
ataxia-myoclonus epilepsy-presenile dementia [208700]	hereditary neuropathy with liability to pressure palsies[2] [162500]
Charcot-Marie-Tooth disease-aplasia cutis congenita [302803]	muscular atrophy-adult spinal [158590]
Charcot-Marie-Tooth disease-deafness [118300]	neuropathy-hereditary sensory radicular [162400]
Charcot-Marie-Tooth disease-deafness [214370]	neuropathy-motor-sensory-deafness-mental retardation [310490]
Charcot-Marie-Tooth disease-Freidreich ataxia [302900]	optic atrophy-deafness, distal neurogenic amyotrophy [258650]
Charcot-Marie-Tooth disease-Guadalajara neuronal type [118230]	optic atrophy-peripheral neuropathy [601152]
Charcot-Marie-Tooth disease- keratoderma [148360]	optic atrophy-polyneuropathy-deafness [311070]
Charcot-Marie-Tooth disease-progressive ataxia-tremor [214380]	Roussy-Levy hereditary areflexic dystasia [180800]
Charcot-Marie-Tooth disease-ptosis-Parkinsonism [118301]	scapuloperoneal atrophy-cardiopathy [181350]
Cowchock syndrome[1] [310490]	scapuloperoneal amyotrophy [181400]
Dejerine-Sottas hypertrophic neuropathy[2,3] [145900]	scapuloperoneal amyotrophy-neurogenic [181405]
Gamstorp-Wohlfart syndrome [137200]	spastic paraplegia-3 [182600]

1: same locus as form X3. 2: same locus as form 1A. 3: same locus as form 1B, another at 8p23.

Genetic Heterogeneity of Corpus Callosum Anomaly (absence, agenesis, partial agenesis).
Severity of anomaly varies among cases, even within families.

Common presenting signs: Newborns: enlarging head.
  (13% are asymptomatic)   Infants: poor growth & development, irritability, periodic vomiting.
                                   Older children & adults: seizures.

Neurological signs vary, even within famlies:
• apneic episodes   • dyskinesias: tremors, athetosis, parkinsonian movements
• hydrocephalus   • periodic hypothermia   • spastic quadriplegia
• mental retardation (2.5% of institutionalized mental retardates have corpus callosum anomaly)
• seizures: infantile spasms (hypsarrhythmia), grand mal, myoclonic, petit mal
• impaired crossed tactile localization, impaired matching of visual patterns in left and right half
  fields (**rare**)
• frequent associations: gyral anomalies (heterotopia, hypoplasia), microcephaly.

Anatomic types of corpus callosum abnormalities [Dobyns WB (1996)]:
1.   Malformations of forebrain occurring prior to corpus callosum anlage, e.g.,
          holoprosencephaly.
2.   Neurons do not form or do not elaborate commissural axons, e.g., lissencephaly.
3.   Massa commissuralis absence: Axons form Probst fiber bundles along medial hemispheric
          walls.
4.   Degeneration or atrophy.

An isolated corpus callosum abnormality is usually either **autosomal recessive** or **x-linked
recessive**. The types are clinically similar and can be differentiated only through genealogy studies.
Apparent autosomal dominant inheritance has also been reported in one family [(Lynn RB et al
(1980)].

Syndromes which have corpus callosum anomaly as part of their signs, though not all cases have it:

Syndrome	Signs in addition to those associated with the corpus callosum anomaly	Etio
Aicardi	Infantile spasms, retinal lacunae, hemivertebrae, scoliosis, absent or malformed ribs, corpus callosum agenesis in 72% (partial agenesis in 28%).	XD
Andermann	Areflexia, paraplegia, anterior horn cell disease, progressive peripheral sensorimotor neuropathy.	AR
da-Silva	Preauricular tags, camptodactyly, poor growth, recurrent pneumonia.	AR
FG	Macrocephaly, prominent forehead, hypotonia, imperforate or anteriorly-placed anus, short stature, contractures, broad thumb and hallux.	XR
Meckel-Gruber	Encephalocoele, polycystic kidneys, polydactyly, hepatic dysplasia.	AR
Neu-Laxova	Intrauterine dwarfism, exophthalmos, ectodermal dysplasia, joint contractures.	AR
Rubinstein-Taybi	Broad angulated thumb, broad hallux, downward eye slant, beaked nose.	?
Taybi-Linder	Intrauterine dwarfism, short bowed limbs.	AR
Toriello	Telecanthus, blepharophimosis, short nose, Pierre Robin anomaly, redundant neck skin, heart malformation, short hands, hypotonia.	AR
Young	Macrocephaly, prominent forehead, deep-set eyes.	AR

<u>Conditions in which corpus callosum anomaly has been reported</u> [Dobyns WB (1996)]: Chromosome aberrations: Deletions (1q, 2q, 4p, 6q, 15q, 16q, 18q, 21q, 21, 21 pq, Xp, Xq), duplications (5p, 6p, 8p, 8, 11q, 13, 14q, 14pq, 18, 19, 19q, 21, 22, triploidy). Metabolic disorders: beta-hydroxyisobutyryl Co A deacylase deficiency, glutaric aciduria 2, Menke syndrome, neonatal adrenoleukodystrophy, nonketotic hyperglycinemia, pyruvate dehydrogenase deficiency, Zellweger syndrome. Syndromes: ACC ectodermal dysplasia, ACC Hirschprung, ACC thrombocytopenia, acrocallosal, Apert, ATRX, basal cell nevus, Buntix-Majewski, C, cleft lip/palate, Cogan, congenital rubella, Curatolo, Delleman, Dincsoy, fetal alcohol, frontonasal dysplasia, Fukuyama, G, genital hypoplasia, HSAS, hydrolethalus, Joubert, leprechaunism, limb malformation, Lowry-Wood, Lyon, Lujan-Frias, macroglossia, MASA, maternal diabetes, micro, MLS, neural tube defects, oro-facio-digital 1, osteodysplasia, Peters plus, pituitary dwarfism, porencephaly, precocious puberty, Proud, renal malformation, sebaceous nevus, Shapiro, Siber, Smith-Lemli-Opitz, tumors of corpus callosum (teratoma, lipoma), tongue malformation, tuberous sclerosis, Vici, Vles, Walker-Warburg, XLIS.

Additional references:

Allan W. Relation of hereditary pattern to clinical severity as illustrated by peroneal atrophy. Arch Intern Med 1939;63:1123-1131.

Dobyns WB. Absence makes the search grow longer. Am J Hum Genet 1996;58:7-16

Hartl DL. *A Primer of Population Genetics*. Sunderland, MA: Sinauer, 1981.

Howell RR. Genetic Disease. The present status of treatment. In: McKusick VA, Claiborne R, (editors). *Medical Genetics*. New York: Hospital Practice Publishing, 1973.

Leahy AM. Nature-nurture and intelligence. Genetic Psychology Monographs 1935;17: 236-308.

Lupski JR. Molecular genetics of inherited primary peripheral neuropathies. Neurogenetic Advances (Genica Pharmaceuticals Worchester, MA 06015) 1994;3:1-5.

Lynn RB, Buchanan DC, Fenichell GM et al. Agenesis of the corpus callosum. Arch Neurol 1980;37:444-445.

McKusick VA. *Mendelian Inheritance in Man. Catalogues of Autosomal Dominant, Autosomal Recessive, and X-linked Phenotypes*, 10th edition. Baltimore: The Johns Hopkins Press, 1992.

Outhit MC. A study of the resemblance of parents and children in general intelligence. Arch Psychol 1933;149:1-60.

Wallace B. *Topics in Population Genetics*. New York: Norton, 1968.

Suzuki DT, Griffiths AJF, Lewontin RC. *An Introduction to Genetic Analysis*, 2nd edition. San Francisco: WH Freeman, 1984.

1. Autosomal dominant inheritance is said to be present when
    *   the phenotype can be inherited from an affected parent,
    *   the phenotype can be found in either sex, and
    *   50% of children of affected parents are also affected.

Inherited from either parent.

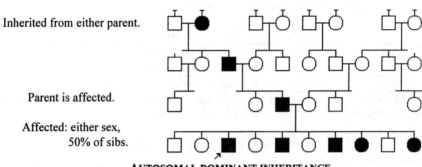

Parent is affected.

Affected: either sex,
50% of sibs.

AUTOSOMAL DOMINANT INHERITANCE

*   New dominant mutation may be responsible for the occurrence of a disease phenotype in a child of normal parents,
    *   usually associated with advanced paternal age.

*   Variable expression is characteristic of dominant alleles,
    *   thought to be due to modifying effects of environment and other genes,
    *   but possibly due to microanatomical variation of the mutant gene:
        *   A mutant APC gene at 5q22 may produce pure adenomatous polyposis of the colon in one relative while producing, in another relative in the same family, Gardner syndrome (adenomatous polyposis of the colon, multiple osteomas, epidermoid cysts, desmoid tumors, congenital hypertrophy of the retinal pigment epithelium).

EXAMPLES OF EXPRESSIVITY

Disorder	Variable	Expression
Huntington disease	Onset age	below 15 years:3%, before 30 years:10%, before 40 years:30%, before 50 years:60%, before 60 years:85%, before 70 years:95%
Neurofibromatosis	Feature	cafe-au-lait spots: 94%, Lisch nodules: 70%, developmental disorder: 30%, plexiform neurofibromas: 27%, optic glioma: 15%, scoliosis: 5%, seizures: 5%, sarcoma: 2%
Multiple exostoses	Area	forearm: 50%, ankle: 45%, knee: 21%, pelvis: 4%, vertebrae: 4%

*   A dominant allele is non-penetrant when
    *   its expression is not detectable under the conditions of the analysis .

*   When both alleles of a heterozygote are expressed, they are codominant.

- Intermediate inheritance is present when
  - the phenotype of the heterozygote is different from those of both homozygotes;
  - i.e., pink-flowering progeny from white-flowering and red-flowering parents,
  - but a semantic problem in human genetics -
  - used as an explanation for the moderate anti-malarial effect of sickle-cell trait.

- Mitochondrial inheritance is through the maternal line, and is quantitative with
  - random distribution of mutant genes,
    - resulting in variable expression of phenotype.

MITOCHONDRIAL DISORDERS

Kearns-Sayre syndrome	External ophthalmoplegia, retinal degeneration, elevated CSF protein, cardiac conduction defect.
Leber optic atrophy	Early onset progressive optic atrophy.
MELAS (Mitochondrial Encephalopathy, Lactic Acidosis, Stroke)	Short stature, sensorineural deafness, encephalomyopathy, lactic acidosis, stroke-like episodes
MERRF (Myoclonic Epilepsy, Ragged Red Fiber)	Myoclonic epilepsy, myopathy, ragged red muscle fibers, lipomas.

- Mitotic mutation may give rise to somatic mosaicism in which a cell or a clone of cells with a mutant gene
  - produces focal genetic disease such as cancer, or
  - localized manifestation of a usually generalized genetic disease, or
  - milder manifestation of a genetic disease
    - if soluble factors mediate the phenotype.

- In germline mosaicism, a mutation occurs prior to gametogenesis
  - during division of a cell whose progeny later form germ cells
  - leading to a segment of germ cells bearing a dominant mutant gene;
  - hence multiple affected children can be born to a normal person.

- Some mutant genes cause meiotic instability of short tandem repeats (STR) of nucleotides:

Disease	STR	Gene	Locus	Normal	Affected
Dentatorubral-pallidoluysian atrophy	CAG	DRPLA	12p	7-23	49-75
Friedreich ataxia	GAA	FRDA	9q13	7-22	200-900
Huntington disease	CAG	IT$_{15}$ near 5' end	4p	11-34	42-100
Machado-Joseph disease	CAG	MJD	14q32	13-36	68-79
Myotonic dystrophy	CTG	untranslated region 3' to myotonin-protein kinase	19q	3-40	50-2000
Spinocerebellar ataxia type I	CAG	SCAI, about 15cm telomeric to HLA	6p	19-36	43-81

- The copy number of unstable short tandem repeats may change during meiosis,
  - increases causing earlier onset in succeeding generations (**anticipation**),
  - decreases causing **reversion** to milder phenotype or to normal.

- The degree of transcription hence degree of expression of some mutant genes
  - is determined by the sex of the parent of origin,
  - a phenomenon called imprinting, due in most cases to
    - differential DNA methylation.
  - MYOTONIC DYSTROPHY IS MORE SEVERE WHEN INHERITED FROM THE MOTHER.
  - HUNTINGTON DISEASE AND SCAI ONSET EARLIER IF INHERITED FROM THE FATHER.

- Either gamete complementation, monosomic conception with subsequent chromosome gain, trisomic conception followed by chromosome loss, or other complex errors around the time of conception, can lead to
  - uniparental disomy of all or part of a chromosome which may cause
    - autosomal recessive disease in a patient with only one heterozygous parent,
    - X-linked disorder transmitted from father to son, or
    - homozygous X-linked disorder in a daughter of a heterozygote.

RELATION of IMPRINTING and UNIPARENTAL DISOMY

Prader-Willi syndrome	2/3 of cases are caused by deletion of paternal 15q11q13 and 1/5 of cases by uniparental disomy of maternal chromosome 15.
Angelman syndrome	Most are caused by deletion of maternal 15q11q13 with only 3% caused by uniparental disomy of paternal chromosome 15.

2. In autosomal recessive inheritance,
   - the phenotype can be found in either sex,
   - parents do not express the phenotype,
   - 25% of all full sibs are affected, and
   - parents are often unknowingly consanguineous.

Parental consanguinity.

Normal parents.

Affected: either sex,
   25% of sibs.

AUTOSOMAL RECESSIVE INHERITANCE

- The rarer the recessive gene,
    - the greater the likelihood that parents of a homozygote are consanguineous;
        - homozygosity for the rarest genes being found only in genetic isolates,
            - all of whose members are related.

- The likelihood of an autosomal recessive disorder in offsprings of consanguineous matings
    - drops rapidly from 14% in parent-child or brother-sister matings
    - to 1% in first cousin matings.

- Incest is reproduction between relatives closer than first cousins.

3. Genes on the sex chromosomes can be either
    - X-linked or
    - Y-linked.

- Visibility of X chromatin in interphase nuclei is due to
    - X chromosome inactivation (lyonization),
    - a process occurring at the 2000 cell stage of the embryo in which
        - DNA methylation starts on Xq then spreads over most loci on either the
        - maternal or paternal X chromosomes at random, leaving one or the other as
        - the single active X chromosome in each cell.

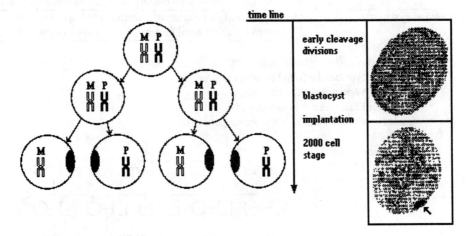

- Results of lyonization include
    - dosage compensation,
    - variability of expression in heterozygous females and
    - mosaicism.

- Meiotic instability of short tandem repeats on the X chromosome causes:
  - Kennedy disease when it results in 40 to 62 CAG repeats (normal 11 to 31) in exon 1 of the androgen receptor gene on Xq,
    - unaffected carriers having gains of 2 to 7 repeats.
  - Fragile X syndrome when it results in greater than 150 CGG repeats in the 5' end of the FMR-1 gene on Xq (mean=30 [range=5-51]), accompanied by
    - methylation of an adjacent CpG island (multiple repeats of 5'-CG-3').
    - Unaffected female carriers ("premutation") have over 57 repeats.

- Genotypic patterns of X-linked inheritance:
  - 50% of the sons of heterozygous females are hemizygous mutant
  - 50% of the daughters of heterozygous females are heterozygous
  - hemizygous mutant males can not father hemizygous mutant sons
  - 100% of the daughters of hemizygous mutant males are heterozygous

- Phenotypic patterns of X-linked recessive inheritance:
  - phenotype is more frequent in males
  - males are affected when hemizygous mutant
  - females are carriers when heterozygous
  - a heterozygous female can be affected if effectively hemizygous due to lyonization
  - a homozygous affected female can be produced by a hemizygous mutant father and a heterozygous mother

Female carriers are heterozygotes

Affected female: heterozygous mother, hemizygous father.

More frequent in males. No male to male transmission.

Progeny of heterozygote: 50% of sons affected, 50% of daughters carriers.

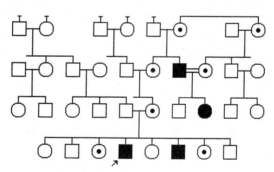

X-LINKED RECESSIVE INHERITANCE

- Phenotypic patterns of X-linked dominant inheritance:
  - phenotype is more frequent in females
  - heterozygous females have milder phenotypes than hemizygous mutant males
  - hemizygosity may be lethal in males
  - homozygosity may be lethal in females
  - genealogy looks like autosomal dominant inheritance in females

More frequent in females.
Milder in heterozygote.
Homozygosity may be lethal.

No male to male transmission.
Hemizygosity may be lethal.

Progeny of heterozygote:
50% affected, either sex.

X-LINKED DOMINANT INHERITANCE

4. Probability, the mathematical expression of chance, is the ratio of the number of
   - occurrences of a specified event to the total number of all possible events.

   - Probability mathematics is used during segregation analysis to assess reliability of
     - observations of mendelian inheritance patterns of phenotypes.

   - Chance is a major determinant of genetic events and
     - most genetic events have independent occurrence.

   - The binomial distribution (discontinuous),
     - a common way to determine the probability of two independent events, is calculated as $(p + q)^n = 1$ where
       - p is the probability of one event,
       - q is the probability of the other and
       - n is the number of trials.

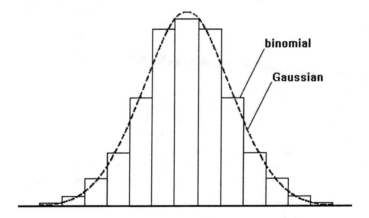

   - When n is large and neither p nor q is close to zero,
     - the binomial distribution approximates the normal or Gaussian (continuous) distribution for which significance testing can be done.

   - When p is small and np = mean = variance,
     - the binomial distribution approximates the Poisson distribution which is
       - typical of natural phenomena that occur in a fixed interval.

   - Significance is the degree to which a data set conforms to a hypothesis.

- Chi square is a statistic often used to determine significance
  - when the distribution of the data is not known:

$$X^2 = \Sigma\left[\frac{(O_i - E_i)}{E_i}\right]$$

- where O=observed value, E=expected value, i = number of (O E) sets.

- The distribution curve of chi square has

$$mean = \nu \quad and \quad variance = 2\nu$$

- and is calculated as:

$$Y = K\left(X^{\nu-s}e^{-0.5X^2}\right)$$

- where

$$\nu = degrees \ of \ freedom = N - 1$$

- N = number of observations (same as number of (O E) sets)
- K is a constant to correct the total area under the curve to 1, and
- e = base of natural logarithms = $(1 + 1/n)^n$= 2.7182818.

- The area under its distribution curve that the chi square value encompasses is a
  - measure of significance of the difference between observed and expected values,
    - the remaining area representing the probability that the difference is due to chance.

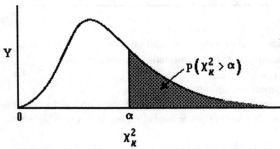

This curve represents the distribution of all values of X^2 for $\nu = 10$. It shows that 25% of all values are above 12. That is the likelihood that the difference is due to chance, $P(H_0)$, while the likelihood that the difference is real is $P(H_1)$ or 75%.

Additional references:

Duke-Elder S. System of Ophthalmology. London: Kimpton, 1964.

Holme E, Larsson N, Oldfors A, et al. Multiple symmetric lipomas with high levels of mtDNA with the tRNA^{lys}A→G$^{(8344)}$ mutation as the only manifestation of disease in a carrier of the myoclonus epilepsy and ragged-red fibers (MERRF) syndrome. Am J Med Genet 1993;52:551-556.

Hsia DY. *Inborn Errors of Metabolism. Part 1. Clinical Aspects.* Chicago: Year Book Medical Publishers, 1966.

Huntington's Disease Collaborative Research Group. A novel gene containing a trinucleotide repeat that is expanded and unstable on Huntington's disease chromosomes. Cell 1993;72:972-983.

LaSpada AR, Roling D, Fischbeck KH. The expanded trinucleotide repeat in X-linked spinal and bulbar muscular atrophy. Abstract 184. Am J Hum Genet 1992;51 (Supplement):A49.

Malcolm S, Clayton-Smith J, Nichols M, et al Uniparental disomy in Angelman syndrome. Lancet 1991;337:694-697.

Mascari MJ, Gottleib W, Rogan PK, et al. The frequency of uniparental disomy in Prader-Willi syndrome. Implications for molecular diagnosis. N Engl J Med 1992;326:1599-1607.

Menkes JH, Phillippart M, Clark DB. Hereditary partial agenesis of corpus callosum. Arch Neurol 1964;11:198-208.

Mettler G, Hunter AGW, O'Hoy K, et al. Clinical correlations of a decrease in CTG trinucleotide repeat amplification with transmission of myotonic dystrophy (DM) from parent to child. Abstract 160. Am J Hum Genet 1992;51 (Supplement):A43.

Nelson DL, Eichler E, King JE, et al. Characterization of the FMR-1 gene at the FRAXA locus of man. Abstract 186. Am J Hum Genet 1992;51 (Supplement):A49.

Nichols RD, Pai GS, Gottlieb W, et al. Paternal uniparental disomy of chromosome 15 in a child with Angelman syndrome. Ann Neurol 1992;32:512-518.

Parrish ML, Roessmann U, Levinsohn MW. Agenesis of the corpus callosum: A study of the frequency of associated malformations. Ann Neurol 1979;6:349-354.

Snow K, Doud LK, Hagerman R, et al. Analysis of a CGG repeat at the FMR-1 locus in Fragile X families and in the general population. Abstract 185. Am J Hum Genet 1992;51 (Supplement):A49.

Warkany J. *Mental Retardation and Congenital Malformations of the Central Nervous System.* Chicago: Year Book Medical Publishers, 1981.

1. The segregation ratio, p, is the
    - expected proportion of affected children in a collection of a very large number of families with known parental genotypes.

- Segregation analysis is the statistical testing of empirical family data for correspondence with a given segregation ratio, and is
    - used to establish the mode of inheritance of phenotypes, e.g.,
        - for autosomal recessive inheritance, expected $p = 0.25$,
        - for autosomal dominant inheritance, expected $p = 0.5$.

- Chi square is used to evaluate the degree to which the observed data (O) conforms to expectations (E).

- E is not equal to p because of the bias of ascertainment,
    - systematic distortion of the segregation ratio due to the fact that
        - the data are ascertained through affected persons hence are non-random.
    - The type of bias is determined by the manner of ascertaining families for study.

- The bias of ascertainment can only be estimated and remains an
    - uncertainty in medical evaluation and counseling.

- A simplex family has one affected person while a
    - multiplex family has multiple affected persons.

- Theoretical complete ascertainment is based on the concept of a random sample in which each category (genotype in this case) has an equal chance of being included in the sample (ascertained); all other type of ascertainment are incomplete.

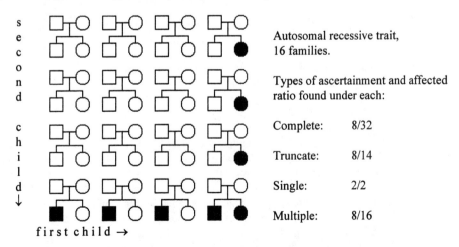

second child ↓

first child →

Autosomal recessive trait, 16 families.

Types of ascertainment and affected ratio found under each:

Complete:	8/32
Truncate:	8/14
Single:	2/2
Multiple:	8/16

- When ascertainment omits the category of families with no affected members but all affected persons are ascertained, this is called truncate ascertainment;
  - each affected person being counted as a proband, resulting in counting of multiplex families several times.

- Prior to 1959, the term, truncate ascertainment, did not exist in the literature of Medical Genetics but a semblance of the same definition was used for complete ascertainment; some confusion remains.

- Single ascertainment means that each sibship is ascertained only once, and there is only
  - one proband per family but
  - the likelihood of ascertaining a family is proportional to the number of affected members.

- Multiple ascertainment means there is only one proband per family
  - but multiplex families may be ascertained more than once, and is
  - closer to clinical data sets.

- The Apert method, one of the methods of calculating E, is also known as the
  - *a priori method* and is based on the binomial distribution:

$$\text{Truncate ascertainment:} \quad E = \frac{sp}{\left(1 - p^s\right)}$$

$$\text{Single ascertainment:} \quad E = 1 + (p(s-1))$$

- where s is sibship size,
- p is the segregation ratio, and
- q = 1 - p

- The Weinberg method of calculating E, also known as the method of
  - discarding the probands, is applicable to
  - truncate ascertainment, the technique being that the
  - probands (P) are removed from both numerator and denominator by calculating
  - (total affected - P) / (total children - P)

- The Li and Mantel method of calculating E, also known as the
  - method of discarding the singles, is applicable to
  - truncate ascertainment, the technique being that the
  - probands that are single cases (J) are removed from both numerator and denominator:
  - (total affected - J) / (total children - J)

- Meiotic drive, a characteristic of mutant genes called Segregation Distorter in Drosophila,
  - distorts the segregation ratio by enhancing transmission of the mutant gene by causing loss of sperm bearing other alleles or inability of those sperm to fertilize.
  - Biologic factors like this may account for odd segregation ratios observed with some human disorders.

A Priori Method

s	Truncate ascertainment		Single ascertainment	
	Expected proportions of affected (E/s) for sibship size s (ideal would be 0.25 for recessive, 0.50 for dominant)			
	recessive	dominant	recessive	dominant
2	0.5714*	0.6667	0.6250!	0.7500
3	0.4324	0.5714*	0.5000#	0.6667
4	0.3267	0.5333	0.4375	0.6250
5	0.3278	0.5161	0.4000	0.6000
6	0.3041	0.5079	0.3750	0.5833
7	0.2885	0.5039	0.3571	0.5714*
8	0.2778	0.5020	0.3438	0.5625
9	0.2703	0.5010	0.3333	0.5556
10	0.2649	0.5005	0.3250	0.5500
11	0.2610	0.5002	0.3182	0.5455
12	0.2582	0.5001	0.3125	0.5417
13	0.2561	0.5001	0.3077	0.5385
14	0.2545	0.5000#	0.3036	0.5357
15	0.2534	0.5000	0.3000	0.5333
16	0.2525	0.5000	0.2969	0.5312

Symbols * ! # indicate confusing results.

Confusion increases as s decreases.

Truncate ascertainment is better with smaller s.

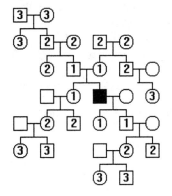

DEGREES OF RELATIONSHIP

First degree: parents, sibs

Second degree: aunts, uncles, nephews, neices, nephews, grandparents, grandchildren

Third degree: great-grandparents, great aunts, great uncles, first cousins, great-granchildren

2. Degree of relationship is used in defining polygenic inheritance; it is
    * the number of steps separating two persons in a genealogy chart.

* The unit of inheritance, or "gene," was initially called "factor."
    * hence, "multifactorial" may be understood as an archaic synonym of "polygenic."
    * It is misused as a term to emphasize the environmental components of polygenic traits.
        * In truth, there are environmental components to all genetic diseases.
            * Environmental factors of polygenic inheritance are more feeble and less identifiable than those of monogenic inheritance.

- Other misuses of "multifactorial" are as a term to:
  - Combine the meanings of phenocopy and genetic heterogeneity.
  - Express that a trait has ill-defined, poorly defined or undefined genetics.

- Metric traits are expressed as measurements.
  - Most metric traits are acquired through polygenic inheritance.
  - Most metric traits represent **normal variation** but
    - extremes of their distributions may account for certain **common genetic diseases**, e.g., hypercholesterolemia, hypertension, obesity and short stature.

- The population frequency distribution of values of a polygenic trait forms a
  - unimodal bell-shaped Gaussian curve, indicating that its factors are <u>very numerous</u> and have <u>equally feeble</u> mathematical effects.
  - The genetic component results from all minor genes that either promote or inhibit expression of the trait.
  - The environmental component results from all minor environmental agents that either promote or inhibit expression of the trait.

- Departures from unimodality cause skewness, kurtosis, or both, indicating the presence of one or more **major** factors which may be either genetic or environmental.

Skewness:

$$g1 = \frac{1}{s^3(n-1)} \Sigma (x - \bar{x})^3$$

left skewness $- \leftarrow 0 \rightarrow +$ right skewness

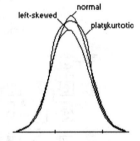

Kurtosis:

$$g2 = \frac{1}{s^4(n-1)} \Sigma (x - \bar{x})^4 - 3$$

platykurtosis $- \leftarrow 0 \rightarrow +$ leptokurtosis

- Presumption of polygenic inheritance of a trait is based on segregation analysis, i.e., the degree to which the
  - frequency of the trait in relatives corresponds to the
  - proportions expected with polygenic inheritance.

- Mathematical expressions of metric polygenic resemblances of relatives are:
  - The frequency of the trait in first degree relatives approximates the
    - square root of the population incidence (proband frequency).
  - The mean values in relatives are shifted toward the mean of probands in an amount proportional to the number of genes shared;
    - for first degree relatives: 1/2, second degree: 1/4, third degree: 1/8.

DEVELOPMENT OF POLYGENIC THEORY FROM DATA ABOUT STATURE.

Among healthy British military conscripts, probands were defined by tallness. Tallness was more frequent among their parents (1° relatives) than among other parents. Distributions were unimodal. Tallness was obviously hereditary, but proportions among relatives were different from proportions that had been observed with traits that had Mendelian inheritance.

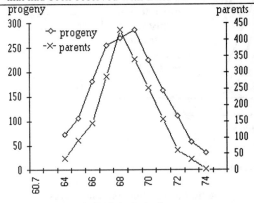

A. Height in inches

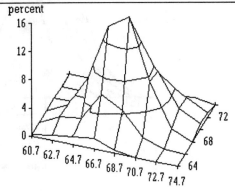

B. Axes of A rotated to form a bivariate surface

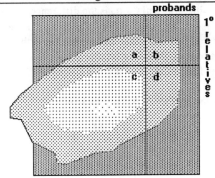

C. Looking down on conical surface of B

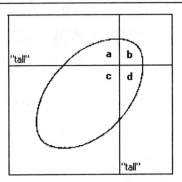

D. Flat surface of r = 0.5 (elliptical)

a,b,c,d = proportions
(in C, partial conical volumes; in D,
partial elliptic areas-density function omitted)

q_g = population incidence
q_{ra} = incidence in 1° relatives

r = correlation coefficient
Note: for 1° relatives, r = 0.5

$$q_g = b+d \qquad q_{ra} = \frac{b}{b+d}$$

$$\ln\frac{bc}{ad} \cong \frac{8}{\pi}z \qquad z = \tanh^{-1}r$$

$$b \cong (b+d)^t \qquad t = 1 + \ln\left(1 + e^{\frac{-8z}{\pi}}\right)/\ln 2$$

$$q_{ra} = (b+d)^{(t-1)} \cong q_g^{1/2}$$

ANALYSIS OF A BIVARIATE NORMAL SURFACE BASED ON PROPORTIONS OF GENES SHARED.

q_g	frequency in general population	$q_g^{3/4}$	frequency in 2° relatives
$q_g^{1/2}$	frequency in 1° relatives	$q_g^{7/8}$	frequency in 3° relatives

EXTENSION OF CALCULATIONS TO OTHER DEGREES OF RELATIONSHIP

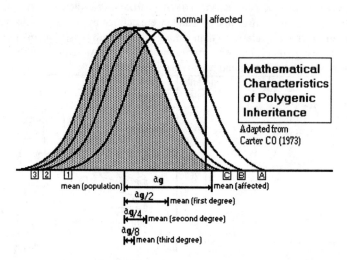

The shaded curve represents the distribution of a polygenic trait in a population. The curves beginning with 1, 2, and 3 are the distributions of the trait in first, second and third degree relatives. The parts of the curves past the affected boundary end with A, B and C. a_g is the difference between the mean of the population and the mean of affected persons. The shift of the mean of $a_g/2$ places a greater proportion of first degree relatives past the affected boundary than the proportion in the population as a whole. With increasing degrees of relationship, there is a smaller proportion affected: Fourth relatives have nearly the same proportion affected as in the population as a whole.

COMPARISON OF MENDELIAN AND POLYGENIC INHERITANCE. A WORKED EXAMPLE:

Both Mendelian and polygenic traits can have bell-shaped distributions in a population but they differ in frequencies among relatives.

Polygenic proportions among relatives are not observed with Mendelian inheritance, and vice versa.

The distribution of "examplase" is bell-shaped and 46 of 925 progeny had an **enzyme level** of 210 or greater (q_g = 0.049). If it were polygenic, the expected frequency among parents would be $\sqrt{q_g}$, or 0.22. Forty five of 884 were found (q_{ra}= 0.051), a deficiency of 87%.

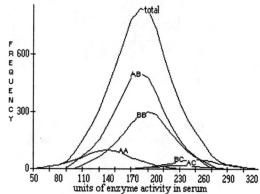

"Examplase" population data. Individual activities are accounted for by combinations of A, B & C subunits.
Modified from Harris H (1975)

Also, as shown in the following analysis, the proportions of **isoenzyme types** in families conform to expectations of Mendelian inheritance (0.999), not polygenic (0.474). Hence, neither the enzyme levels nor the isoenzyme types conform to expectations of polygenic inheritance.

Progeny $(p+q+r)^2$

No.	Parents	AA	AB	BB	CC	AC	BC	Total	
13	AA|AA	22						22	
50	AA|AB	65	48					113	
27	AA|BB		65					65	
6	AA|AC	4				5		9	
10	AA|BC		5			14		19	
94	AB|AB	40	91	54				185	
109	AB|BB		106	96				202	
16	AB|AC	14	9			6	4	33	
16	AB|BC		10	7		6	10	33	
55	BB|BB			141				141	
12	BB|AC		12				20	32	
24	BB|BC			33			25	58	
5	AC|BC		2		1	2	3	8	
5	BC|BC				1		4	5	
	Obs	145	348	331	2	33	66	925	
	Exp	138	359	326	3	33	66	924	0.999
		(p^2)	$(2pq)$	(q^2)	(r^2)	$(2pr)$	$(2qr)$		
	q_{ra}	0.157	0.376	0.358	0.002	0.036	0.071	1.000	
	q_g	0.135	0.429	0.319	0.000	0.044	0.074		
	$\sqrt{q_g}$	0.396	0.613	0.598	0.046	0.189	0.267	2.110	0.474

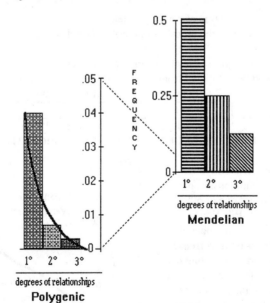

Polygenic

Mendelian

degrees of relationships

Frequencies of typical polygenic traits among relatives are an order of magnitude less than frequencies of Mendelian traits among relatives. The **distribution** of affected relatives is discrete for Mendelian traits while it is continuous for polygenic traits.

- Heritability (h^2) is the proportion of the variance of a trait that is due to
  - the genetic component (s_G^2), the remainder being due to
    - the environmental component (s_E^2).

Heritability	Standard deviation	Variance	
$h^2 = \dfrac{s_G^2}{s_G^2 + s_E^2}$ <u>Genetic =1 ↔ 0 = Environmental</u> **difficult to parameterize**	$s = \sqrt{s^2}$	$s^2 = \dfrac{\Sigma(x_i - \bar{x})^2}{N-1}$ x_i = **individual trait value** $\bar{x}$ = **mean**	
Covariance	Correlation coefficient	q	h^2
$s_{xy}^2 = \dfrac{\Sigma\left[(x_i - \bar{x})(y_i - \bar{y})\right]}{N-1}$ **probands: x, relatives: y**	$r = \dfrac{s_{xy}^2}{s_x - s_y}$ **parameterizable**	<u>MZ twins</u> <u>Sibs</u> <u>Uncles</u> 1ˢᵗ cousins	r <u>2r</u> <u>4r</u> <u>8r</u>

HERITABILITY CALCULATION

- Variance (s^2) is the average squared deviation of the observations (x_i) from the mean; its square root is the standard deviation (s).

- The covariance (s_{xy}^2) of p and q is the sum of the products of the
  - deviations of each observation among probands (x_i) of p from their mean
  - deviations of each observation among relatives (y_i) of q from their mean
  - divided by the number of observations (N) minus 1.

- The correlation coefficient (r) of p and q is their
  - covariance divided by the product of their standard deviations.

- Taking q as various degrees of relationship to probands p,
  - heritability can be calculated from r.

q	h^2	stature	finger ridge count	IQ
Sibs	2r	.56	.50	.58

Adapted from Fraser-Roberts JA (1961)
EXAMPLES OF HERITABILITIES OF METRIC TRAITS

- Genetic biases in heritability:
  Parental consanguinity pushes phenotypes of progeny toward one or other end of the population distribution resulting in
  - more frequent abnormal phenotypes.
  Parental phenotypes often correlate because of assortative mating but
  - one is usually closer to the population mean, lessening the predicted effect of genes in common on the phenotypes of relatives of all degrees,
  - a phenomenon known as **regression to the mean.**

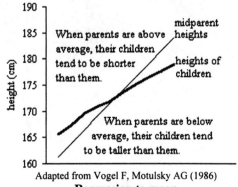

Adapted from Vogel F, Motulsky AG (1986)
Regression to mean

- Environmental biases in heritability
    - National effects: different trait frequencies in progeny of immigrants.
    - Familial effects: different trait frequencies in adoptees.
    - Maternal effects: different trait frequencies in progeny of different mothers.
    The contribution a mother makes to the phenotype of an offspring over and above that which results from the genes that she contributes to the zygote: Transcription of maternally derived active mRNA's, maternal nutrition either via the egg or via pre- or post-natal supplies of food, transmission of pathogens and antibodies through the prenatal blood supply or by postnatal feeding, imitative behavior, interaction between sibs either directly with one another or through the mother.

- Genealogical characteristics that suggest polygenic inheritance of a **disease**:
    - frequency of phenotype in relatives is greater than the population rate,
    - risk to unborn increases with the number of affected relatives,
    - risk to unborn is inversely proportional to population rate
    (populations with higher rates have lower relative risks).

Rate in population (Risk of first)	Risk of second	Risk of third	Risk of fourth	Risk to mother's sister's children	Risk to children of affected person
.003 (U.K.)	.05 (17X)	.1 (33X)	.2 (66X)	.006 (2X)	.03 (10X)
.001 (U.S.)	.032 (32X)				

The data have the genealogic characteristics of polygenic inheritance: frequency in relatives is greater than the population rate, risk to unborn increases with number of affected relatives, risk to unborn is inversely proportional to population rate.

DATA ABOUT NEURAL TUBE DEFECTS

- Distributions of common diseases and malformations among relatives conform to expectations of threshhold polygenic inheritance,
    with theoretical underlying continuous distributions that cannot be discerned,
    - the phenotype becoming evident only when it reaches sufficient magnitude to disturb subsequent developmental steps.

THE THEORY OF POLYGENIC THRESHHOLD INHERITANCE: The distribution is continuous but the phenotype is evident only in part of the distribution.

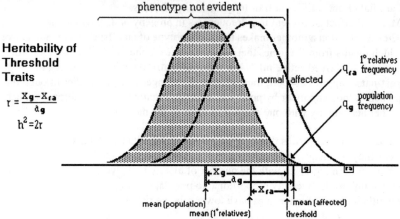

X_{ra} is the deviation of the threshhold from the mean of 1° relatives, a_g is the deviation of the mean of affecteds from the population mean, X_g is the deviation of the threshold from the population mean.

Only q_g and q_{ra} are measurable but they are proportions of normal curves so the other factors can be derived or obtained from tables in Emery AEH (1986).

- Under polygenic threshhold inheritance theory,
  Relatives are closer to the threshold and the risk to unborn is higher when
  - the proband has a severe case (see data on Hirschsprung disease),
  - there are multiple cases in the family (see data on Club foot) or
  - the proband is of the seldom affected sex (see data on Pyloric stenosis).

- Careful, extensive studies of large numbers of probands of a disease trait may reveal extensive genetic heterogeneity,
  - a large proportion of cases due to polygenic inheritance,
  - others cases due to
    - classical Mendelian inheritance of a major gene,
    - complex forms of inheritance of a major gene,
    - oligogenic inheritance,
    - new mutations of a wide variety of types.

COMMON DISEASES AND MALFORMATIONS WHOSE DISTRIBUTIONS
CONFORM TO EXPECTATIONS OF POLYGENIC THRESHHOLD INHERITANCE

Disorder	Rate (%)	h^2	Sex ratio M:F	Normal parents Rate of second affected child (%)	Affected parent Rate of having affected child (%)	Affected parent Rate of second affected child (%)
Ankylosing spondylitis	.2	.70				
Asthma	4	.80				
Cleft lip/palate	.1	.76		2		
bilateral				6		
Club foot	0.1	.68	2:1	3	3	10
Congenital heart defect	.5	.35		2 (same type)	14 (if mother)	
additional risk				4 (other type)		
Coronary heart disease	3	.65				
Hip dislocation	0.07	.60	1:6	6	12	36
Hirschsprung disease	0.02		4:1			
short segment				3	2	
long segment				12		
Hypertension	5	.62				
Hypospadias (males)	0.2			10	10	
Neural tube defect	.5	.60		4	4	8
Peptic ulcer	4	.37				
Pyloric stenosis	0.3	.75	5:1			
male proband				2	4	13
female proband				10	17	38
Renal agenesis bilateral	0.01		3:1			
male proband				3		
female proband				7		
Schizophrenia	1	.85				
Scoliosis adolescent	0.22		1:6	7	5	
Tracheoesophageal fistula	0.03		1:1	1	1	

Adapted from Nora JJ, Fraser CF (1989), Emery AEH (1986)

- The extensive genetic heterogeneity of many disease traits may yield population data that are consistent with polygenic theory but not representative of individual families.
  - Careful genealogical evaluation is required to determine if the disease has a Mendelian inheritance pattern.
  - Laboratory testing is required for diseases that may not be distinguishable by physical examination, e.g., 22q11.2 deletion testing in conotruncal heart defects.
  - Careful examination of each case is required to ensure that the disease is an isolated problem rather than a syndrome due to a major factor.
  - If those steps reveal no discrete cause for the disease, actuarial figures based on population data may be offered as provisory risks, but only after ensuring that the consultand understands the concepts of genetic heterogeneity and risk.

- The quantitative trait locus (*QTL*) research model extends techniques of linkage analysis by the use of anonymous DNA markers throughout the genome.
  - It has identified oligogenes, previously unknown loci for common disease traits such as affective disorders, asthma, and diabetes.
    - Oligogenes are incompletely penetrant genes with a strength of effect between that of major and minor genes.
    - Uses of the term, oligogene, in the literature imply extended co-dominance or confined additiveness, reflecting the fact that the concept is still developing.
    - Oligogenes may produce disorders either alone, additively, or in concert with polygenic or environmental components.
  - Though of great heuristic importance, the oligogene concept may not significantly alter actuarial risk figures nor medical management principles in the foreseeable future.

The current most popular *QTL* method is the total genome search. Markers throughout the genome at regular intervals less than 10 centimorgans are typed in sibs. Analysis is done by the Haseman-Elston, or sib-pair, method based on Fisher's work. A computation is done at each marker locus to determine the difference in trait value between a pair of sibs. It is squared and graphed on the Y axis. Sibs must share either 0, 1, or 2 marker alleles by descent. This status is graphed on the X axis. If the slope of the resulting line is negative (as in the panel at the right) the marker is near an oligogene. Finer resolution studies can identify the gene.

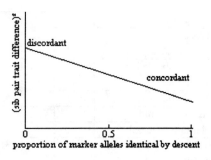

Additional references:

Carter CO. Multifactorial Genetic Disease. In: McKusick VA, Claiborne R (editors). *Medical Genetics*. New York: Hospital Practice Publishers, 1973.

Craddock N, Khodel V, Eerdewegh PV, et al. Mathematical limits of multilocus models: The genetic transmission of bipolar disorder. Am J Hum Genet 1995;57:690-702.

Edwards JH. Familial predisposition in man. Brit Med Bull 1969;25:58-64.

Elston RC. Algorithms and inferences: The challenge of multifactorial diseases. Am J Hum Genet 1997;60:255-62.

Emery AEH. *Methodology in Medical Genetics. An Introduction to Statistical Methods*. New York: Churchill Livingstone, 1986.

Fraser-Roberts JA. Multifactorial inheritance in relation to normal and abnormal human traits. Brit Med Bull 1961;17:241-246.

Harris H. *An Introduction to Human Biochemical Genetics. Eugenics Laboratory Memoirs 37*. New York: Cambridge, 1955.

Harris H. The Principles of Human Biochemical Genetics. New York: Elsevier, 1975.

Harrison GA, Weiner JS, Tanner JM, et al. *Human Biology*, 2nd edition. Oxford: Oxford University Press, 1977.

Johannsen W. *Elemente der exaten Erblich-keitslehre*. Jena: G Fischer, Jena, 1926.

Morton NE. Significance levels in complex inheritance. Am J Hum Genet 1998;62:690-697.

Nora JJ, Fraser FC. *Medical Genetics. Principles and Practice*, 3rd edition. Philadephia: Lea & Febiger, 1989.

Plomin R, Owen MJ, McGuffin P. The genetic basis of complex human traits. Science 1994;264:1733-1739.

Toriello HV, Higgins JV. Occurrence of neural tube defects among first, second and third degree relatives of probands: Results of a United States study. Am J Med Genet 1983;15:601-606.

Wright S. Coefficients of inbreeding and relationship. Am Nat 1922;56:330-8.

1. Marked decreases of infectious and nutritional diseases have focused attention on genetic disorders.

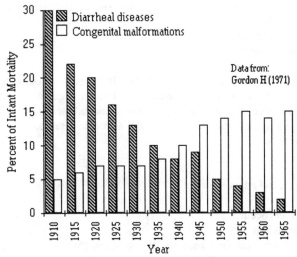

*   Two factors causing a slight rise in the prevalence of genetic disorders are:
    *   modern medical treatment which
        *   allows persons with genetic diseases to reproduce
    *   increased longevity which
        *   allows time for genetic diseases to manifest themselves.

*   Between implantation and the 8th week of gestation,
    *   about 62% of fetuses dies spontaneously;
    *   95% are visibly malformed;
    *   62% have a chromosome aberration.

*   Between the 9th week of gestation and term,
    *   about 24% of fetuses dies spontaneously;
    *   50% between 9 and 16 weeks have a chromosome aberration;
    *   15% between 21 and 40 weeks have a chromosome aberration.

*   At least 2% of liveborns have a genetic disorder, many of which
    *   require laboratory procedures for diagnosis or confirmation of diagnosis.

*   About 1/3 of pediatric inpatients are hospitalized for a genetic disorder while
    *   about 1/3 more are there for conditions with a genetic basis.

*   At least 20% of persons will develop a disorder with a genetic basis at some time during their lives.

2. Single gene disorders have frequencies of less than 1:1000 and each is
   - caused by a gene which has a mutation that decreases its ability
   - to control the effect of a <u>strong</u> environmental factor,
     - resulting in one of many types of diseases, typically a metabolic error,
     - treatable through
       - metabolic alterations
       - gene replacement

- Polygenic disorders have frequencies of greater than 1:1000 and are thought to be
  - caused by the co-occurrence of many mutations that decrease genetic ability
  - to control the collective effect of many <u>weak</u> environmental factors,
    - typically resulting in a congenital anomaly or a chronic disease,
    - treatable through
      - surgery
      - habilitation
      - environmental adjustment

- Chromosomal disorders occur
  - in 7:1000 liveborns and
  - over 500:1000 spontaneous first trimester abortions, and are
  - due to physical changes in the genetic material rather than mutant genes
    - affecting either embryogenic or stem cell functions,
    - typically resulting in multiple congenital anomalies or malignancy,
    - treatable through
      - surgery
      - habilitation
      - environmental adjustment

- There are so many genetic disorders that
  - each physician may not encounter more than one case of some of them, so
  - diagnosis and management require learning the principles of genetics rather than learning the characteristics of specific disorders.

- No genetic disorder is more significant:
  - each genetic disorder is relatively uncommon and of
  - relatively similar frequency to genetic disorders with the same basis and
  - each genetic disorder is of relatively similar genetic impact.

- Genetic nosology, the study of genetic disorders through classification and categorization, is
  - the binding link in the circle of knowledge of medical genetics.
  - The first link is characterization of the phenotype.

3.   Characterization of the phenotype is a medical service.
It requires medical decision making based on
- data about the proband that are obtained by a physician from
- a medical evaluation consisting of
  - a history which characterizes the proband's condition or malfunctions,
  - physical examination which detects physical abnormalities, and
  - laboratory testing for biochemical, karyotype and DNA abnormalities.

Administrative Aspects of Phenotype Characterization

CODING OF LEVEL OF SERVICE (also see section of this same name in *Genetic Counseling*)
Phenotype characterization by a physician is an encounter that is covered by Evaluation and Management definitions in *Physician's Current Procedural Terminology* (CPT). Principles are the same as for any other type of encounter between physician and patient.

DIAGNOSIS CODING (also see section of this same name in *Genetic Counseling*)
Page ix of the *International Classification of Diseases*, *Clinical Modification*, ninth edition (ICD-9-CM) emphasizes that modifying codes are to be used in brackets after the disease code to indicate the manifestation of the disease if the manifestation is not explicit in the disease code. There are either specific or general codes for all diseases that affect probands. The modifying code for female consultands is 629.8 and for male consultands, 608.81. Those are the codes for *specified disorders of the genital organs* of which production of genetically abnormal gametes is definitely one. In systems that do not have room for modifying codes, only the code of the basic disease is used for consultands.

- An abnormal phenotype may be recognizable,
  - because of findings identical to those of other cases in the medical literature,
  but in many cases, data are suggestive or consistent rather than definitive, so
  - diagnosis is usually tentative (a medical opinion).

- An unrecognizable abnormal phenotype is frequently
  - unprecedented in the medical literature,
  - usually unique to the patient ("private" condition),
  - rarely a new category of disorders.

- History data obtained by interview is tentative, to be interpreted only
  - in connection with physical and laboratory data;
  - if there has been prior evaluation, actual medical data must be obtained as part of the history-taking process.

A form used in practice to record medical history data is in Appendix 2.

- Age of parents when proband was born
  - may help differentiate mutation from other etiologies:
    - chromosome mutation frequency increases with maternal age and
    - single gene mutation frequency increases with paternal age.

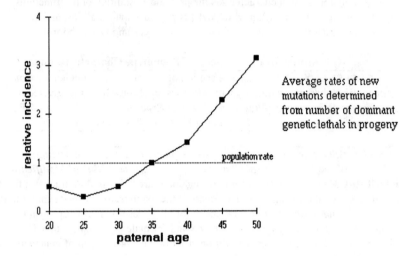

Average rates of new mutations determined from number of dominant genetic lethals in progeny

- It is important to determine the age of onset of the problem because
  - some types of genetic diseases are of prenatal (congenital) onset while
  - other types are of postnatal onset.

Category	Estimated percentages	
	Congenital	Non-congenital
Polygenic	50	60
Monogenic	19	29
Chromosomal	15	0.5
Exogenous	16	10.5

- Detailed history of gestation may disclose teratogenic influences; however,
  - false positive information is obtained with great frequency due to
    - societal paranoia about teratogens;
  - false negative information is also frequent and is usually due to either
    - ignorance or
    - denial.

Hence, teratogen exposure data are acceptable only when verified and quantitated.

- Weight and other measurements at birth, when compared to length of gestation,
  - may help to determine if a disorder was present but not noticed at that time,
    - since many congenital disorders cause poor fetal growth and development.

- Physical examination produces
  - quantitative data (measurements) and
  - qualitative data (observations).

A form used in practice to record physical examination data is in Appendix 2.

- If range statistics, such as percentile charts, are available for comparison,
  - quantitative physical data are of value in nearly all cases,
    - but are of little value otherwise.

Selected range statistics are in Appendix 1.

- Qualitative data are of value only if evaluated by an
  - examiner who has acquired a gestalt (mental image) of the patient's disorder
    - through reading or experience.

The monologue on Multiple Congenital Anomalies in Appendix 3 is helpful.

- Photographs are valuable for recording physical data if
  - taken with non-distorting technique and a
  - measurement scale is included.
  Among their uses are
  - record-keeping when words fail to adequately describe findings
  - consultation
  - future diagnosis of indeterminate cases.

4.   Dermatoglyphics aberrations reflect either
   • specific or non-specific alterations of the first 16 weeks of fetal development.
   • See Appendix 1 for norms.

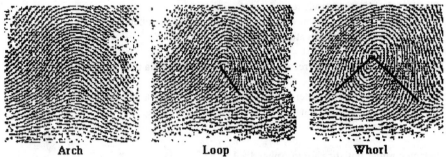

Arch   Loop   Whorl

Dermatoglyphics fingertip patterns. The ridge count is the number of ridges crossed by a line from the triradius to the center of the pattern. A loop has one triradius. A whorl has several triradii so several ridge counts. By convention, only the largest is used in the total ridge count calculation.

   • Accurate evaluation of the significance of dermatoglyphics aberrations requires
      • examination of first degree relatives because
         • any aberration may be due to rare familial variation.

   • Incomplete or disturbed differentiation of the fingertips causes arch patterns; hence
      • lower ridge count
      but, when the fingertips are fully formed,
      • excessive numbers of arch patterns suggest chromosome aberrations,
         • especially chromosome 18 trisomy and XXXXY.

   • Excessive numbers of whorl patterns are found in
      • Turner syndrome and
      • Smith-Lemli-Opitz syndrome

   • A single flexion crease (simian crease) on the palm,
      • instead of the expected two creases suggests chromosome aberrations,
         • especially Down syndrome, as do
      • distal axial triradius of palm,
      • halluceal arch tibial and
      • radial loops on fingertips 4 & 5.

   • Lack of hypothenar ridges suggests Cornelia De Lange syndrome.

5. A genealogical chart is part of the medical history even though genealogy data are often obtained after the physical examination which is required to indicate worthwhile paths of genealogical inquiry.
   * Functions of the genealogical chart include
     * efficient summarization of genetic data and
     * analysis of the genetic mechanism that produces a phenotype.

* The Germanic chart is used most commonly;
  * terminology is so variable that a legend should always be included on the chart.

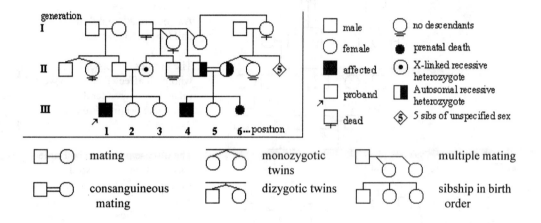

* Public records of marriages, births, deaths and successions
  * are the most accurate source of genealogical data but
  * recollections of family members are the most commonly used;
  * the Catholic Church and the Mormon Church are also good sources of data.

Forms used in practice to record genealogical data are in Appendix 2.

- Pedigree is a term used for a type of genealogy chart that is
  - used to detect consanguinity; and consists of
  - the full names of the direct ancestors
    (parents in each generation prior to the proband);
  if completed for ten generations, it establishes
  - the likelihood of autosomal recessive inheritance of a phenotype
  - and the genetic risks of that type of transmission.

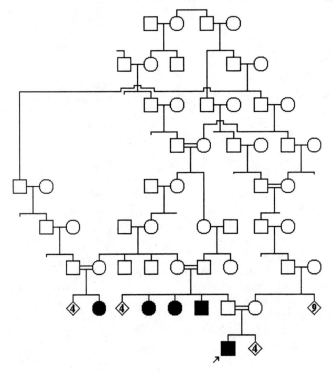

An "outbreak" of deformed children in Kinder, LA.

The brother and sister through whom all affected children were related were grandchildren of one of the original French-Acadian pioneers.

The disease proved to be Bardet-Biedl syndrome, a disorder shown in 1920 to be inherited as an autosomal recessive trait in French families.

None of the parents of the affected children was aware that they were related to each other until their genealogies were traced.

- Collateral relatives is a term used for the
  - descendants of the sibs of persons in the pedigree chart.

- Data about the pregnancies of all of the proband's relatives,
  - especially the ultimate medical condition of each conceptus,
  - including pregnancies of collateral relatives,
  are needed to
  - establish the likelihood of dominant, X-linked or polygenic inheritance, and to
  - calculate genetic risks.

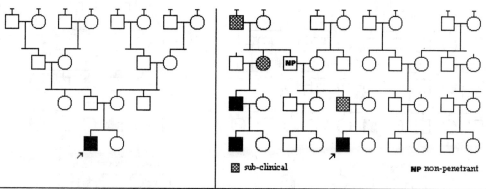

Initial family history.	**Genealogy.**
Autosomal recessive?	Note affected collateral relatives, and relatives with
Polygenic?	sub-clinical cases revealed by medical evaluations.
Teratogenic?	Typical autosomal dominant.
New mutation?	

- To reinforce the accuracy of genealogical data obtained by interview, it is often necessary to obtain data about relatives, including
  - medical records,
  - photographs, or
  - physical examination.

- Due to "privacy" laws and regulations, data about relatives may be available
  - only to the proband or a legal agent of the proband who must obtain the data
  - and submit it to the physician for analysis.

- Examination of a relative of a proband by a physician is a service to the relative
  - to determine if the relative has the same condition as the proband,
  - with the usual physician-patient responsibilities,
  - for which records, fees and coding are the same as for the proband.

- Most informative data from a medical genealogy is found in the
  - descendants of the proband's great-grandparents, and is often
  - limited to a small section of the genealogy.

- Limiting factors include:
  - Non-paternity.
  - Distant consanguinity.
    - Bilateral ancestry among a pioneer group may be the only clue.

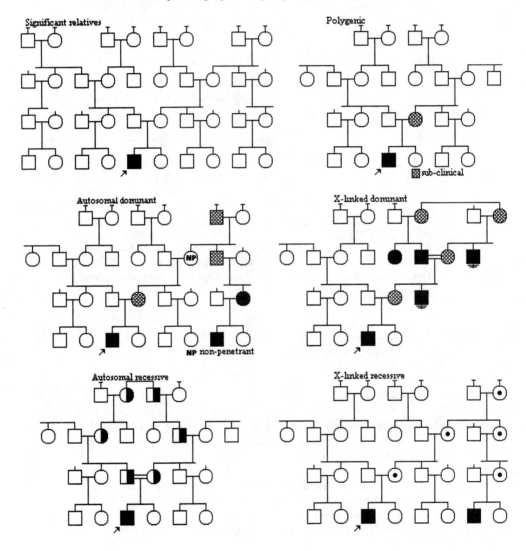

Additional references:

American Medical Association. *Physician's Current Procedural Terminology. 4th Edition.* Chicago: American Medical Association, Chicago, 1992.

Bergsma D, Lowry RB (editors). *Numerical Taxonomy of Birth Defects and Polygenic Disorders.* Birth Defects Original Article Series XIII (3A). New York: Alan R. Liss, 1977.

Boue J, Boue A, Lazar P. Retrospective and prospective epidemiological studies of 1500 karyotyped spontaneous human abortions. Teratology 1975;12:11-26.

Byrne JM. Fetal Pathology: *Laboratory Manual.* Birth Defects Original Article Series 19 (2). White Plains: March of Dimes Birth Defects Foundation, 1983.

Byrne JM, Warburton D, Kline J, et al. Morphology of early fetal deaths and their chromosomal characteristics. Teratology 1985;32:297-315.

Carr DH, Gedeon M. Population cytogenetics of human abortuses. In: Hook EB, Porter IH (editors). *Population Cytogenetics: Studies in Humans.* Academic Press, New York: Academic Press, 1977.

Creasy MR, Crolla JA, Alberman D. A cytogenetic study of human spontaneous abortions using banding techniques. Hum Genet 1976;31:177-196.

Fantel AG, Shepard TH, Vadheim-Roth C, et al. Embryonic and fetal phenotypes: Prevalence and other associated factors in a large study of spontaneous abortions. In Porter IH, Hook EB (editors). *Human Embryonic and Fetal Death.* New York: Academic Press, 1980.

Gordon H. Genetic counseling. Considerations for talking to parents and prospective parents. JAMA 1971;217:1215-25.

Hall JG, Froster-Iskenius UG, Allanson JE. *Handbook of Normal Physical Measurements.* New York: Oxford, 1989

Harlap S, Shiono PH, Ramcharan S. A life table of spontaneous abortions and the effects of age, parity and other variables. In Porter IH, Hook, EB (editors). *Human Embryonic and Fetal Death.* New York: Academic Press, 1980.

Hassold T, Chen N, Funkhouser J, et al. A cytogenetic study of 1000 spontaneous abortions. Ann Hum Genet 1980;44(Pt 2): 151-78.

Kajii T, Ferrier A, Nikawa N, et al. Anatomic and chromosomal anomalies in 639 spontaneous abortuses. Hum Genet 1980;55(1): 87-98.

Loesch DZ. *Quantitative Dermatoglyphics.* Oxford Monographs on Medical Genetics No. 10. New York: Oxford, 1983.

Milunsky A. The Prevention of Genetic Disease and Mental Retardation. Philadelphia: Saunders, 1975.

Munne S, Griffo J, Cohen J, et al. Chromosome abnormalities in human arrested preimplantation embryos: A multiprobe FISH study. Am J Hum Genet 1994;55:150-159.

Penrose LS. *Memorandum on dermatoglyphic nomenclature.* Birth Defects Original Article Series 4(3): 1-13. White Plains: March of Dimes Birth Defects Foundation, 1968.

Schaumann B, Alter M. *Dermatoglyphics in Medical Disorders*. New York: Springer-Verlag, 1976.

Stein Z, Kline J, Susser E, et al. Maternal age and spontaneous abortion. In: Porter IH, Hook, EB (editors) *Human Embryonic and Fetal Death*. New York: Academic Press, 1980.

U.S. Department of Health and Human Services. *The International Classification of Diseases, 9th revision. Clincal Modification*, 2nd edition. DHHS Publication No. (PHS) 80-1260. Washington, DC: U S Government Printing Office, 1980.

Vogel F, Ratherberg R. Spontaneous mutation in man. Adv Hum Genet 1975;5:223-318.

Warburton D, Kline J, Stein Z, et al. Cytogenetic abnormalities in spontaneous abortions of recognized conceptions. In: Porter IH, Hatcher NH, Willey AM (editors). *Perinatal Genetics: Diagnosis and Treatment*. New York: Academic Press, 1986.

Warkany J. *Congenital Malformations. Notes and Comments*. Chicago: Year Book Medical Publishers, 1971.

1. Molecular genetic diagnostic techniques allow
    *   **prenatal diagnosis of some genetic diseases** as well as
    *   **testing for the carrier state of some recessive genes** and
    *   **premorbid diagnosis of some late-onset genetic diseases**.

*   A mutation that transforms a normal gene into a disease gene
    *   may result in an additional restriction enzyme cleavage site,
        *   causing a shorter than normal DNA fragment to be diagnostic,
    *   or may obliterate a cleavage site,
        *   causing a longer than normal DNA fragment to be diagnostic.

*   One of the effects of a disease gene may be to cause
    *   amplification of a distant segment of DNA, resulting in
        *   a new marker if one site is within the segment,
        *   increased concentration of a marker if two sites are within the segment,
        *   or combinations of these results.

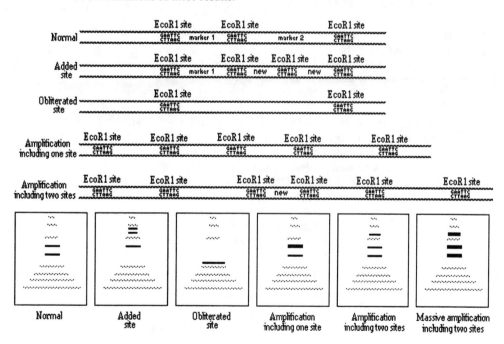

*   Often, a cleavage site may be found so close to a disease gene
    *   that they are usually not separated by crossovers during meiosis,
        *   which is called linkage.

- Loci on the same chromosome are syntenic, and,
  - when close together, they are said to be linked, which means that
  - they occur together after cross-over more frequently than expected.

- The frequency that two linked genes are found together should equal
  - the product of the frequencies of the two genes in the population.

- When linked genes are found together much more frequently than expected,
  - this is called linkage disequilibrium and is usually due to
    - natural selection,
    - recent mutation,
    - recent population admixture, or
    - chromosome inversion.

- Efficient linkage studies in small human families requires that
  - the loci must be polymorphic (no allele with frequency greater than 0.99) and
  - the linkage phase must be known.

- The most frequent procedure used to determine if two human genes are linked is
  - analysis for lod score which is the
    - logarithm of the odds favoring linkage, used because it is
    - permissible to add the scores from multiple small human families,
    - a total score (Z) of 3 (1000:1) arbitrarily accepted as significant.

- In the chart, there is no test for a hypothetical disease, XYZ disease,
  and one can only await its appearance for diagnosis.
  - Homozygotes have short stature, no eyes and die in childhood.
  - Heterozygotes develop incapacitating dementia around age 25.
  - A gene for an easily detectable DNA marker is known through cell
    hybridization to be syntenic ("wild type" = B = marker absent, b = marker present)

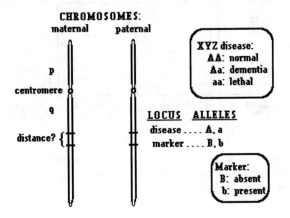

CHROMOSOMES:

maternal   paternal

p

centromere

q

distance? {

XYZ disease:
AA: normal
Aa: dementia
aa: lethal

LOCUS ALLELES
disease .... A, a
marker .... B, b

Marker:
B: absent
b: present

- The next chart illustrates a family in which the father has developed the heterozygous form of the disease after fathering two children.
  - We pick up the story years later after both of the children have also developed the disease.
  - Our object is to determine if the disease gene is close enough to the marker gene to allow diagnosis of the presence of the gene prior to reproduction.

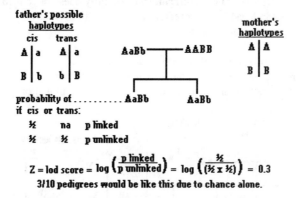

father's possible haplotypes

cis   trans

A | a   A | a
B | b   b | B

AaBb —————— AABB

mother's haplotypes

A | A
B | B

AaBb   AaBb

probability of .... AaBb
if cis or trans:

½   na   p linked
½   ½   p unlinked

$$Z = \text{lod score} = \log\left(\frac{\text{p linked}}{\text{p unlinked}}\right) = \log\left(\frac{\frac{1}{2}}{(\frac{1}{2} \times \frac{1}{2})}\right) = 0.3$$

3/10 pedigrees would be like this due to chance alone.

- We find *fortuitously* that the
  - father and both children are heterozygous for the marker.
  In reality, it could take years of searching to find an "informative" family like this.

- In the lod technique, we draw up probabilities of
  - the genotypes of the children based on the genotypes of the parents.

- In the father, the dominant gene, A, and the wild type, B, could be on
  - same member of the chromosome pair
    - which is called cis linkage phase or coupling;
  - or they could be on opposite members
    - which is called trans linkage phase or repulsion.

- If in trans and far enough apart, there could be crossovers between the chromosomes during meiosis, resulting in a cis arrangement in the gamete.
  - This is called recombination.
  - If they are in trans and linked, recombination would not occur.

- A child who has a combination of linked genes that is different from either parent is a recombinant, and
  - the proportion of those is called the recombination fraction.

- Fortuitously, the mother is homozygous normal for the disease gene and lacks the marker gene;
  - hence, she can contribute only one type of allele.

- The total lod score in this family is the log of the overall probability,
  - there being a probability of 1/2 if the disease and the marker are linked
  - and a 1/2 x 1/2 probability if they are not.
  - the final lod score of .3 means that this family pattern would occur
    - 3 out of 10 times simply due to chance.

- A lod score of 3 (p<0.001) is significant so this family does not contribute much.
  - Lod scores can be added, so a search for similar families may eventually prove that the genes are linked

- The next chart shows the family of a similar couple.
  - There are 3 affected children, one of whom lacks the marker.
  - We want to use this family to calculate theta, the recombination fraction.

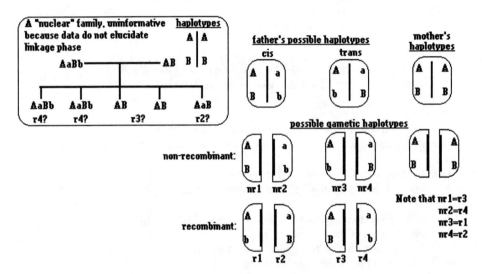

- From a practical standpoint,
  - the recombination fraction is the error rate when using linkage for diagnosis.

- Since we do not know the cis-trans arrangement, it is possible that the father could
  - have produced one of 4 types of non-recombinant gametes
  - or one of 4 types of recombinant gametes.
  - each of the affected children could be one of the recombinants so our study comes to naught.

Problems of Paternity

DNA polymorphisms allow very accurate parentage testing. Non-parentage will be exposed in the course of linkage analysis for clinical purposes. Non-maternity is rare, and usually stems from accidental exchange of newborns in hospital nurseries. Non-paternity is much more frequent; studies indicate an average of 15%. The repercussions of disclosure must be considered prior to clinical testing.

- In the next chart, we study the grandparents and find, fortuitously, that their mating was informative, i.e.,
  - only one possibility existed for the parent's phenotype.
  - The paternal grandfather had no eyes but otherwise mild expression of homozygosity for the gene so he married a school-mate from the School for the Blind and produced 3 children prior to developing the dementia at age 20. He died at age 25. His case came to the attention of a geneticist who froze some of his cells for future analysis. Studies now reveal homozygosity for the marker.
  - All three of his children had eyes but later developed dementia.

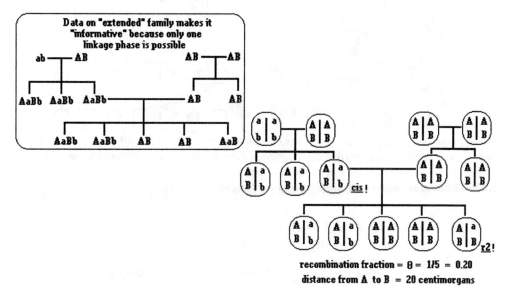

recombination fraction = θ = 1/5 = 0.20
distance from A to B = 20 centimorgans

- The data from the fortuitously informative extended family now prove that the father in our original nuclear family was in cis.
  - Hence, the affected child lacking the marker was a recombinant.

- Theta in this family is 1/5 or 0.20.
  - If corroborated by studies of other families, that means that there would be a 20% error rate in using the marker for detecting the disease gene.

- Theta also represents the "genetic distance" between genes,
  - classically measured in centimorgans (100 x theta):
  - roughly 1 million base pairs = 1 centimorgan.

- For closely linked genes, theta averages 5% but is much higher for syntenic genes,
  - which limits accuracy of synteny tests for mutations like those of BRCA1 only to situations in which large numbers of family members can be tested.

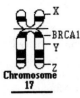

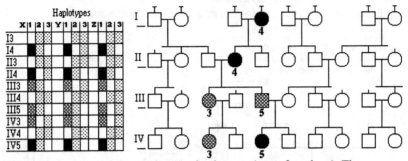

One variety of breast cancer results from a heritable mutation in the BRCA-1 gene on 17q. There are many types of those mutations so one patient may not have the same type as another patient. A mutation increases the age-specific breast cancer risk by a factor of about 12. Testing for one type of mutation will not detect other types but syntenic marker genes on chromosome 17 can be used to trace inheritance of the whole chromosome.

Chromosomes are paired so each person has two haplotypes (sets of markers). The women with breast cancer in this genealogy (darkened symbols) share the X1 Y1 Z1 haplotype as does the intervening male. That haplotype identifies the chromosome that bears the mutant BRCA1 gene. III3 and IV3 (shaded symbols) have the gene but have not yet sustained a breast cancer.

2. Older diagnostic genetic marker techniques utilize
    • enzymatic digestion of native DNA or total cDNA
    • followed by electrophoresis
        • (see table, Technical Aspects of DNA and Chromosome Analysis).

• Newer DNA diagnostic electrophoresis methodology detects nucleotide changes through
    • amplification of specific segments of DNA
       (see table, Amplification of DNA), followed by either
        • denaturation/renaturation with wild-type DNA,
            • base pair mismatches in hybrid DNA segments changing mobility, or
        • SSCP (denaturation to single-stranded DNA),
            • DNA sequence alterations changing mobility.

- Fluorescence in-situ hybridization (FISH) can diagnose disorders caused by
    - specific DNA sequence differences, currently, mostly deletions.
    - Reliability correlates with size of segment and specificity of hybridization.
    - Reliable tests are currently available for
        - Angelman syndrome.
        - DiGeorge syndrome.
        - Miller-Dieker syndrome.
        - Prader-Willi syndrome.
        - Smith-Magenis syndrome.
        - Velo-cardio-facial syndrome
        - Williams syndrome.

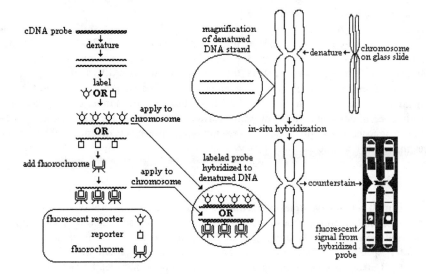

3. Mutations of over 2000 genes that cause human diseases have been identified but
    - few analyses are commercially practicable for clinical use because of
        - the rarity of the individual mutations,
        - variability in clinical expression,
        - genetic heterogeneity.
        - Extensive DNA polymorphisms associated with no phenotypic abnormality limits use of most DNA tests to biological relatives of cases that have been tested already.

See table, Commercial Laboratories offering DNA Diagnostic Tests.

Helix, a subscription service on the Internet, maintains a list of testing sources: http://www.hslib.washington.edu/helix/

If there is only one mutation (a) of a gene (A), the frequency of A may be denoted as p and the frequency of a may be denoted q and the frequency of phenotypes, $(p+q)^2$:

frequency: p^2 $2pq$ q^2

phenotype: AA   Aa   aa

If there were n mutations, the frequency of phenotypes would be $(p+q+r \ldots n)^2$

EXAMPLE: The most common mutation causing cystic fibrosis, delta F508, accounts for 67% of cystic fibrosis mutations but there are at least 400 other disease-causing mutations of the cystic fibrosis gene and new ones are found frequently. As a simplifying assumption, call delta F508 a and say that there were only 3 other mutant genes, b, c, and d. The equation would then be $(p+q+r+s+t)^2$ which expands to:

frequency: t^2 $2st$ s^2 $2rt$ $2rs$ r^2 $2qt$ $2qs$ $2qr$ q^2 $2pt$ $2ps$ $2pr$ $2pq$ p^2

phenotype: dd   cd   cc   bd   bc   bb   ad   ac   ab   aa   Ad   Ac   Ab   Aa   AA

The frequencies of the disease phenotypes:

phenotype	**dd**	**cd**	**cc**	**bd**	**bc**
frequency	1.367×10^{-4}	2.735×10^{-5}	1.367×10^{-4}	2.735×10^{-5}	2.735×10^{-5}
phenotype	**bb**	**ad**	**ac**	**ab**	**aa**
frequency	1.367×10^{-4}	1.914×10^{-4}	1.914×10^{-4}	1.914×10^{-4}	6.7×10^{-4}

Diagnosis of the presence of each gene mutation requires a separate procedure. This over-simplification may be difficult to follow but the true situation is even more complex and indicates that the direction of development is toward the particular, i.e., each case requiring a mini-research project for diagnosis. The implications are very important. Erroneous diagnosis of non-paternity has been made when a child and mother were probe positive only for delta F508, and the father, with an undiscovered mutation, was negative.

- Congenital adrenal hyperplasia illustrates others of these considerations:
    - Seemingly identical cases have differing genetic bases and seemingly identical mutations produce different types of the disorder, requiring complex diagnosis:
        - Specific CYP21B probes (diagnoses 15% of classic patients)
        - Linkage analysis (patient and both parents minimum: ideally, an unaffected sib and all four grandparents also).
            - Direct probes for both CYP21 genes
            - HLA-B probe
            - HLA-DR probe

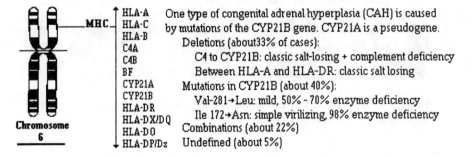

MHC
HLA-A
HLA-C
HLA-B
C4A
C4B
BF
CYP21A
CYP21B
HLA-DR
HLA-DX/DQ
HLA-DO
HLA-DP/Dz

Chromosome 6

One type of congenital adrenal hyperplasia (CAH) is caused by mutations of the CYP21B gene. CYP21A is a pseudogene.

Deletions (about 33% of cases):
C4 to CYP21B: classic salt-losing + complement deficiency
Between HLA-A and HLA-DR: classic salt losing

Mutations in CYP21B (about 40%):
Val-281→Leu: mild, 50% – 70% enzyme deficiency
Ile 172→Asn: simple virilizing, 98% enzyme deficiency

Combinations (about 22%)

Undefined (about 5%)

DNA Analysis

1. Collect 20 ml blood in EDTA.
2. Add 30 ml distilled water, centrifuge, discard supernate.
3. Wash pellet sucessively with Nonidet, NaCl/EDTA
4. Digest with proteinase.
5. Extract successively with phenol/chloroform, chloroform.
6. Precipitate DNA with 0.3 M NaCl or sodium acetate in ethanol.
7. Dissolve DNA in water and measure concentration as 260 nm absorbance.
8. Digest DNA with 10 units enzyme from commercial supplier.
9. Load 5 ug into well of agarose gel, electrophorese 16 hours.
10. Stain for DNA fragments with ethidium bromide, photograph.
11. Soak gel successively in 0.25 N HCl 15 minutes, 0.5 N NaOH 30 minutes, 0.6 M NaCl 30 minutes, then in SSC buffer 30 minutes.
12. Overlay gel with nitrocellulose/nylon filter, transfer overnight.
13. Obtain DNA probes from commercial supplier, label with ^{32}P reagent.
14. Remove nitrocellulose filter, bake 2 hours at 80^0 2 hours, add probe.
15. Incubate 16 hours.
16. Remove filter, wash multiple times to remove excess probe.
17. Overlay filter with photographic film.
18. Incubate at -80^0 16 hours.
19. Remove film and develop.
20. Compare autoradiograph to original photo of gel to determine which DNA fragments hybridized with the probe.

Chromosome Analysis

1. Collect 2 ml blood in heparin.
2. Sediment and remove buffy coat
3. Add buffy coat to culture medium.
4. Incubate 72 hours.
5. Add colchicine to culture.
6. Incubate 3 hours.
7. Add water until hypotonic.
8. Incubate 10 minutes.
9. Wash twice with acetic/methanol fixative.
10. Spread cell suspension onto slides, air dry.
11. Age slides 1 to 7 days, or partially denature.
12. Stain. Geimsa is standard but chromosome "paints" differentiate quicker, and probes can be used for parts of many chromosomes.
13. Examine for well spread sets of chromosomes.
14. Count and sort 10 to 60 sets of chromosomes, photograph representative sets.
15. Develop and print photos.
16. Cut and mount chromosome images.

Steps 14 - 16 may be done with a computer using digitized images.

Technical Aspects of DNA and Chromosome Analysis

Note: this is for analysis of white blood cells. Marrow cells can be processed for chromosome analysis without culturing. Other cells must be cultured long enough for confluency in a 25 ml tissue culture flask, then start at step 2 (DNA) or 5 (chromosomes). The time for culture to confluency averages about a month. Special rapid culture techniques are used for amniocytes.

Amplification of DNA

When the structure of a gene is known, it can be purified and amplified by many orders of magnitude prior to analysis through the use of simple elegant techniques.

1. RNA isolation. The tissue of interest is homogenized in guanidium thiocyanate plus 2-mercaptoethanol. Total cellular RNA is obtained by ethanol precipitation.

2. cDNA synthesis. Random deoxynucleotide hexamers ("random primers") are added to total cellular RNA, followed by reverse transcriptase, then hydrolysis with NaOH. cDNA is precipitated with ethanol.

3. Polymerase chain reaction (PCR): annealing to cDNA of short sequences (oligonucleotide primers) of nucleotides with a free 3' end allows covalent extension of a chain of nucleotides complementary to the cDNA. The primers are synthesized to be complementary only to beginning sequences of the gene of interest so only it is produced.

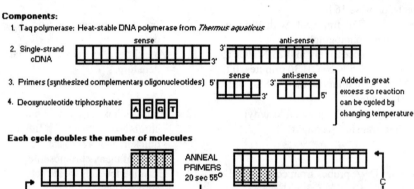

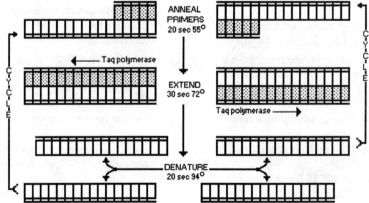

Commercial Laboratories offering DNA Diagnostic Tests

Code	Name	Location	Telephone
A	Athena Diagnostics	Worchester, MA	(800) 394-4493
Bd	Baylor DNA Diagnostic Laboratory	Houston, TX	(800) 226-3624
Bk	Baylor Kleberg Cytogenetics Laboratory	Houston, TX	(800) 411-4363
Bo	Boston University Human Genetics	Boston, MA	(617) 638-7083
C	Corning Nichols Institute	San Juan Capistrano, CA	(800) 642-4657
J	Jefferson Institute of Molecular Medicine	Philadelphia, PA	(215) 955-4830
L	Laboratory Corporation of America	Research Triangle Park, NC	(800) 334-5161
M	Mayo Medical Laboratories	Rochester, MN	(800) 533-0567

Disorder	A	Bd	Bk	Bo	C	J	L	M
Achondrogenesis II						+		
Achondroplasia		+						
Adrenal hypoplasia			+					
Amyloidosis								+
Amyotrophic lateral sclerosis	+							
Angelman syndrome		+	+	+	+		+	+
Canavan disease		+						
Charcot-Marie-Tooth 1A			+		+			
Chondrodysplasia						+		
Chronic granulomatous disease				+				
Citrullinemia				+				
Colorectal cancer							+	
Cystic fibrosis		+		+	+		+	+
Dentatorubral pallidoluysian atrophy		+		+				
DiGeorge syndrome			+	+	+		+	
Duchenne/Becker muscular dystrophy	+	+		+	+			+
Fragile X syndrome		+		+	+		+	
Friedreich ataxia				+				
Gaucher disease		+		+			+	
Hemophilia A		+		+				+
Hereditary neuropathy	+		+					
Huntington disease	+	+		+				
Kallman syndrome			+					
Kearns-Sayre syndrome	+							
Kennedy spinal bulbar atrophy	+	+						
Kneist syndrome						+		
Leber optic atrophy	+							
Leigh syndrome	+							
Machado-Joesph syndrome	+	+		+				
MELAS	+							
MERRF	+							
Miller-Dieker syndrome			+	+	+		+	

Commercial Laboratories offering DNA Diagnostic Tests
(continued)

Disorder	A	Bd	Bk	Bo	C	J	L	M
Multiple endocrine neoplasia 2				+				+
Myelogenous leukemia				+				+
Myotonic dystrophy		+		+				+
Neurofibromatosis 1				+			+	
Neurofibromatosis 2	+							
Norrie disease	+							
Ornithine transcarbamalase deficiency				+				
Phenylketonuria				+				
Polycystic kidney disease				+				
Polyposis coli				+			+	+
Prader-Willi syndrome		+	+	+	+		+	+
Sickle cell/SC anemia		+		+			+	
Smith-Magenis syndrome			+		+		+	
Spinal muscular atrophy				+				
Spinocerebellar ataxia 1	+	+		+				+
Spondyloepiphyseal dysplasia						+		
Stickler syndrome	+					+		
Tay-Sachs disease		+		+			+	
Thalassemia alpha							+	+
Uniparental disomy							+	
Vas deferens absence				+				
Velocardiofacial syndrome			+	+			+	
Von-Hippel-Lindau disease				+				
Waardenburg syndrome 1				+				
Williams syndrome			+	+			+	
Wilson disease				+				
Y chromosome DNA				+		+		+

Additional references:

Bernstam VA. *Pocket Guide to Gene Level Diagnostics in Clinical Practice*. Boca Raton: CRC Press, 1993.

Davis KE. *Human Genetic Diseases. A Practical Approach*. Washington, DC: IRL Press, 1986.

Huntington's Disease Collaborative Research Group. A novel gene containing a trinucleotide repeat that is expanded and unstable on Huntington's disease chromosomes. Cell 1993;72:972-983.

LaSpada AR, Roling D, Fischbeck KH. The expanded trinucleotide repeat in X-linked spinal and bulbar muscular atrophy. Abstract 184. Am J Hum Genet 1992;51 (Supplement):A49.

McKusick VA. *Mendelian Inheritance in Man. Catalogues of Autosomal Dominant, Autosomal Recessive, and X-linked Phenotypes*, 10th edition. Baltimore: The Johns Hopkins Press, 1992.

Mettler G, Hunter AGW, O'Hoy K, et al. Clincal correlations of a decrease in CTG trinucleotide repeat amplification with transmission of myotonic dystrophy (DM) from parent to child. Abstract 160. Am J Hum Genet 1992;51 (Supplement):A43.

Nelson DL, Eichler E, King JE, et al. Characterization of the FMR-1 gene at the FRAXA locus of man. Abstract 186. Am J Hum Genet 1992;51 (Supplement):A49.

Snow K, Doud LK, Hagerman R, et al. Analysis of a CGG repeat at the FMR-1 locus in Fragile X families and in the general population. Abstract 185. Am J Hum Genet 1992;51 (Supplement):A49.

Verma RS, Babu A. *Human Chromosomes. Principles and Techniques*, 2nd edition. New York: McGraw-Hill, 1995.

Wong Z, Wilson V, Patel I, et al. Characterization of a panel of highly variable minisatellites cloned from human DNA. Ann Hum Genet 1987;51:269-288.

1. Chromosome analysis is used for **diagnosis of etiology** of
    *   <u>**congenital anomalies**</u>,
    *   <u>**sex identity problems**</u>,
    *   <u>**reproductive problems**</u> (infertility, spontaneous abortions),
    *   <u>**behavioral disorders**</u>,
    *   <u>**mental retardation**</u> and
    *   <u>**neoplasms**</u> (also used to evaluate therapeutic response).

*   Chromosome analysis of a tissue requires that a
    *   large percentage of the cells be in metaphase, found naturally only in
        *   bone marrow and
        *   chorionic villus which yield
            *   preliminary results within 24 hours and final results within a week.

*   BUCCAL MUCOSA CELLS ARE NOT USED FOR CHROMOSOME ANALYSIS;
    *   they were once used for Barr body or sex chromatin analysis
        *   an archaic and anecdotal study of no clinical value under any circumstance.

*   Short term cell culture combined with mitotic synchronization allows
    *   chromosome analysis of lymphocytes, which yields
        *   preliminary results within a week and final results within 2 weeks.
    *   THIS IS THE MOST COMMONLY USED TYPE OF CHROMOSOME ANALYSIS.
    *   Special types of short-term cultures are used for amniocytes.
    The basic technique is outlined in the section, *Technical Aspects of DNA and Chromosome analysis*, in the chapter on *Laboratory Diagnosis: Molecular Genetics*

*   Long term culture combined with mitotic synchronization allows
    *   chromosome analysis of fibroblasts which yields
        *   preliminary results within 3 weeks and final results within 4 weeks.

*   Toxins can be used to block division of cultured cells in S phase allowing
    *   chromosome analysis in prophase or prometaphase which reveals that
        *   each chromosome sub-band is itself composed of other sub-bands,
        *   but greatly extends the time until results are available.
    *   This is also called high-resolution chromosome analysis because it may reveal
        *   chromosome aberrations not visible in metaphase chromosomes.

*   Cell culture done under conditions of thymidine deprivation which reveals fragile site heteromorphisms where chromosome arms may fracture, most associated with
    *   no perceptible phenotypic abnormality, but excessive frequency of fractures
    *   at the fragile site on Xq27 is found with the *fragile X syndrome*

2.   The frequencies of some chromosome aberrations,
-    especially chromosome 21 trisomy, are associated with maternal age but
   -    their basic cause is not known;
-    mechanisms that cause them experimentally do not appear to cause actual cases.

-    Chromosome aberrations are frequent among spontaneous abortuses and the types
   -    differ from those found in liveborns but are associated with
      higher risk of aneuploidy in subsequent conceptuses of the mother.
   -    Some result from segregation of a chromosome aberration in a parent who has a
      high risk of related chromosome aberrations in subsequent conceptuses.

Aberrations	Abortuses		Newborns	
	percent	frequency	percent	frequency
trisomy 13			0.005	1/20,000
trisomy 14	2.2	1/45		
trisomy 15	2.5	1/40		
trisomy 16	9.8	1/10		
trisomy 18	1.8	1/56	0.0125	1/8000
trisomy 21	5.0	1/20	0.143	1/700
trisomy 22	3.4	1/29		
XXY			0.1 males	1/1000
XYY			0.1 males	1/1000
45,X	5.4 (females)	1/19	0.01 females	1/10,000
XXX			0.1 females	1/1000
balanced translocations			0.2	1/500
unbalanced translocations	1.8	1/56	0.05	1/2000
triploidy	10.2	1/10		
tetraploidy	3.6	1/28		
other	10.4	1/10	0.11	1/900

-    Duplication or deletion of chromosomes or parts of them during gametogenesis
   -    causes phenotypic abnormalities of the conceptus formed by that gamete;
      -    the manner of production of the phenotypes is not known.

-    Duplication of a whole set (n) of chromosomes results in polyploidy
   -    triploidy being 3N (e.g., 69,XXX) and
   -    tetraploidy being 4N (e.g., 92,XXXX).

-    Conditions associated with polyploidy include: poor or aberrant fetal growth
                                                           spontaneous abortion

3.   Characteristics common to the phenotypes produced by chromosome aberrations include:
         poor growth and development
         multiple dysmorphic features
         close resemblance to other persons with same aberration.

- Chromosome 21 trisomy, the most frequent autosome aberration at birth, is due to
  - duplication of 21q, and causes a characteristic syndrome:
    - hypotonia,
    - short broad hands,
    - widely separated first and second toes.
    - brachycephaly,
    - midfacial hypoplasia, which causes slant-eyed facies and
      - small oropharynx which in turn causes tongue protrusion.

- The syndrome of Chromosome 18 trisomy
  - is associated with duplication of 18q and includes the following specific phenotype characteristics:
    - hypertonia,
    - dolichocephaly,
    - micrognathia,
    - small poorly formed ears,
    - short sternum,
    - heart malformation,
    - index finger overlaps middle finger and little finger overlaps ring finger
    - dorsiflexed hallux giving rocker bottom appearance to feet.

- The syndrome of Chromosome 13 trisomy
  - is associated with duplication of 13q and includes the following specific phenotype characteristics:
    - receding forehead
    - hypertelorism,
    - microphthalmia,
    - cleft lip and palate,
    - postaxial polydactyly,
    - flexion contracture of fingers,
    - vertical talus which inverts arch, giving rocker bottom appearance to feet,
    - penile scrotum.

- The syndrome of Chromosome 5p deletion includes the following specific phenotype characteristics:
  - microcephaly,
  - midfacial prominence,
  - hypertelorism,
  - faint mewing cry (cri du chat).

- Characteristic syndromes have been associated with a large number of other chromosome aberrations that are random mutations and occur at basal frequencies,
  - concentrations of cases being observed only in family distributions,
  - most often due to translocations or inversions.
  - Most are described in Appendix 3.

DOWN SYNDROME: A FACT SHEET. First named *"furfuraceaous idiocy"* - Sequin, 1846. The term, *"mongolian idiocy,"* was originated by Down, 1866. The chromosome aberration was described by Lejeune, 1959. *"Down syndrome"* is a recent term.

Etiology: *Spontaneous mutation.* Exogenous causes have not been proven.

Cytogenetics: *Simple trisomy: 92%* - due to a germ cell mutation in a parent (5% are paternal). *Translocation: 5%* - mostly Robertsonian; over half are due to germ cell mutation in a parent; the remainder due to segregation of a mutant chromosome in a parent. *Mosaicism: 3%* - a normal cell line arises due to reversion in the early trisomic embryo.

Pathogenesis: *Unknown.* Several genes are located on chromosome 21. Homozygosity of a disease allele or a 1.5 X dose effect of a normal allele may cause Alzheimer disease, cataract, hyperuricemia and leukemia. Similar effects for genes of band 21q22 may cause the malformations.

Incidence: 1/20 abortuses, 1/700 births. Sex ratio: 3 male/2 females.

Mean maternal age: 34.4 (N=28.2). Mean gestation length: 270 days (N=282).

Mean birth weight: 6 lb 6 oz (N=7 lb 8 oz). Birth length slightly decreased.

Mean head circumference at birth: 12 1/2 in. (N=13 1/2).

Average IQ drops with age: 60 @ 1 yrs, 50 @ 3 yrs, 40 @ 6 yrs, 24 @ 21 yrs.

Growth is slow: Mean adult height is 56 2/3 in. (female), 60 1/2 in. (male).

Reproductive: Puberty may be slightly delayed. Libido and secondary sexual characteristics are weakly manifested. Males are usually impotent. Females are usually fertile, and produce equal numbers of trisomic and euploid children. The euploid children are often mentally retarded for unknown reasons.

Life expectancy: 70% survive past 1 year, 50% past 5, 8% past 40, 3% past 50

Anomalies: *Brain:* Fusion of walls of fissures; irregular, infantile gray matter pattern; underdevelopment of myelin in cortex and cerebellum.

> *Eye:* Most have refractive errors, keratoconus, and cataracts. Cataract surgery is often complicated due to the generally anomalous eye. Strabismus - 20%. Glaucoma - rare.

> *Heart:* Most have malformation - 60% are clinically significant. Heart surgery may be non-beneficial or fatal unless done in the first few months of life.

> *Intestinal:* Duodenal atresia - 1%.

> *Midface hypoplasia:* Lends characteristic appearance and causes nasal obstruction with resultant respiratory infections.

> *Oral:* Small throat pushes tongue forward making it appear large. Hypodontia is frequent.

> *Skeletal:* Instability of upper neck vertebrae - 20%. Can lead to spinal injury and paraplegia if it dislocates during exercise. Most have other loose joints which also tend to dislocate.

> *Skin:* Most have dry scaly skin which becomes rough in pressure areas.

> *Urinary:* 5% have anatomic malformations that may cause infections.

Illnesses: *Blood:* Various types of leukemia are more common than in normal children, the most common being lymphocytic leukemia which eventually affects about 1%.

> *Brain:* Seizures - 5% (a few have hypsarrhythmia). Most over age 40 years have Alzheimer disease.

> *Endocrinologic:* Thyroid function dwindles (1/3 are hypothyroid by age 21 years).

> *Immunologic:* All have poor T-cell function (recurrent, prolonged infectious diseases).

> *Urinary:* Some are hyperuricemic (kidney stones & gout).

Reference: Pueschel, S.M., Steinberg, L. ***Down Syndrome. A Comprehensive Bibliography***. Garland STPM Press, New York, 1980. 6000 references on all aspects.

Chromosome 13 Aberrations
Deletions

del(13)(q14->qter):

Head & face	microcephaly, holoprosencephaly, large ears, flat face, hypotelorism, strabismus, retinoblastoma
Skeletal	synostosis of metacarpals 4 & 5, hypoplastic thumbs, focal lumbar vertebral agenesis
Visceral	heart, urinary tract malformation, and genital malformation
Functional	mental retardation
Mechanism	usually a spontaneous mutation

del(13)(q21):

Head & face	prominent maxilla, retinoblastoma
Skeletal	short hypoplastic thumbs, hypoplastic phalanges, polydactyly
Visceral	
Functional	mental retardation, motor impairment
Mechanism	dominant transmission from parent or spontaneous mutation

del(13)(q31->q32)

Head & face	microcephaly, trigonocephaly, frontal bossing, low-set ears, prominent maxilla, hypertelorism, epicanthus, eye malformation
Skeletal	absent thumbs, hypoplastic phalanges, metacarpal 1 hypoplasia, metacarpal 4-5 fusion
Visceral	urinary tract, and genital malformation
Functional	poor growth, mental retardation
Mechanism	usually a spontaneous mutation

del(13)(q32->q34) and r(13)(p11q32) cause the same phenotype:

Head & face	microcephaly, trigonocephaly, large ears, protruding central incisors, eye malformation
Skeletal	
Visceral	imperforate anus; urinary tract, and genital malformation
Functional	poor growth, mental retardation
Mechanism	usually a spontaneous mutation

Duplications

dup(13)(pter->q14):

Head & face	microcephaly, prominent forehead, microstomia, retrognathia
Skeletal	clinodactyly, simian crease
Visceral	persistent fetal hemoglobin
Functional	mental retardation
Mechanism	segregation from balanced translocation or spontaneous mutation

dup(13)(q13->qter):

Head & face	microcephaly, prominent forehead, capillary hemangioma, low-set malformed ears, curly eyelashes, microphthalmia, epicanthus, delayed dentition
Skeletal	polydactyly, simian crease
Visceral	persistent fetal hemoglobin, hernias, renal malformation
Functional	mental retardation
Mechanism	segregation from balanced translocation or spontaneous mutation

4. Mitotic instability syndromes are characterized by chromosome fragility,
    - fractures of chromosome arms during preparation for analysis, and by
    - excessive rates of intrachromosome recombinations, and
    - increases or decreases of copy numbers of short tandem repeats.

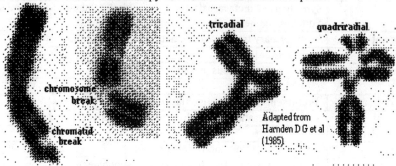

Adapted from Harnden D G et al (1985)

MITOTIC INSTABILITY SYNDROMES
CLASSIC

SYNDROME	CLINICAL FEATURES	GEN	CYTOGENETIC	CANCERS
Ataxia telangiectasia	Progressive cerebellar ataxia, oculocutaneous telangiectasia, immunodeficiency	AR	Gaps, breaks, pseudo-diploid clones with rearrangements of chromosomes 7 & 14	Lymphomas, lymphocytic leukemia
Bloom syndrome	Gestational dwarfism, photosensitive telangiectatic erythroderma, long face, malar hypoplasia	AR	Excessive sister chromatid exchanges, breaks and rearrangements	Non-lymphocytic leukemias
Fanconi anemia	Radial malformations, progressive pancytopenia, hyperpigmentation, poor growth	AR	Chromatid breaks & gaps, mitomycin sensitivity	Leukemia, hepatocellular carcinoma, squamous cell carcinoma
Werner syndrome	Premature aging, scleropoikiloderma, juvenile cataracts, short stature with thin limbs and stocky trunk	AR	Variegated translocation mosaicism	Sarcomas, meningiomas
Xeroderma pigmentosum	Photosensitivity, neurologic deficits	AR	UV & UV mimetic sensitivity no spontaneous chromosome instability	Basal cell carcinoma, squamous cell carcinoma

MITOTIC INSTABILITY SYNDROMES
OTHERS

Basal cell nevus syndrome	Multiple nevoid basal cell carcinomas, odontogenic cysts, variegated rib and vertebral anomalies	AD	Chromatid and isochromosome gaps and breaks, acentric fragments, dicentrics, quadriradials	Basal cell carcinoma, melanoma
Familial polyposis coli	Polyps of colon	AD	Aberrations of all types in lymphocytes	Colon carcinoma, instestinal carcinoma
Gardner syndrome	Polyposis of stomach, small intestine and colon, osseous & soft tissue tumors, sebaceous & epidermoid cysts, congenital retinal pigment epithelium hypertrophy	AD	Aneuploidy, random loss & gain of chromosomes, tetraploidy	Periampullary carcinoma, thyroid carcinoma, adrenal carcinoma, malignant changes in polyps
Glutathione reductase deficiency	Hemolytic anemia, decreased leukocyte bacteriocidal activity, cataract	AR	Breakage, more in homozygote, mitotic chiasmata	Leukemia
Incontentia pigmenti	Marbled skin pigmentation, eye malformations, heart, teeth and skeleton	XL	Gaps, rearrangements in lymphocytes	Acute myelogenous leukemia, pheochromo-cytoma
Inflammatory bowel disease	Crohn disease, ulcerative colitis	?	Breaks, fragments, rings, dicentrics, rearrangements	Colorectal carcinoma
Kostman agranulocytosis	Severe neutropenia	AR	Aberrations in bone marrow cells	Acute monocytic leukemia
Multiple endocrine adenomatosis II		AD	Gaps and chromatid aberrations	Medullary thyroid carcinoma, pheochromo-cytoma
Nimegen breakage syndrome	Microcephaly, cafe-au-lait spots, poor growth, mental retardation, immunodeficiency	AR	Rearrangements involving chromosomes 7 & 14 at specific break points	Lymphyoblastic leukemia, mediastinal malignancies, lymphoma
Porokeratosis of Mibelli	Keratoatrophoderma, crater-like skin lesions	AD	Abormalities in skin fibroblasts from lesions	Squamous cell carcinoma

MITOTIC INSTABILITY SYNDROMES
OTHERS (continued)

Scleroderma (Progressive systemic sclerosis)	Thickening & tightness of skin, Raynaud phenomenon, esophageal dysfunction, pulmonary fibrosis	?	Chromatid breaks & gaps, rings, acentric fragments, dicentrics, rearrangements	5% have malignancies
Sezary syndrome	Infiltrative erythroderma with pruritis and alopecia; palmar & plantar hyperhidrosis, onychodystrophy, Sezary cells in skin & blood	?	Aneuploidy, hypodiploidy, translocations with centromere breakpoints	Skin lesion which looks like mycosis fungoides on EM

5. Chromosome aberrations of most neoplasms involve all chromosomes, and
   - occur near oncogenes; well known examples:
     - t(9q;22q) ("Philadelphia chromosome"): chronic myelogenous lukemia
     - t(8q;14q): Burkitt lymphoma
     - 13q14- : retinoblastoma
     - 3p14-23- : small cell carcinoma of lung
     - 11p15- : aniridia-Wilms tumor (WAGR) syndrome.
   - Certain neoplasms appears to have aberrrations of only certain chromosomes:
     - Non-lymphocytic leukemias, special type: 2-15, 17, 19, 21, X, Y
     - Neoplasms of unspecified histiogenesis: 7

Neoplasms in which chromosome aberrations have been found:

DISORDERS	**SUBTYPES**
Hematologic disorders	
Acute lymphocytic leukemias	
NOS	special type
FAB types L1 to L3	
Acute nonlymphocytic leukemias	
NOS	FAB type M4-M5
FAB types M1 to M7	FAB types 5a to 5b
FAB type M1-M2	special type
Chronic lymphoproliferative disorders	
chronic lymphocytic leukemia	Sezary syndrome
adult T-cell leukemia/lymphoma	Waldenstrom macroglobulinemia
prolymphocytic leukemia	multiple myeloma
hairy cell leukemia	plasma cell leukemia/plasmacytoma
cutaneous T-cell leukemia	NOS
mycosis fungoides	special type
Chronic myeloid leukemias	
t(9;22)	Ph[1] negative
aberrant translocation	special type

Neoplasms in which chromosome aberrations have been found (continued):

DISORDERS	SUBTYPES
Myelodysplastic disorders	
NOS	chronic monomyelocytic anemia
refractory anemia	aplastic anemia
refractory anemia with ringed sideroblasts	paroxysmal nocturnal hemoglobinuria
refractory anemia with excessive blasts	special type
RAEB and RAEB-T	
Myeloproliferative disorders	
polycythemia vera	idiopathic thrombocytopenia
idiopathic myelofibrosis	NOS
angiogenic myeloid metalpasia	special type
Nonlymphocytic leukemias, special type	
basophilic leukemia	special type
eosinophilic leukemia	
Undifferentiated and special leukemias	
acute	special type

Lymphomas

Hodgkins disease	
NOS	lymphocytic depletion
lymphocytic predominance	nodular sclerosis
mixed cellularity	
Non-Hodgkins lymphomas	
NOS	follicular, small cleaved cell
diffuse	follicular, mixed small cleaved and large cell
follicular	follicular, large cell
lymphocytic	diffuse, small cleaved cell
immunocytoma	diffuse, mixed small cleaved and large cell
centrocytic	diffuse, large cell
centroblastic-centrocytic, diffuse	large cell, immunoblastic
centroblastic-centrocytic, follicular	lymphoblastic
centroblastic, diffuse	small non-cleaved cell
centroblastic, follicular	miscellaneous
lymphoblastic, unclassified	other
lymphoblastic, Burkitt type	malignant histiocytosis
lymphoblastic, convoluted type	angioimmunoblastic lymphadenopathy
immunoblastic	Lennert lymphoma
small lymphocytic	special type

Solid tumors

Benign epithelial neoplasms	
adenoma	special type
papilloma	
Benign mesenchymal neoplasms	
fibroma	hemangioma
fibromatosis	lymphangioma
desmoid tumor	chondroma
myxoma	chondroblastoma
lipoma	chondromyxoid fibroma

Neoplasms in which chromosome aberrations have been found (continued):

DISORDERS	SUBTYPES
leiomyoma	special type
Benign neurogenic neoplasms	
meningioma	neurofibroma
mengioma atypical	neurinoma
Germ cell neoplasms	
seminoma	gonadal stroma tumors
dysgerminoma	NOS
teratoma mature and immature	special type
combined tumors	
Malignant epithelial neoplasms	
carcinoma in situ NOS	adenocarcinoma
carcinoma NOS	squamous cell carcinoma
carcinoma undifferentiated	transitional cell carcinoma
carcinoma undifferentiated large cell	basal cell carcinoma
carcinoma undifferentiated small cell	carcinoma special type
Malignant mesenchymal neoplasms	
sarcoma NOS	giant cell tumor of bone
fibrosarcoma	synovial sarcoma
malignant fibrous histiocytoma	clear cell sarcoma
myxofibrosarcoma	epithelioid cell sarcoma
liposarcoma	Kaposi sarcoma
leiomyosarcoma	special type
rhabdomyosarcoma	Ewing sarcoma
chondrosarcoma	Askin tumor
osteosarcoma	mesothelioma
Malignant neurogenic neoplasms	
astrocytoma NOS	malignant glioma NOS
astrocytoma grades I-II and III-IV	neuroblastoma
astrocytoma juvenile	retinoblastoma
oligodendroglioma	neuroepithelioma
medulloblastoma	neurofibrosarcoma
ependymoma	special type
Melanocytic neoplasms	
nevus NOS	dysplastic nevus
benign nevus	malignant melanoma
Neoplasms of unspecified histiogenesis	
benign neoplasm special type	malignant neoplasm NOS

6. Yp is required for male differentiation of the fetus,
    *   particularly the testicular determining region (TDR).

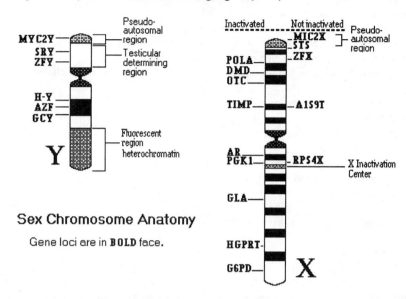

Sex Chromosome Anatomy

Gene loci are in **BOLD** face.

*   Yq has heritable variability in length and due to
    *   repetitive sequences that are responsible for visibility of
        *   Y chromatin in fluorescent stained interphase nuclei.

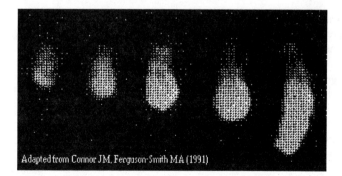

Adapted from Connor JM, Ferguson-Smith MA (1991)

*   Recombination in meiosis I results in cross overs between X and Y in the
    *   pseudoautosomal region of the short arms;
    *   aberrant cross overs may extend into the TDR and result in either
        *   XY females with insufficient TDR for male differentiation or
        *   XX males who have a functional TDR on Xp.

- Randomness of lyonization is disturbed in certain situations:
    - structurally abnormal X chromosomes are preferentially inactivated,
    - balanced X;autosome translocations result in
        - preferential inactivation of the normal X,
    - unbalanced X;autosome translocations result in preferential inactivation of the
        - translocation product which bears the X inactivation center,
    - the paternal X chromosome is preferentially inactivated in amnion and chorion.

- Klinefelter syndrome is characterized by
    - small head,
    - difficulty of verbal expression,
    - submissive personality,
    - inadequate pubertal testicular growth and a
    - tendency toward tallness and
    - gynecomastia.

- Over 10 varieties of abnormal karyotypes have been associated with Klinefelter syndrome but
    - 80% are 47,XXY.

- In cases of Klinefelter syndrome with more than two X chromosomes there is there is a tendency toward
    - midfacial hypoplasia,
    - short stature and
    - radioulnar synostosis
proportional to the number of X chromosomes.

- Cases of Klinefelter syndrome with 46,XX chromosomes
    - may represent 47,XXY/46,XX mosaics
        - in which the trisomic cell line is difficult to detect.

- Excessive numbers of X chromosomes (XXX, etc) in females produce
    - menstrual disorders and
    - phenotypic abnormalities similar to Klinefelter syndrome.

- Cases of Klinefelter syndrome with 48,XXYY
    - have a combination of the characteristics of 47,XXY and 47,XYY.

- The Chromosome XYY syndrome is characterized by
    - excessive prepubertal growth
    - difficulty in learning language-related subjects,
    - explosive behavior, and
    - impulsiveness
the psychological characteristics predisposing to
        - delinquency

- Turner syndrome is characterized by
  - neonatal edema,
  - coarctation of aorta,
  - redundant skin and subcutaneous tissue cuffing the neck, or webbed neck,
  - sexual infantilism, and
  - short stature.

- Over 20 varieties of abnormal karyotypes have been associated with the Turner syndrome, with
  - 45,X accounting for 55%,
  - X isochromosomes of various types: 20%,
  - mosaicism: 10%, and
  - Y chromosome aberrations, X deletions and X rings 5% each.

- Either primordial (streak) or hypoplastic ovaries are characteristic of the Turner syndrome and
  - cases with a Y chromosome tend to develop ovarian carcinoma.

- True hermaphrodites have gonads with both male and female structures
  - but about 66% appear masculine externally.

- Over 10 varieties of abnormal karyotypes have been associated with true hermaphroditism with
  - 46,XX accounting for 50%,
  - mosaics of various types: 30%, and
  - 46,XY: 20%

- Male pseudohermaphrodites have male gonadal tissue but ambiguous genitalia.

- Over 12 varieties of abnormal karyotypes have been associated with male pseudohermaphroditism
  - but most are 46,XY/45,X.

- Female pseudohermaphroditism is due to one of several autosomal recessive genes
  - that produce failure of synthesis of cortisol by the adrenals,
    - feedback elevation of ACTH leading to adrenal hyperplasia and excessive adrenal androgen production which masculinizes the female fetus;
      - the karyotype is normal.

- Testicular feminization has a 46,XY karyotype and is due to
  - an X-linked recessive gene that causes absence of androgen receptor which causes female differentiation; characteristics include
    - blind vagina,
    - inguinal testes,
    - lack of axillary and pubic hair and
    - voluptuous feminine pubertal development

Additional references:

Anneren G, Karlsson B, Gustafsson J, et al. Thyroid function in children and adolescents with Down syndrome in relation to age, sex, growth velocity and thyroid autoantibodies. 4th Joint Clinical Genetics Meeting, Ft Lauderdale, 1997: Abstract 184.

Bartram CR, Koske-Westphal T, Passarge E. Chromatid exchanges in ataxia telangiectasia, Bloom Syndrome, Werner Syndrome, and xeroderma pigmentosum. Ann Hum Genet 1976;40:79-86.

Borgaonkar DS. *Chromosomal Variation in Man. A Catalogue of Chromosomal Variants and Anomalies.* New York: Wiley-Liss, 1991.

Boue J, Boue A, Gropp A. Cytogenetics of pregnancy wastage. Adv Hum Genet 1985;14:1-57.

Braekeleer MD, Smith B, Lin CC. Fragile sites and structural rearrangements in cancer. Hum Genet, 1985;69:112-16.

Daneshbod-Skibba G, Therman E, Shahidi NT. A boy with congenital malformations and chromosome breakage. Am J Med Genet 1980;5:315-320.

Darlington GJ, Dutkowski R, Brown WT. Sister chromatid exchange frequencies in progeria and Werner Syndrome patients. Am J Hum Genet 1981;33:762-766.

Delhanty JDA, Davis MB, Wood J. Chromosome instability in lymphocytes, fibroblasts and colon epithelial-like cells from patients with familial polyposis coli. Cancer Genet Cytogenet 1983;8:27-50.

Di Lernia R, Magnani I, Doneda L, et al. Cytogenetic instability in a family with gastric cancer Recurrence. Cancer Genet Cytogenet 1987;27:299-310.

Emerit I, Emerit J, Levy A, et al. Chromosomal breakage in Chron's disease: Anticlastogenic effect of D-Penicillamine and L-Cysteine. Hum Genet 1979;50:51-57.

Emerit I. Chromosomal breakage in systemic sclerosis and related disorders. Dermatologica 1976;153:145-156.

Emerit I, Emerit J, Tosoni-Pittoni A, et al. Chromosome studies in patients with ulcerative colitis. Humangenetik 1972;16:313.

Epstein CJ. The Consequences of Chromosome Imbalance. Cambridge: Cambridge University Press, 1986.

Epstein CJ (editor). The Neurobiology of Down syndrome. New York: Raven Press, 1986.

Gardner EJ, Woodward SR, Hughes PJ. Evaluation of chromosomal diagnosis for hereditary adenomatosis of the colorectum. Cancer Genet Cytogenet 1985;15:321-34.

Groden J, German J. Bloom's syndrome. XVIII. Hypermutability at a tandem-repeat locus. Hum Genet 1992;90:360-367.

Hecht F, Kaiser McCaw B. Chromosome instability syndromes. In: Mulvihill JJ, Miller RW, Fraumeni JF (editors). *Genetics of human cancer.* New York: Raven Press, 1977:105-23.

Hsu TC, Pathak S, Samman N, et al. Chromosome instability in patients with medullary carcinoma of the thyroid. J A M A 1981;18:2046-48.

Koskull von H, Aula P. Non-random distribution of chromosome breaks in Fanconi's anemia. Cytogenet Cell Genet, 1973;12:423-434.

Loesch DZ, Hay DA. Clinical features and reproductive patterns in fragile X female heterozygotes. J Med Genet 1988;25:407-14.

Mandel JL, Hagerman R, Froster U, et al. Fifth International Workshop on the Fragile X and X-Linked Mental Retardation. Am J Med Genet 1992;43:5-27.

Mark J, Dahlenfors R, Ekedahl C, Stenman G. Chromosomal pattern in a benign human neoplasm, the mixed salivary gland tumor. Hereditas 1982;96:141-48.

Meyn MS. High spontaneous intrachromosomal recombination rates in ataxia-telangiectasia. Science 1993;260:1327-1330.

Mitelman F. *Catalogue of Chromosome Aberrations in Cancer*. New York: Wiley-Liss, 1991.

Moore KL, Barr ML. Smears from the oral mucosa in the determination of chromosomal sex. 1955;Lancet 2: 57-58.

Neibuhr E. Partial trisomies and deletions of chromosome 13. In: Yunis JJ (editor). *New Chromosomal Syndromes*. New York: Academic Press, 1977.

Nishimura H, Okamoto N (editors). *Sequential Atlas of Human Congenital Malformations. Observations of Embryos, Fetuses and Newborns*. Baltimore: University Park Press, 1976.

Nordenson I. Increased frequencies of chromosomal abnormalities in families with a history of fetal wastage. Clin Genet 1981;19:168-173.

Passarge E. Spontaneous chromosomal instability. Humangenetik 1972;16:151-7.

Runger TM, Sobotta P, Dekant B, et al. In-vivo assessment of DNA ligation efficiency and fidelity in cells from patients with Fanconi's anemia and other cancer-prone hereditary disorders. Toxicol Letters 1993;67:309-324.

Shiraish Y. Cytogenetic studies in 12 patients with Itai-Itai disease. Humangenetik 1975;27:31-44.

Sutton EH. *An Introduction to Human Genetics*. Philadelphia: Saunders, 1980.

Swift M. Malignant neoplasms in heterozygous carriers of genes for certain autosomal recessive syndromes. In Mulvihill JJ, Miller RW, Fraumeni JF (editors). *Genetics of Human Cancer*. New York: Raven Press, 1977.

Taylor AMR, Harnden DG, Fairburn EA. Chromosomal instability associated with susceptibility to malignant disease in patients with porokeratosis of Mibelli. J Natl Cancer Inst 1973;51:371-378.

Tamaren J, Spuhler K, Sujansky E. Risk of Down syndrome among second and third degree relatives of a proband with Trisomy 21. Am J Med Genet 1983;19:393-403.

Weemaes CMR, Hustinx TWJ, Scheres JMJC, et al, A new chromosome instability disorder: The Nijmegen breakage syndrome. Acta Paediat Scand 1981;70:557-564.

Yunis JJ, Soreng AL. Constitutive fragile sites and cancer. Science 1984;226:1199-204.

1.   Hereditary disorders of biochemical origin are very numerous
- many being the purview of specific medical specialties,
  - especially those with physically identifiable features
    (see table, Other Hereditary Disorders of Biochemical Origin),
- while others exemplify Garrod's original designation of inborn errors which
  - are difficult to characterize physically (discussed here).

- There are many types of inherited metabolic diseases (inborn errors) and
  - it is likely that each case can be traced to different mutations; hence,
  - individual cases of each type are exceedingly rare,
  - concentrations of cases being observed only in family distributions;
  - however, the overall frequency of all types together approaches 1%.

2.   Severe *disorders of amino acids, urea cycle and organic acids* occur mainly in the <u>**newborn**</u> and typically cause either
- <u>**fulminant disease**</u> indistinguishable from
  - *asphyxia, sepsis, or respiratory distress*
- <u>**involutional symptoms**</u> such as
  - vomiting
  - hypotonia
  - hypertonia
  - seizure
  - lethargy
  - anorexia.

- Patients who survive the newborn forms and
  - children with milder forms
    - <u>**develop fluid & electrolyte problems when ill**</u>, and have
    - <u>**susceptibility to infectious diseases**</u> and
    - <u>**poor growth and development,**</u>
    - culminating in adulthood in
      - <u>**short stature**</u> and
      - <u>**mental retardation,**</u>
    - and some have <u>**epilepsy**</u>.
  - Carnitine depletion may occur whenever systemic organic or fatty acids are excessive.

Carnitine deficiency symptoms may be due to organic acid toxicity or CoA deficiency. Characteristic are **muscle weakness and hypotonia, cardiomyopathy** and **hepatic steatosis**, which may be intermittent and may be accompanied by **hypoglycemia** and **hyperammonemia**. Diagnosis is through determination of plasma free carnitine level and analysis of types of urinary acylcarnitines.

Deficiency syndrome	Gen	Mechanism
Systemic	?	Defective biosynthesis ? (most cases were actually MCAD)
Fanconi renal	AD	Excessive urinary loss
Propionic acidemia	AR	Depletion due to overproduction of propionyl CoA
Valproate toxicity	?	β-oxidation blockade

Carnitine synthesis is mainly in the kidney and carnitine is transported to other tissues, especially muscle. Liver synthesizes some carnitine and brain may have its own carnitine synthesis system.

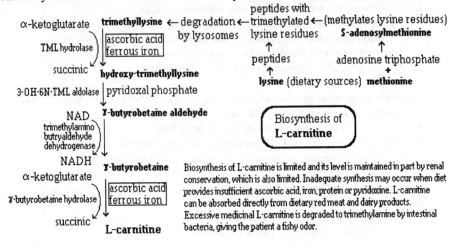

Biosynthesis of L-carnitine is limited and its level is maintained in part by renal conservation, which is also limited. Inadequate synthesis may occur when diet provides insufficient ascorbic acid, iron, protein or pyridoxine. L-carnitine can be absorbed directly from dietary red meat and dairy products. Excessive medicinal L-carnitine is degraded to trimethylamine by intestinal bacteria, giving the patient a fishy odor.

Carnitine metabolism is through detoxification of organic acids. Excessive formation of organic acids may deplete carnitine. Characteristic urinary acylcarnitine types may be present. Metabolic blocks may cause formation of abnormal acylcarnitines which trap carnitine in mitochondria, reversing the free carnitine:acyl carnitine ratio and causing relative insufficiency although the total amount of carnitine may be normal. The mechanisms of carnitine lowering by TPN, soy-based infant formulas and vegetarian diets are unclear.

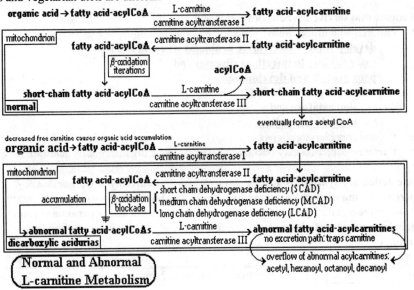

- Prominent factors interfering with diagnosis include:
  - Substrate deprivation in patients receiving only electrolyte solution which causes
    - failure of excretion of diagnostic metabolites of some disorders.
  - Many of the disorders lack recognizable clinical signs until their late stages,
    - and some have no clinical signs that allow recognition of the disorder.
  - There are intermittent forms, so some of the disorders are present only
    - when exacerbated by other diseases or trauma.

- Diagnosis in the newborn (see table, Diagnosis of Disorders of Amino Acids, Urea Cycle and Organic Acids in the Newborn)
  - utilizes an initial set of screening tests
    - blood: NH_3^+, Ca^{++}, Mg^{++}, pH, CBC, electrolytes, ketones, sugar.
      - Hyperammonemia must be managed while diagnosis proceeds (see table, Neonatal Hyperammonemia).
    - urine: reducing substances, ketones, sugar
  - a second level of qualitative tests to verify a metabolic disorder
    - urine: thin layer chromatography of amino acids, organic acids, sugars
  - a third level of definitive tests to plan therapy
    - blood: amino acid column chromatography
    - urine: orotate, amino acid column chromatography, organic gas chromatography/mass spectroscopy

3. *Lysosomal storage disorders* may cause
    - **hydrops fetalis,**
    - **progressive coarsening of features, particularly hands and feet,**
    - **growth failure when onset before completion of growth,**
    - **deterioration of mental functions,**
    - **liver and/or spleen enlargement when onset in infants and children,**
    along with other findings which may allow clinical recognition.

- Laboratory diagnosis of lysosomal disorders requires
  - screening evaluations:
    - x-rays of skull, hands and spine for dysostosis multiplex,
      - a coarsening of bone outlines that parallels the coarsening of features,
    - GAG (mucopolysaccharide) screening: quantitation and TLC,
    - oligosaccharide screening by TLC: poorly characterized but affected patients have bands that are darker and in positions different from normals.
  - enzyme determinations based on clinical abnormalities and screening results.

4. *Peroxysomal enzyme disorders* may produce a recognizable syndrome:
   - **hypotonia of prenatal onset,**
   - **apnea or inadequate respiration at birth**
   - **odd face with high forehead and full cheeks**

   - Laboratory diagnosis of peroxisomal disorders requires
     - screening evaluations:
       - x-rays for stippled epiphyses
       - plasma very long chain fatty acids
       - plasma pipecolic acid
       - serum cortisol response to ACTH injection
     - enzyme determinations based on clinical abnormalities and screening results.

5. Between 2% and 15% of patients with **mental retardation** or **epilepsy**
   - have an inherited metabolic disease which either has no other manifestation or may have typical symptoms that have escaped medical attention.
   - Laboratory testing of patients with these disorders is justified
     - to treat some cases that will benefit from it
     - to allow more accurate genetic counseling of relatives
     - to dispel erroneous popular notions of etiology of these problems
   - Tests for certain metabolites are practical in nearly all cases:
     - blood:
       - amino acids by TLC or HPLC
       - very long chain fatty acids
     - urine:
       - amino acids by TLC or HPLC
       - organic acids by TLC or GC/MS
       - sugars by TLC
       - GAG (mucopolysaccharide) quantitation & TLC
       - oligosaccharides by TLC
       (Lack of TLC in some laboratories may make it necessary to use column chromatography for amino acids and gas chromatography/mass spectroscopy for organic acids)
   - Chromosome analysis is also required.

AMINO ACID DISORDERS

DISORDER	PLASMA	URINE	ENZYMES	TREATMENT
β-alaninemia	β-alanine γ-aminobutyric	β-alanine β-aminoiso- butyric	x	x
biopterin defi- ciency*	phenylalanine	phenylalanine phenylpyruvic phenyllactic o-hydroxy- phenyllactic	dihydropteridine reductase, dihydropteridine synthetase	low phenyl- alanine diet, L- DOPA, 5- hydroxy- tryptophan, ascorbate
carboxypropyl- cysteinuria*	x	S-(2-carboxy- propylcysteine), S-(2-carboxy- propyl- cystamine)	3-hydroxybutyryl CoA reductase	x
carnosinemia	carnosine	carnosine	carnosinase	x
histidinemia	histidine	histidine, imidazoleacetic, imadazole- pyruvic	histidase	low histidine diet ?
homocystinuria	methionine, homocystine, homocystine- cysteine disulfide	methionine, homocystine, homocystine- cysteine disulfide	cystathionine synthetase, methylene tetrahydro- folate reductase	low methionine high cystine diet, folate, B6, dipyridamole?
hyperprolinemia I	proline	proline, glycine, hydroxyproline	proline oxidase	low proline diet
hyperprolinemia II	proline	proline, glycine, hydroxyproline, δ-pyrroline-5- carboxylate	δ'-pyrroline-5- carboxylic acid dehydrogenase	low proline diet
lactic acidemia*	alanine, citrulline, lysine, lactate, proline, pyruvate	alanine, citrulline, lysine, proline	pyruvate carboxylase, pyruvate dehydrogenase	B12, biotin, lipoic acid
lysinemia	lysine	homoarginine, homocitrulline, ε-N-acetyl lysine	lysine α- ketoglutarate reductase, saccharopine reductase	x
phenylketonuria	phenylalanine	phenylalanine, phenylpyruvic, phenyllactic, o-hydroxy phenylacetic	phenylalanine hydroxylase	low phenyl- alanine diet

AMINO ACID DISORDERS (continued)

DISORDER	PLASMA	URINE	ENZYMES	TREATMENT
tyrosinemia, * hepato-renal	tyrosine	p-hydroxy phenylacetic, p-hydroxy phenyllactic, tyrosine	fumaroaceto-acetase	low methionine phenylalanine tyrosine diet
tyrosinemia, * oculo-cutaneous	tyrosine	p-hydroxy phenylacetic, p-hydroxy phenyllactic, tyrosine	tyrosine amino-transferase	low phenyl-alanine diet

* newborn form known

UREA CYCLE DISORDERS

DISORDER	PLASMA	URINE	ENZYME	TREATMENT
argininosuccinic aciduria*	argininosuccinic	argininosuccinic, alanine, glutamate, lysine, orotic	argininosuccin-ase	arginine, benzoate, low protein diet
citrullinemia*	citrulline	citrulline, acidic amino acids, neutral amino acids	argininosuccinic synthetase	arginine, benzoate, low protein diet
CPS deficiency*	alanine, glutamate, lysine	(orotic normal)	carbamyl phosphate synthetase	peritoneal dialysis, low protein diet, benzoate, phenylacetate, keto analogues
hyperarginemia	arginine	arginine, cystine, lysine, ornithine	arginase	low protein diet
hyperornithin-emia	ornithine	homocitrulline, ornithine	x	x
lysinuric protein intolerance	ornithine	arginine, cystine, lysine, citrulline	dibasic amino acid transport	citrulline
ornithinemia with gyrate atrophy	ornithine	ornithine	ornithine amino transferase	creatine, low protein diet
OTC deficiency*	alanine, glutamate, lysine	orotic increased	ornithine transcarbamy-lase	creatine, low protein diet

* newborn form known

ORGANIC ACID DISORDERS

DISORDER	PLASMA	URINE	ENZYME	TREATMENT
3-hydroxy-3-methyl glutaric aciduria*	alanine, glutamate, isoleucine, leucine, lysine, valine ketones low	3-methyl crotonic, 3-methyl glutaconic, 3-hydroxy-3-methyl glutaric, 3-hydroxy-3-methylbutyric, methyl-glutaric	3-hydroxy-3-methyl glutaryl-CoA lyase	high carbohydrate low protein diet
α-ketoadipic aciduria	α-amino adipic, phenylalanine	α-amino adipic, α-hydroxy adipate	α-ketoadipate dehydrogenase	x
α-methyl acetoacetic aciduria	x	α-methyl-b-hydroxy butyric, α-methyl-acetoacetic, tigylglycine, n-butanone	β-ketothiolase	low protein diet
β-methyl crotonyl glycinuria*	β-methyl crotonyl glycine, hydroxy isovalerate	β-methyl crotonic, β-methyl crotonyl glycine, β-hydroxy-isovaleric	β-methyl crotonyl-CoA carboxylase	biotin
D-glyceric acidemia*	glyceric, glycine	cysteine, glyceric, glycine, lysine	D-glycerate dehydrogenase	bicarbonate
formimino-glutamic aciduria	formimino-glutamic	formimino-glutamic, hydantoin-5-hydroxy-propionic	glutamate-formimino transferase	folate
glutaric aciduria I	glycine, glutaric	β-hydroxy-glutaric, glycine, glutaric, glutaconic	glutaryl-CoA dehydrogenase	riboflavin, 4-amino-3-butyric
glutaric aciduria II*	x	adipic, butyric, ethylmalonic, glutaric, isobutyric, isovaleric, sebacic, suberic	multiple CoA dehydrogenase	x

ORGANIC ACID DISORDERS (continued)

DISORDER	PLASMA	URINE	ENZYME	TREATMENT
holocarboxylase deficiency*	isoleucine, leucine, valine	β-hydroxyiso-valerate, β-methyl crotonic, β-methyl crotonyl glycine, hydroxy-propionic, propionic, methyl citrate	holocarboxylase deficiency	biotin
hyperglycinemia	glycine, threonine	butanone, glycine, hexanone	x	x
isovaleric acidemia*	glycine, isovaleric	β-hydroxyiso-valeric, isovaleryl glycine	isovaleryl-CoA dehydrogenase	low protein diet, glycine 250 mg/day
maple syrup urine*	isoleucine, leucine, valine	keto acids, alloleucine	α-keto decarboxylases	B6 100 mg/day, peritoneal dialysis
methylmalonic aciduria*	glycine, methylmalonic	β-hydroxy-propionic, β-hydroxy-n-valeric, long chain ketones, methyl citrate, methylmalonic, propionic	methylmalonyl mutase or racemase	prenatal B12
propionic aciduria*	glycine, propionic	3-hydroxy-propionate, butanone, glycine, hexanone, methyl citrate, pentanone, propionate, propionyl glycine	propionyl-CoA-carboxylase	biotin, low protein diet
pyroglutamic aciduria*	5-oxyproline, proline, tyrosine	5-oxyproline	glutathione synthetase	x
remethylation defect*	x	cystathionine, homocystine, methylmalonic	x	B12

* newborn form known

Diagnosis of Disorders of Amino Acids, Urea Cycle and Organic Acids in the Newborn

Clinical features:	→ →	Initial tests:	→ →	Disorders diagnosed by initial tests:
anorexia vomiting hypotonia hypertonia seizures lethargy		Blood: NH_3^+, Ca^{++}, Mg^{++}, CBC, pH, electrolytes, ketones, sugar Urine: ketones, sugar, reducing substances		hypocalcemia hypomagnesemia hyponatremia hypernatremia
Results that require level 2 tests:	→ →	Level 2 tests:	→ →	Disorders diagnosed by level 2 tests:

leukopenia
thrombocytopenia
mellituria
hypoglycemia
		Urine (TLC):
		    sugars
		    amino acids
		    organic acids
				fructosuria
				galactosemia

ketosis
metabolic acidosis
respiratory alkalosis
hyperammonemia

Results that require level 3 tests:	→ →	Level 3 tests:	Disorders that cause clinical features like newborn metabolic disorders but have normal initial or level 2 tests:

aminoaciduria
organic aciduria
 	
(Level 3 tests are also
required if initial tests
are positive but level
2 tests are unavailable)
		Blood:
		    lactate
		    amino acid analysis
		Urine:
		    orotate
		    amino acid analysis
		    organic acid analysis
			asphyxia
			brain anomaly
			brain hemorrhage
			infection
			trauma

	Interpretation of results of level 3 tests	

SEVERE ACIDOSIS
citrulline 100-300
    lactate elevated
    high lactate/pyruvate
	Congenital lactic acidosis: pyruvate dehydrogenase deficiency
	                                       pyruvate decarboxylase deficiency	

glycine>700	β-alaninemia β-methylcrotonylglycinemia glutaric acidemia hyperglycinemia maple syrup urine methylmalonic acidemia propionic acidemia	β-ketothiolase deficiency dicarboxylic acidemias hydroxymethyl glutaric acidemia isovaleric acidemia methionine malabsorption multiple carboxylase deficiency tyrosinemia

MILD OR NO ACIDOSIS		*(Note: Severe disorders requiring urgent therapy are listed here. Other*
citrulline	orotate	* disorders in preceding tables are also diagnosed by these procedures.)*
0-trace	low >500	NAGS or CPS deficiency OTC deficiency
6-20		newborn transient hyperammonemia: NH_3^+ 2000-4000 if symptoms
100-300	low >500	argininosuccinic acidemia arginase deficiency
>1000		citrullinemia

Neonatal Hyperammonemia
An exercise in the use of the laboratory

See flow chart: <u>Diagnosis of Disorders of Amino Acids, Urea Cycle and Organic Acids in the Newborn</u>

A. Suggestive symptoms: correlated with ammonia level
    - 50-100 micromolar: asymptomatic
    - 100-200 micromolar: anorexia, vomiting, ataxia, irritability/hyperactivity
    - 200-250 micromolar: stage II coma (vomiting, lethargy, combative, stuporous)
    - 300-500 micromolar: stage III coma (responsive only to pain)
    - >500 micromolar: stage IV coma (decerebrate but responsive to pain, increased CSF pressure)

B. Differential diagnosis:
    - Neonatal asphyxia, symptoms before 24 hours age:
        - newborn transient hyperammonemia
    - Normal apgar, symptoms onset 24-48 hours age:
        - congenital lactic acidosis
        - organic acidemias
        - urea cycle disorders

C. Prognosis is related more to duration of coma than to peak ammonia level.
    Less than 15% survive the first year on nitrogen restriction alone.
    Data from a recent study of aggressive treatment of urea cycle disorders:
    - Figures for all babies who had >100 micromolar ammonia:
        - 8% had fulminant course and neonatal death despite treatment.
        - An additional 16% died over the first year of life
        - Condition of treated survivors:
            - 46% have cerebral palsy
            - 17% have seizures
            - 5% are blind
            - average IQ is 43 (100% with coma over 120 hours are mentally retarded)
            - 21% have normal IQ (80% with coma of less than 48 hours have normal IQ)

D. Treatment prior to specific diagnosis:
    - Withhold nitrogen from diet whenever ammonia>100 micromolar.
    - 100 kcal/kg/day as IV glucose.
    - If acidotic, biotin & B12.
    - If not acidotic, sodium benzoate & sodium phenyl acetate, both 0.25 g/kg, and arginine 0.21 g/kg, IV over 90 minutes, followed by the same doses per day.
    - If beyond stage II coma, hemodialysis or peritoneal dialysis. Rebound may require repeat.
        - Ammonia>500 micromolar causes cerebral edema (visible on CT), cytoxicity of liver & brain, slow delta wave activity on EEG.
        - At physiologic pH, 98% of ammonia is NH_4^+ which permeates membrane poorly.
        - Elevated pH changes ammonia to NH_3 which permeates lipid membranes (brain).
        - Hyperventilation treatment is contraindicated because it elevates cerebral pH>7.4.

Neonatal Hyperammonemia (continued)

E.   Clinical Notes
- Congenital lactic acidosis: seizures, hypotonia, posturing, lethargy, poor feeding.
    - Increased lactate:pyruvate ratio (both elevated).
    - Treatment: thiamine & lipoic acid stimulate residual pyruvate dehydrogenase, biotin stimulates residual pyruvate carboxylase.
    - Both enzymes are in amniocytes.
- Organic acidemias: severe metabolic acidosis (pH 6.9-7.2, bicarbonate<10 meQ/L, anion gap>20 meQ/L, bone marrow depression, carnitine depletion).
    - Mild or partial: intermittent vomiting, lethargy, metabolic derangements.
    - Severe or complete: Respiratory distress, poor feeding, hypotonia, lethargy, coma.
    - Treatment: bicarbonate, carnitine, biotin for propionic acidemia & multiple carboxylase deficiency, B12 for methylmalonic acidemia.
    - Most of the enzymes are in amniocytes, some of the organic acids are in amniotic fluid.
- Newborn transient hyperammonemia: unknown etiology.
    - Asymptomatic hyperammonemia occurs in half of infants<2500 grams birth weight.
        - Normalizes spontaneously in 6-8 weeks.
        - Arginine p.o. normalizes ammonia in 24 hrs but produces no clinical improvement.
    - Symptomatic: usually in prematures with respiratory distress.
        - Arginine does not decrease ammonia level.
        - Rebound after dialysis is rare.
        - Mortality during coma is 30%-50%.
- Urea cycle disorders: 60% had a sib who died in neonatal period.
    - Partial defects may cause mild disease in newborn or may occur with dietary protein protein increase as with switching from formula to cow's milk: anorexia, cyclic vomiting, irritability, occasionally coma. Repeated episodes cause neurological deterioration.
    - Complete defects: coma.
    n-Acetyl glutamate synthetase (NAGS) deficiency or carbamyl phosphate synthetase (CPS) deficiency: decreased arginine, increased glutamine & alanine.
    - Fetal CPS is in liver, rectum, duodenum; NAGS in liver, neither in amniocytes.
    - Treat with sodium benzoate, sodium phenyl acetate, and arginine as in D above.
    Ornithine carbamyl transcarbamyl (OTC) deficiency: X-linked.
    - Fetal OTC is in liver, none in amniocytes. RFLP informative in fetus in 60% of matings.
    - Similar to partial defect in most expressing heterozygote females.
    - Females with milder defects may have modest IQ deficit, and may have vomiting, migraine headache after protein loading.
    - Treat with sodium benzoate, sodium phenyl acetate, and arginine as in D above.
    Argininosuccinase (AL) deficiency, argininosuccinic aciduria: usual onset 5-7 days age
    - argininosuccinic acid (ASA) co-chromatographs with isoleucine in plasma but anhydride derivitization or urine chromatography will resolve.
    - Arginine 0.66 g/kg/day IV treats trichorrhexis nodosa & erythematous maculopapular rash.
    - AL is present in amniocytes. Increased ASA in amniotic fluid of affected fetus. skin rash. Hepatomegaly remains in treated patients.

Neonatal Hyperammonemia (continued)

Argininosuccinate synthetase (AS) deficiency, citrullinemia: 3 forms:

- Newborn form causes coma in first week of life.
- Partial defect causes intermittent disease like other urea cycle disorders.
- Adult type: bizarre behavior, dysarthria, weakness, lethargy, irritability.
  - Many had attacks of recurrent vomiting, lethargy, irritability during childhood.
- Treat with sodium benzoate, sodium phenyl acetate, and arginine as in D above, except that the arginine dose is 0.66 g/kg.
- AS is present in amniocytes. Increased citrulline in amniotic fluid of affected fetus.

LYSOSOMAL STORAGE DISORDERS

Onset: n=early infancy, i=late infancy, c=early childhood, p=late chldhood

Disease, onset, enzyme	Some early signs	Some late signs
Galactosialidosis I*, (n), neuraminidase, β-galactosidase	Hydrops fetalis, cloudy cornea	
Gaucher disease II, (n), glucocerebrosidase	Hepatosplenomegaly, dysphagia	Lung infections, hypertonia
GM1 gangliosidosis I, (n), β-galactosidase	Coarse face, hypotonia	Gingival hypertrophy, cherry red spot of retina
I-cell disease* (mucolipidosis II), (n), N-acetylglucosamine-1-phospho-transferase	Narrow forehead, coarse face, gingival hyperplasia	Stiff joints, thick skin, heart failure, mental retardation
Niemann-Pick A, (n), sphingomyelinase	Hepatosplenomegaly, dysphagia	Spasticity, cherry red spot of retina
Sialidosis I*, (n) neuraminidase	Hydrops fetalis, hepatosplenomegaly	Recurrent infections
Aspartylglycosaminuria* (i), N-aspartyl-β-glucosaminidase	Recurrent infections, coarse face with wrinkled skin, hoarse voice, hypotonia	Speech defect, crystalline lens opacities, macroglossia, loose joints, fractures
Farber disease, (i), ceramidase	Hypotonia	Hoarseness, joint pain, soft tissue nodules
Fucosidosis*, (i), α-fucosidase	Sweating	Thick skin, spasticity, high sweat chloride
GM1 gangliosidosis II*, (i), β-galactosidase	Hypotonia	Coarse face, stiff joints
Hurler syndrome, (i), α-iduronidase	Noisy respiration	Coarse face, stiff joints, cloudy cornea
Krabbe disease, (i), galactocerebrosidase	Irritability, vomiting	Rigidity, blindness
Mannosidosis*, (i), α-mannosidase	Hepatosplenomegaly	Macrocephaly, coarse face, macroglossia, gibbus, deafness
Metachromatic leukodystrophy, (i), aryl sulfatase A	Hypotonia, weakness	Rigidity, spasticity

LYSOSOMAL STORAGE DISORDERS (continued)

Pompe disease*, (i), acid maltase	Hypotonia, macroglossia	Heart failure
Sandhoff disease*, (i), hexosaminidase A & B	Hyperacusis	Hypotonia, cherry red spot of retina
Sialidosis II*, (i), neuraminidase	Coarse face, hepatosplenomegaly	Stiff joints, mental retardation
Sly syndrome, (i), β-glucuronidase	Coarse face, hernia	Stiff joints, cloudy cornea
Tay-Sachs disease, (i), hexosaminidase A	Hyperacusis	Macrocephaly, blindness, cherry red spot of retina
Gaucher disease III, (c), glucocerebrosidase	Hepatosplenomegaly	Myoclonic epilepsy, incoordination
Maroteaux-Lamy syndrome, (c), aryl-sulfatase B	Coarse face, cloudy cornea	Heart failure, stiff joints
Niemann-Pick C, (c), cholesterol esterification	Hepatosplenomegaly	Seizures, ataxia
Pompe disease II*, (c), acid maltase	Hypotonia, weakness	
Pseudo-Hurler polydystrophy* (mucolipidosis III), (c), N-acetylglucosamine-1-phosphotransferase	Stiff joints, coarse face	Cloudy cornea, mental retardation, aortic insufficiency
Sanfilippo syndrome, (c), α-glucosaminidase	Coarse face, hirsutism, hyperactivity	Hepatosplenomegaly, stiff joints
Sialidosis III* (mucolipidosis I), (c), neuraminidase	Coarse face, hepatosplenomegaly	Stiff joints, mental retardation
Fabry disease, (p), ceramide trihexosidase	Angiokeratoma, abdominal pain attacks	Corneal dystrophy, nephropathy
Galactosialidosis II*, (p), neuraminidase, β-galactosidase	Coarse features, cloudy cornea	Cherry red spot of retina, mental retardation
Gaucher disease II, (p), glucocerebrosidase	Hepatosplenomegaly, thrombocytopenia	Bone pain, fractures
Metachromatic leukodystrophy, (p), aryl sulfatase A	Movement & posture disorder	Schizophrenia, non-visualizing gall bladder
Niemann-Pick B, (p), sphingomyelinase	Hepatosplenomegaly, short stature	Lung infiltrates
Sialidosis IV*, (p), neuraminidase	Myoclonic epilepsy	Cherry red spot of retina

* abnormal oligosaccharide in urine

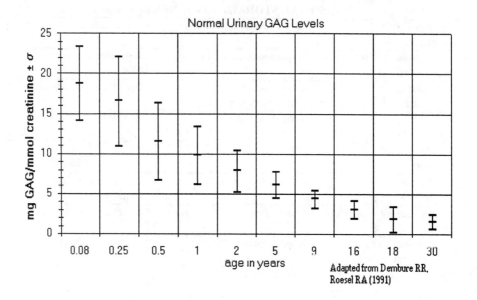

Adapted from Dembure RR, Roesel RA (1991)

Type	Eponym	dermatan sulfate	heparan sulfate	chondroitin 6-sulfate	keratan sulfate
MPS I	Hurler/Scheie	+++	++	+	0
MPS II	Hunter	+++	0	+	0
MPS III	Sanfilippo A - D	0	+++	+	0
MPS IV A	Morquio A	0	0	+++	++
MPS IV B	Morguio B	0	0	+	+++
MPS VI	Maroteaux-Lamy	++	0	+	0
MPS VII	Sly	++	0	++	0
Normal		0	0	+	0

Adapted from Dembure RR, Roesel RA (1991).

Types and Amounts of Urinary GAG

Some patients may have normal or near normal quantities but abnormal types.

Peroxisomal Enzyme Disorders

Group 1: Peroxisomes reduced or absent, multiple enzyme defects
- **ZS**: Zellweger syndrome
- **NALD**: neonatal adrenoleukodystrophy
- **IRD**: infantile Refsum disease
- Hyperpipecolic acidemia

Group 2: Peroxisomes normal, single enzyme defect
- **XLD**: X-linked adrenoleukodystrophy (adrenomyeloneuropathy)
- Acatalasemia
- Hyperoxaluria I
- 3-Oxoacyl-CoA thiolase deficiency (pseudo-Zellweger)
- Acyl CoA oxidase deficiency
- Bifunctional enzyme deficiency
- **ARD**: adult Refsum disease

Group 3: Peroxisomes structurally abnormal, multiple enzyme defects
- **RCDP**: rhizomelic chrondrodysplasia punctata
- Zellweger variants

Features	ZS	NALD	XALD	IRD	ARD	RCDP
Dysmorphism: high forehead, flat face, full cheeks, flat occiput, hypotonia	+++	++	-	-	-	++
Hepatomegaly	++	++	-	++	-	-
Pigmentary retinopathy	+++	+++	-	?	++	++
Renal cortical cysts	+++	-	-	-	-	-
Chondrodysplasia calcificans	+	-	-	+	-	+++
Plasma very long chain fatty acids elevated	++	++	+	+	-	-
Pipecolic acids elevated in plasma	++	+	-	+	-	-
Plasmalogens decreased in fibroblasts	+	+	-	+	-	+
Adrenal cortex atrophy	++	+++	+++	-	-	-
Abnormal neuronal migration	+++	++	-	-	-	-

Adapted from Scriver CR, Beaudet AL, Sly WS, Valle DW, Eds (1989)

OTHER HEREDITARY DISORDERS OF BIOCHEMICAL ORIGIN

BILIRUBINOPATHIES
- Crigler-Najjar syndromes
- Gilbert diseases

CARBOHYDRATE DISORDERS
- Fructosrias
- Galactosemias
- Glycogen storage diseases
- Lactic acidoses
- Malabsorptive enzymopathies
- Oxaluria
- Pentosuria

COLLAGEN DISORDERS
- Osteogenesis imperfectas
- Ehlers-Danlos syndromes
- Marfan syndrome
- Cutis laxa
- Epidermolysis bullosa

ENTEROKINASE DEFICIENCY

ERYTHROCYTE ENZYMOPATHIES
- Glycolysis enzymopathies
- Hexose monophosphate shunt enzymopathies
- Glutathione reductase deficieency
- Pyrimidine nucleotidase deficiency

HEMOGLOBINOPATHIES
- Hemoglobinopathies C
- Hemoglobinopathies E
- Methemoglobinemias
- Sickle hemoglobinopathy
- Thalassemias
- Unstable hemoglobins

HYPOPHOSPHATASIAS

LIPID DISORDERS
- Apoprotein A defects
- Apoprotein B defects
- Apoprotein CII defects
- Apoprotein E defects
- LDL receptor defects
- Remnant receptor defects
- Lipoprotein enzyme defects

METAL DISORDERS
- Copper malabsorption
- Copper storage
- Hemachromatosis
- Magnesium malabsorption
- Molybdenum deficiency
- Zinc malabsorption

NUCLEOTIDE DISORDERS
- Adenylosuccinase deficiency
- Adenosine deaminase deficiency
- Adenosine phosphoribosyltransferase deficiency
- Hyperurcemias
- Lesch-Nyhan syndrome
- Myoadenylate deaminase deficiency
- Orotic aciduria
- Purine nuceoside phosphorylase deficiency
- Xanthine oxidase deficiency

PANCREATIC ENZYMOPATHIES
- Pancreatic lipase deficiency
- Combined peptidase deficiency

PORPHYRIAS
- Hepatic porphyrias
- Erythropoetic porphyrias

PSEUDOCHOLINESTERASE DEFICIENCY

STEROID DISORDERS
- Adrenogenital syndromes
- Aldosterone deficiencies
- Androgen resistances
- Testosterone deficiencies

THYROID DISORDERS
- Iodine transport defect
- Iodotyrosine coupling defect
- Iodotyrosine deiodinase defect
- Pendred syndorme
- Plasma iodoprotein defect
- Thyroglobulin synthesis defects
- Thyroid hormone unresponsiveness
- Thyroid peroxidase defect

VITAMIN D DEPENDENCIES

Additional references:

Batshaw ML. *Hyperammonemia*. Current Problems in Pediatrics 14 (11). Chicago: Year Book Medical Publishers, 1984.

Benson PF, Fensom AH. *Genetic Biochemical Disorders*. Oxford Monographs on Medical Genetics No. 12. New York: Oxford, 1985.

Davis KE. Human Genetic Diseases. A Practical Approach. Washington, DC: IRL Press, 1986.

Dembure PP, Roesel RA. Screening for mucopolysaccharidoses by analysis of urinary glycosaminoglycans. In: Hommes FA (editor). *Techniques in Diagnostic Human Biochemical Genetics. A Laboratory Manual*. New York: Wiley-Liss, 1991.

Hill RE. Carnitine. Jour Intl Fed Clin Chem 1991;3:66-71.

Holton JB. *The Inherited Metabolic Diseases*. New York: Churchill Livingstone, 1987.

Lee BY, Thurmon TF. Clinical amino acid screening by thin-layer chromatography. LC-GC 1991;9:494-497.

Lee BY, Thurmon TF. Practical clinical screening for organic acid disorders. LC-GC 1992;10:884-887.

Scriver CR, Beaudet AL, Sly WS, et al (editors). *The Metabolic and Molecular Bases of Inherited Disease. 7th Edition*. New York: McGraw-Hill, 1995.

Sewell AC. Urinary oligosaccharides. In: Hommes FA (editor). *Techniques in Diagnostic Human Biochemical Genetics. A Laboratory Manual*. New York: Wiley-Liss, 1991.

Sweetman L. Organic acid analysis. In: Hommes FA (editor). *Techniques in Diagnostic Human Biochemical Genetics. A Laboratory Manual*. New York: Wiley-Liss, 1991.

1.   HLA (human lymphocyte antigen) gene products are
   - cell membrane proteins of all cells except erythrocytes and are
   - called tissue types.

   The MHC (major histocompatibility complex) on chromosome 6p contains
   - HLA-A, HLA-B, HLA-C, and HLA-D, as well as the
   - complement genes Bf, C2, C4A and C4B, and a gene for
   - congenital adrenal hyperplasia (CYP21).

HLA-A, -B, and -C genes produce protein moieties of glycoproteins that are located in the cell membrane of all cells and are used by T lymphocytes to identify "self" cells. HLA-D and -DR genes produce polypeptides that are located on the surfaces of B lymphocytes and macrophages and are used by T-helper lymphocytes to recognize "self" and communicate with other cells of the immune response. Some recognized alleles:

HLA-A	HLA-B	HLA-C	HLA-D	HLA-Dr
A1-A3, A9-11	B5, B7-8	Cw6-8	Dw1-12	Dr1-5, Dr7
A28, A29	B12-15, B17-18			Drw6, Drw8-10
Aw19, Aw23-26	B27, B37, B40			
Aw30-34, Aw36	Bw4, Bw6			
Aw43	Bw16, Bw21-22			
	Bw35, Bw38-39			
	Bw41-42,			
	Bw44-63			

   - HLA genes are described as haplotypes
   (list of HLA alleles in each MHC complex),
     - one haplotype for each chromosome 6, with such close linkage
       - within the complex that less than 2% of zygotes are recombinants.

   - Several HLA genes are in linkage disequilibrium
     - which means that the frequency with which they are found to be associated
     - is much greater than its random likelihood
       - (product of their individual gene frequencies).

   - HLA genes may represent a fine tuning of the immune system such that
     - there are so many immunologic differences among humans that
     - no invading organism could simulate human immune characteristics
     - well enough to permit it to enter a significant percentage of humans.

   - The close association of HLA and autoimmune diseases implies that
     - the fine tuning is sometimes overdone and certain tissues (e.g., thyroid)
       - begin to be treated as invading organisms.

- HLA genes were unknown until attempts were made at grafting (transplanting) human tissues and it was found that
  - autografts (from self) and
  - isografts (from MZ twin) were accepted but
  - allografts (from same species) and
  - xenografts (from different species) were rejected.

- An allograft is initially accepted but B and T cell immunity
  - rapidly develops against the HLA antigens of the graft
    - and it is rejected (host versus graft).

- If immunocompetent bone marrow is grafted into an immunodeficient host, it develops
  - graft versus host immunity, which may be fatal or may develop into a
    - chronic sickness known as runt disease.

- The fetus is an allograft which is tolerated because of a
  - poorly defined type of immune supression that can be breached by
    - overt spillage of fetal erythrocytes into maternal circulation

- Maternal IgG crosses the placenta (a major protective mechanism of the newborn),
      but, though a foreign protein, does not stimulate an immune response until
  - after birth when the infant slowly develops antibodies against Gm,
    - one of the antigenic sites on the IgG molecule.

2. Blood group phenotypes were unknown until
  - early attempts at blood transfusion showed agglutination of erythrocytes when they were transfused into a person whose blood group alleles were different
      from the donor,
    - a form of graft rejection.

- Antigens similar to blood group antigens occur widely in plants, animals and microorganisms and
  - contacts with them lead to development in blood of
    - antibodies to non-self antigens.

- The clinically important blood group antigens are
  - protein components of the erythrocyte cell membrane,
    coded by gene loci as follows:
  - ABO is on 9q
  - Rh is on 1p
  - Duffy is on 1q
  - Kell is on Xp
  - Kidd is on 2p
  - Lutheran is on 19p
  - MNSs is on 4q

- For ABO,
  Rh or
  MNSs,
  - precursor proteins must be processed by enzymes into actual blood group antigens.

- Autosomal recessive precursor deficiency can cause a situation in which the blood group gene is present but not detectable by blood typing for
  - O_h',
  - Rh_{null} or
  - M^k

- The dominant gene Se (secretor) produces blood group antigens in body secretions;
  - its recessive allele, se causing lack of blood group secretion.

- About 10 blood groups are "public" while about 11 others are
  - "private," neither being polymorphisms.

- Seven blood groups including over 100 individual antigens are of clinical importance;
  - only ABO and Rh are routinely tested prior to transfusion therapy,
  - the others being detected by cross-matching.

- Current aspects of clinical importance of blood groups include
  - transfusion and transplantation of other tissues,
  - hemolytic disease of the newborn, and
  - parentage testing.

- The criterion of importance to transfusion, transplantation and hemolytic disease of the newborn is
  - strength of adverse reactions

- Blood groups capable of producing strong adverse reactions include
  - ABO
  - Rh
  - Duffy
  - Kell
  - Kidd
  - Lutheran

Type	Locus	processed from precursor	precursor deficiency type	adverse transfusion reactions	parentage testing
ABO	9q	x	Oh'	x	x
Rh	1p	x	Rhnull	x	x
Duffy	1q			x	x
Kell	Xp			x	x
Kidd	2p			x	x
Lutheran	19p			x	
MNNs	4p	x	M^k		x

- Criteria of importance for parentage testing include
  - availability of antisera,
  - reliable methodology,
  - well-defined genetics including population frequencies,
  - adequate probability of exclusion, and
  - accepted validity

- Blood groups important for parentage testing include
  - ABO
  - Rh
  - Duffy
  - Kell
  - Kidd
  - MNSs

3. Parentage testing starts with blood typing;
  - if no exclusion is found, HLA typing follows. This allows a 92% likelihood of one of the following types of exclusions for non-relatives:
    - Type 1: Consultand lacks an antigen which is present in child.
    - Type 2: Child lacks an antigen that must be transmitted by consultand.

- Exclusions for relatives are complicated by the necessity to consider recombination.
  - Blood types and tissue types have a significant rate of failure to exclude relatives.
  - See "Parentage Testing" at the end of this chapter for likelihood calculatiuons.

- Some racially limited antigens and
  - some sexually limited antigens allow exclusions.

- Numerous special cases interfere with parental exclusion so parentage testing must be done in a laboratory certified for that purpose.

- DNA techniques have largely supplanted blood typing for parentage testing (see the chapter on Laboratory Testing: Molecular Genetics) but
  - blood typing is still required in some cases and
    - the techniques are valuable as vehicles for study.

- An outline, Parentage ("Paternity") Testing, is at the end of this chapter.

- Digestion of DNA by a restriction enzyme results in
  - pieces of DNA called restriction fragments.

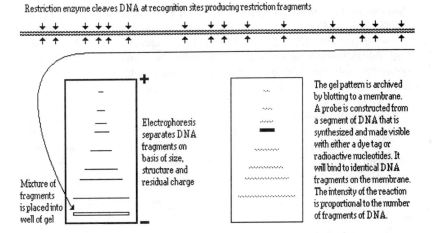

Restriction enzyme cleaves DNA at recognition sites producing restriction fragments

Mixture of fragments is placed into well of gel

Electrophoresis separates DNA fragments on basis of size, structure and residual charge

The gel pattern is archived by blotting to a membrane. A probe is constructed from a segment of DNA that is synthesized and made visible with either a dye tag or radioactive nucleotides. It will bind to identical DNA fragments on the membrane. The intensity of the reaction is proportional to the number of fragments of DNA.

- Mutations cause DNA from different people to have
  - differences in lengths of DNA segments because some
  - cleavage sites are present in some people and absent in others.

EcoR1 site   EcoR1 site   EcoR1 site   Normal or "wild type" gene
GAATTC / CTTAAG

EcoR1 site   EcoR1 site   Mutant gene
GAATTC / CTTAAG   GACTTC / CTGAAG   GAATTC / CTTAAG

An A→C mutation in the sense strand obliterates an EcoR1 cleavage site

Homozygous normal   Heterozygous   Homozygous mutant

Each person should have 2 copies of each gene (diploid). If there is only one mutant type, the possible DNA marker patterns are:

- The terms, restriction fragment length polymorphism (RFLP) or
  - DNA marker, are used to describe the DNA cleavage site differences,
  - most of which are not associated with discernible disease.
  - RFLP's are heritable and many are unique.

- Restriction fragment length polymorphisms are very numerous and may be used to establish parentage and identity when neither blood types nor tissue types show an exclusion, but
  - frequency data are not available for some **local populations**,
  - **meiotic instability** of length polymorphisms make interpretation problematical,
  - inexpert technique can cause errors from **band-shifting** and
  - inbreeding in local populations can cause errors from **band-sharing**.
  - Most often useable are:
    - sequence polymorphisms: HLA (DP, DQ, DR).
    - length polymorphisms of satellite DNA: (SSLP and VNTR).
      - In British whites, VNTR's 33.6 and 33.15 used together can exclude parentage with 99.999996% likelihood for non-relatives and 99.92% likelihood for relatives.

											Sample	DQα type
ASO probes		1 2 3 4	1 2 3									
		1.1 1.2 1.3	4 1.1	4 1.1 1.2								
1	2	3 4 1.3	1.1	1.3	1.3	1.2						
		● ● ◉		●		●				Husband	3, 4
●	●		●		●					Wife	1.2, 2
●			●		●	●	●			Child	1.2, 1.3

**Allele specific oligonucleotide Dqα
typing in a case of non-paternity**

- Parentage exclusion is **absolute** while proof of parentage is **relative**, always leaving a margin of error. Persons outside of a local population have a near zero likelihood of parenting a child in a local population so it is meaningless to compare the phenotype of a putative parent to the national frequency. Local population data are required for plausibility.

4. Dizygotic twining is the most common form of multizygosity and is due to
    - fertilization of 2 ova by 2 sperms and
    - there may be fusion to form one placenta (40%) which may have vascular connections leading to
      - blood group chimerism
    - fusion at the zygote stage leading to complete chimerism

- A chimera is an individual with at least two cell lines of genetically different origin;
  - a mosaic has at least two cell lines originating from the same zygote.

- Dizygotic twinning is familial due to
  - polygenic inheritance of multiple ovulation or
  - dominant inheritance of superfetation (discordant gestational age)
  - and also increases with maternal age.

- Multizygosity rates vary in ethnic groups:
    - dizygotic twins, 1:20 (African Yorubas), 1:125 (Europeans), 1:500 (Asians)
    - triplets, 1:10,000
    - quadruplets, 1:100,000

- The rate of monozygotic twinning is 1:250, varying little among ethnic groups,
    - 1/400 being conjoined twins (1:120,000).

- Monozygotic twinning has little hereditary tendency but is associated with
    - induction of ovulation by gonadotrophins.

- Monozygotic twins are due to division of the conceptus at some stage during the first 14 days after fertilization,
    - dichorionic, diamniotic if at the two-cell stage (1/3),
    - monochorionic, diamniotic if the early blastocyst inner cell mass splits (2/3),
    - monochorionic monoamniotic if the bilaminar germ disk splits before appearance of the primitive streak (rare).

- Conjoined twins are monozygotic twins in which the division of
    - either the inner cell mass or the
    - embryonic disk is incomplete, are classified as either
    - thoracoomphalopagus (28%), thoracopagus (18%), omphalopagus (10%), parasitic (10%), craniopagus (6%) and
    - cannot be produced by chemicals in experimental animals.

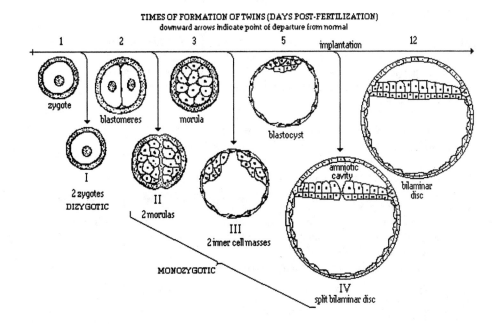

TIMES OF FORMATION OF TWINS (DAYS POST-FERTILIZATION)
downward arrows indicate point of departure from normal

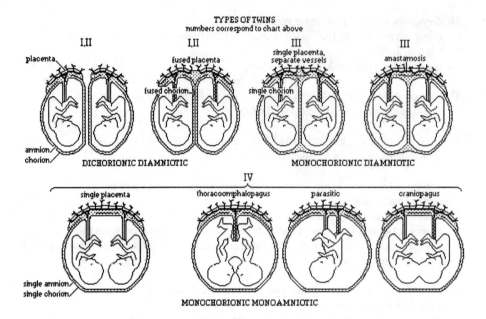

TYPES OF TWINS
numbers correspond to chart above

I,II — placenta, amnion, chorion — **DICHORIONIC DIAMNIOTIC**

I,II — fused placenta, fused chorion — **DICHORIONIC DIAMNIOTIC**

III — single placenta, separate vessels, single chorion — **MONOCHORIONIC DIAMNIOTIC**

III — anastamosis — **MONOCHORIONIC DIAMNIOTIC**

IV — single placenta, single amnion, single chorion — thoracoomphalopagus — parasitic — craniopagus — **MONOCHORIONIC MONOAMNIOTIC**

- Information about twins is steeped in mysticism and misconception;
  - determination of zygosity from fetal membranes is often impossible;
  - most phenotypic characteristics are polygenic and poorly objectified as
    - concordant if apparently identical or
    - discordant if different.

- Monozygotic twins due to early division of the conceptus may have identical monogenic phenotypes initially but they and all other types of twins
  - develop extensive genetic differences during embyrogenesis due to haphazard
    - developmental rearrangements in their genomes and
    - somatic mutations.

- Monozygotic twins can have different karyotypes if
  - an abnormality of an early post-zygotic cell division leads to
    - mitotic non-disjunction or
    - reversion of an aneuploidy to normal.

7. Human gestational mechanisms are not well suited for twins so they have
  - have a fetal death rate 4X and neonatal death rate 6X singleton rates, and many surviving twins of both types suffer from many adverse environmental factors before and during birth and
    - may have similar disorders due to this.

- Twinning is teratogenic and leads to frequent disorders:
  - dizygotic
    - chromosome aneuploidy
  - monozygotic
    - anencephaly
    - artery-artery twin disruption
    - artery-vein transfusion
    - exstrophy of cloaca
    - holoprosencephaly
    - sacrococcygeal teratoma
    - sirenomelia
    - VATER association
  - monozygotic twin anomalies related to death of co-twin:
    - aplasia cutis
    - gastroschisis
    - hydranencephaly
    - intestinal atresia
    - intravascular coagulation
    - limb amputation
    - porencephalic cyst
- conjoined twins: 15% incidence major anomalies not at juncture site.

ARTERY-VEIN TWIN TRANSFUSION

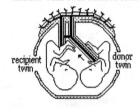

ARTERY-ARTERY TWIN DISRUPTION

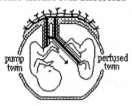

Recipient twin	Donor twin
larger	smaller
high hematocrit	low hematocrit
hypervolemia	hypovolemia
large kidneys	small kidneys
large heart	small heart
polyhydramnios (if diamniotic)	oligohydramnios (if diamniotic)

Pump twin	Perfused twin
normal karyotype	50% abnormal karyotype
large heart, heart failure	rudimentary heart "acardius"
normal head	rudimentary head "acephalus"
no anomalies	multiple anomalies
50% mortality	100% mortality

32. Though studies of twins do not differentiate genetic from environmental factors as well as is popularly thought,
    - accurate heritability studies can be done using the formula:

$$h^2 = \frac{s_{dz}^2 - s_{mz}^2}{s_{dz}^2}$$

environmental $0 \leftarrow \; \rightarrow 1$ genetic

Additional references:

Aickin M. Some fallacies in the computation of paternity probabilities. Am J Hum Genet 1984;36:906-915.

Alford RL, Hammond HA, Coto I, et al. Rapid and efficient resolution of parentage by amplification of short tandem repeats. Am J Hum Genet 1994;55:190-195.

American Medical Association, American Bar Association. Joint AMA-ABA guidelines: present status of serologic testing in problems of disputed parentage. Family Law Quarterly 1978;10:247-285.

Austad SN. Forensic DNA typing. Science 1972;255:1050.

Bellamy RJ, Inglehearn CF, Jalili IK, et al. Increased band-sharing in DNA fingerprints of an inbred population. Hum Genet 1991;87:341-347.

Bever RA, DeGuglielmo M, Staub RW, et al. Forensic DNA typing. Science 1992;255:1050-1052.

Budowlc B. Population genetic issues in DNA fingerprinting: Reply to Green. Am J Hum Genet 1992;50:441-443.

Chakraborty R, Kidd KK. Forensic DNA typing. Science 1992;255:1052-1053.

Green P. Population genetic issues in DNA fingerprinting. Am JHum Genet 1992;50:440-441.

Holland HA, Jin L, Zhong Y, et al. Evaluation of 13 short tandem repeat loci for use in personal identification. Am J Hum Genet 1994;55:175-189.

Jeffreys AJ, Wilson V, Thein SL. Individual-specific "fingerprints" of human DNA. Nature 1985;316:76-79.

Lewontin RC, Hartl DL. Forensic DNA typing. Science 1992;255:1054-1055.

McCabe ERB. Applications of DNA fingerprinting in pediatric practice. J Pediatr 1992;120:499-509.

Moore KL. *The Developing Human. Clinically Oriented Embryology*, 3rd Edition. Philadelphia: Saunders, 1982.

Patten BM. *Human Embryology*. New York: McGraw-Hill, 1968.

Plachot M, DeGrouchy J, Cohen J, et al. Chromosome abnormalities of the fertilized human egg. Reproduction, Nutrition and Developpement. 1990;Supplement 1:83-88.

Risch NJ, Devlin B. The probability of matching DNA fingerprints. Science 1992;255:717-720.

Schwartz TR, Schwartz EA, Mieszerski L, et al. Characterization of deoxyribonucleic acid (DNA) obtained from teeth subjected to various environmental conditions. J Forensic Sci 1991;36:979-90.

Van Allen MI, Smith DW, Shepard TH. Twin reversed arterial perfusion (TRAP) sequence: A study of 14 twin pregnancies with acardius. Seminars in Perinatology 1983;7:285-93, 1983.

Weiss ML. DNA fingerprints in physical anthropology. Am J Hum Biol 1988;1:567-759.

Wills C. Forensic DNA typing. Science 1992;255:1050.

Wong Z, Wilson V, Patel I, et al Characterization of a panel of highly variable minisatellites cloned from human DNA. Ann Hum Genet 1987;51:269-288.

Yarbrough LR. Forensic DNA typing. Science 1992;255:1052.

PARENTAGE ("Paternity") TESTING
Examples based on blood types:
principles & calculations are the same for other markers.

Exclusion of Parentage

Type 1: Consultand lacks an antigen which is present in child.
Type 2: Child lacks an antigen that must be transmitted by consultand.

Racially limited antigens allowing exclusions

RACE	BLOOD GROUP	TYPES
Black	Rh	V (0.5% in whites)
		e variants
	Kell	J_s^a, J_s^b
	Duffy	Fy (rare in whites)
		Fy(a-b-)
	MNSs	H_u+, H_e+
		S-s-U (S^uS^u)
Orientals, Caribs, Chippewas	Diego	D_ia

Sexually limited antigens allowing exclusions

The Xg blood group gene is on the X chromosome. An Xg(a+) man cannot father an Xg(a-) daughter. If both mother and putative father are Xg(a-), this excludes paternity of an Xg(a+) girl.

Choice of systems for parentage exclusion

1. Antisera must be available in multiple laboratories.

2. The testing methodology must be reliable and reproducible.

3. The genetics of the system must be well defined, including population frequencies.

4. The probability of exclusion must be appreciable.

5. The validity of the system must be accepted by the scientific and legal communities.

<u>American Medical Association-American Bar Association</u>
<u>Recommended Systems for Parental Exclusion</u>

Note: Blood groups, enzymes, proteins and tissue types comprise 62 systems that can be used. If six blood group systems are used, the cumulative probability of exclusion is 68%. If HLA is added, it is 92%. The remaining 55 systems would have to be added to bring the probability up to 98%.

	System	Black Mean	White Cumulative	Japanese Mean	Cumulative	Mean	Cumulative
1	ABO	.1774	.1774	.1342	.1342	.1917	.1917
2	Rh	.1859	.3303	.2746	.3719	.2050	.3574
3	MNSs	.3206	.5450	.3095	.5663	.2531	.5200
4	Kell	.0049	.5472	.03554	.5817	.0000	.5200
5	Duffy	.0420	.5663	.1844	.6568	.1159	.5756
6	Kidd	.1545	.6337	.1869	.7226	.1573	.6424
7	HLA	.7900	.9121	.7900	.9334	.7900	.9142

<u>Special Cases that Interfere with Parental Exclusion</u>

ABO 1. h/h or Bombay phenotype. Usually occurs in offspring of consanguineous unions. Can be discerned by testing both erythrocytes and serum.

2. A_m types as "O" but has no anti A in serum. Secretor consultand will have A and H antigens in saliva. Elution tests will show that the cells absorb anti A but do not clump.

3. A_x has no anti A_1 in serum, otherwise like A_m and secretes only H in saliva (if secretor).

4. Acquired B type occurs rarely with cancer and chronic colon disorders.

MNSs 1. M_g does not react with anti M so allows incorrect exclusions:

Father		Mother	Child	
genotype	phenotype	genotype	genotype	phenotype
M_gM	M	MN	N	M_gN
M_gM	M	NN	N	M_gN
M_gN	N	MM	M	M_gM
M_gN	N	MN	M	M_gN

2. M^k behaves like h/h producing absence of MNSs.

Rh 1. Complex locus requiring best of personnel and materials.

2. Rare variant antibodies may be present in some antisera producing false exclusions. Avoid by testing parents and child with same antisera.

3. Suppressed antigens may test negative in parent, be transmitted to child and produce weak positive tests in child yielding false exclusions. Unexplained Rh+ children from Rh- parents. Usually found in children of consanguineous unions. Can be detected by testing with appropriate "incomplete" sera.

4. Rh_{null} is similar to M^k and h/h producing no Rh type at all. Can pass as Rh- if testing is not careful. Usually found in children of consanguineous unions.

5. Variant e in Blacks does not react with usual anti e so can yield false exclusions.

Proof of Parentage

1. Extremely rare phenotype combinations can indicate a very high likelihood of parentage if present only in consultand and child. Combination of B, NS, C^{w}D^{u}e/cde, Lu(a+), K+ yields only 1 chance in 10,000,000 that the consultand is not a parent of the child. HLA haplotypes have similar likelihoods.

2. Rare single types which, if present in consultand and child, leave less than 1 chance in 10,000 that consultand is not a parent of the child:

System	Type	System	Type	System	Type
ABO	AB	Rh	cDe	Rh	C^{w}DE
MNSs	Mg		C^{w}De		C^{w}dE
	M^k		cdE		C^{x}De
	M^u		Cde		cDE^w
Lutheran	Lu(a-b-)		CDE		CD^{w}e
Kell	K(a+)		C^{w}de		cD^{w}e
	K$_o$		CdE		

3. "Private" types which, if present only in consultand and child, leave less than 1 chance in 10,000 that consultand is not a parent of the child: Bishop, Evans, Good, Griffiths, Radin, Swann, Torkildsen, Traversu, Webb, Wright, Wolfsberg.

4. If consultand is male, his male relatives must be ruled out. Also, the denominator may be much less impressive *if the case is from an inbred population* in which rare phenotype frequency is higher.

Bayesian Calculations of Likelihood of Parentage

Types B, cde, N, Fy^b shared only by consultand and child and not by the other parent. Likelihood of non-parentage is equivalent to the population frequency of the phenotype (also see #4 above). Any part of the phenotype shared by consultand and other parent would halve the likelihood of that part, e.g. if both were A / B, the likelihood in that row would be 0.5 instead of 1.0.

State of Nature	Likelihoods	
	Non-Parentage	Parentage
Prior probability:		
1. Likelihood of parentage	0.5	0.5
Conditional probability		
2. A/B	0.03	1.0
3. cDE/cde	0.37	1.0
4. M/N	0.22	1.0
5. Fy^a/Fy^b	0.20	1.0
Joint probability (1x2x3x4x5 each column)	0.0002442	0.5
Marginal probability (sum of joint probabilities)	0.5002442	
Posterior probability (joint/marginal each column)	0.0004884	0.99951

Conclusion: chances are greater than 999 out of 1000 that the consultand has the same phenotype as the child because of parentage and less than 1 out of 1000 because of random occurrence.

1. Each immunoglobulin gene family is composed of
    *   over 100 Variable genes, as well as
    *   a small number of Joining genes,
    *   Diversity genes and
    *   Constant genes

*   Immunoglobulin genes are located as follows:
    *   kappa light chain on 2p,
    *   lambda light chain on 22q,
    *   heavy chain on 14q.

*   During differentiation from hematopoetic stem cells to B lymphocytes,
    *   one V gene in each cell is translocated to a position adjacent to a
    *   D gene and intervening introns are excised,
    *   followed by a similar process that translocates the
    *   VD complex to a position adjacent to a J gene.

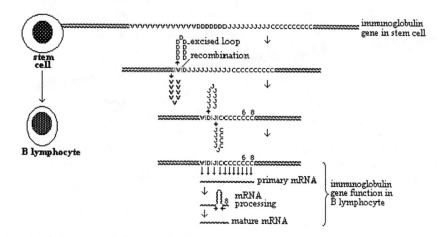

*   During mRNA processing in B lymphocytes,
    *   before the mRNA is translated into light or heavy chains,
    *   the nucleotides between the J gene and one of the C genes are
    *   transcribed but deleted and
    *   the cell produces immunoglobulin M (IgM).

*   Membrane-bound polysomes fabricate a complete immunoglobulin molecule by forming
    *   sulfide bridges between chains (HL), (L2), (H2), then forming
    *   sulfide bridges between these precursors to arrive at (H2L2).

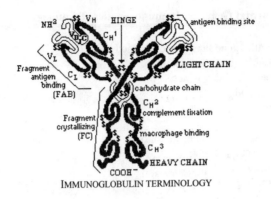

IMMUNOGLOBULIN TERMINOLOGY

- If an antigen attaches to the immunoglobulin receptor site, it stimulates cell division,
  - younger cells appearing larger and lighter staining (plasma cells), and differentiation
  - continues as the VDJ complex is translocated to a position adjacent to another C gene,
  - "class switch" (a genetic switch), and the cell begins producing immunoglobulin G (IgG).

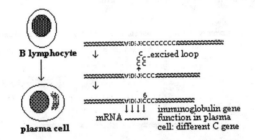

- Allelic exclusion occurs for immunoglobulin genes in that each cell has
  - 2 alleles each for heavy chain, kappa light chain and lambda light chain but,
  - during differentiation, commits to synthesis of only one heavy chain
  - and either one kappa or one lambda light chain (functional hemizygosity).

- Cells involved in immune function differentiate from bone marrow stem cells.
  - Macrophages wander in tissues, engulf antigens, and present them to T lymphocytes.
  - T lymphocytes, the majority of those in peripheral blood, mature in thymus and skin,
    - are activated by presented antigens into helper T cells (cellular immunity).
  - B lymphocytes mature in gut-associated lymphoid tissues. When stimulated by
    - helper T cells, they differentiate into plasma cells (humoral immunity).
  - Many immunodeficiencies arise from abnormalities of differentiation.

Disorder [McKusick number]	Differentiation Abnormality	Inheritance
Bruton agammaglobulinemia [300300]	Src tyrosine kinase deficiency causing differentiation failure of B cells	X-linked, Xq21
Common variable immunodeficiency	Differentiation failure of B cells into plasma cells.	Heterogeneous
Hyperimmunoglobulinemia M [308230]	CD40 ligand deficiency prevents the genetic switch to IgG	X-linked, Xq26
IgA deficiency	Differentiation failure of B cells into IgA secreting plasma cells.	Heterogeneous
Reticular dysgenesis [267500]	Failure of initiation of stem cell differentiation	Autosomal recessive
SCID (Severe combined immunodeficiency) [202500]	Abnormal recombination pattern of D-J heavy chain	Autosomal recessive, chromosome 8q11
SCID (Severe combined immunodeficiency) [300400]	Differentiation failure primarily of T cells and B cells to lesser degree	X-linked, Xq11
ZAP-70 protein kinase deficiency causing SCID [176947]	Differentiation failure of T cell receptor	Autosomal recessive, chromosome 2q12

- Other components of immune function include phagocytes and the complement system.
  - Macrophages and T cells produce cytokines which cause neutrophil proliferation.
    - Neutrophils opsonize (adhere to) bacteria, ingest and digest antigens.
  - Complement proteins in serum act sequentially when activated by
    - Antigen binding with antibody (classical pathway):
      - C1qrs → C4 → C2 → C3 → C3a
    - Foreign cell membrane (alternate pathway):
      - D → C3 → B + properdin + I + H → C3b
    - C3a + C3b → opsonization, mast cell degranulation, and
      - membrane attack complex (C5, C6, C7, C8, C9) → lysis of cell
  - Immunodeficiencies may arise from abnormalities of these components.

Disorder [McKusick number]	Phagocytosis Abnormality	Inheritance
Chronic granulomatous disease [306400]	Cytochrome b beta chain deficiency	X-linked, Xp21
Chronic granulomatous disease [233690]	Cytochrome b alpha chain deficiency	Autosomal recessive, chromosome 16q24
Infectious diseases proclivity [116920]	Leukocyte adhesion defect	Autosomal recessive, chromosome 21q22.3
Kostmann syndrome. Infantile agranulocytosis.[202700]	Deficiency of cytokine (granulocyte colony-stimulating factor receptor)	Autosomal dominant, chromosome 1p35

Disorder [McKusick number]	Complement Abnormality	Inheritance
Infectious diseases proclivity [134370], [134350], [120950], [120700]	Deficiencies of H, D, C8, or C3	Autosomal dominant
Infectious diseases proclivity [217070]	Deficiencies of I, or C7	Autosomal recessive
Systemic lupus erythematosis [216950], [120970]	Deficiencies of C1r, C1q, or C4	Autosomal recessive Autosomal dominant
Infectious diseases proclivity [312060]	Properdin P deficiency	X-linked, Xp 21.1

EXAMPLES OF INBORN ERRORS CAUSING IMMUNODEFICIENCY

Disorder [McKusick number]	Abnormality	Inheritance
Adenosine deaminase deficiency causing SCID [102700]	Toxic purine metabolites accumulate and destroy T cells	Autosomal recessive, chromosome 20q13
Purine nucleoside phosphorylase deficiency causing defective cellular immunity [164070]	Toxic purine metabolites accumulate and destroy T cells	Autosomal recessive, chromosome 14q13.1

EXAMPLES OF DYSMORPHIC SYNDROMES ASSOCIATED WITH IMMUNODEFICIENCY

Syndrome: abnormality	Findings	Etiology [McKusick number]
Ataxia telangiectasia: thymus hypoplasia.	Oculomotor apraxia, telangiectasia of conjunctiva appearing between 3 and 5 years, truncal ataxia preceding appendicular ataxia, choreoathetosis and/or dystonia, loss of deep tendon reflexes by age 8, lymphomas, lymphocytic leukemia.	Autosomal recessive, chromosome 11q22.23 [208900]
Chédiak-Higashi syndrome: natural killer lymphocyte membrane defect.	Decreased pigmentation of hair and eyes, photophobia, nystagmus, lymph adenopathy, hepatosplenomegaly, large eosinophilic peroxidase-positive inclusion bodies in myeloblasts and promyelocytes, neutropenia, large lysosomal granules in leukocytes, giant melanosomes in melanocytes, lymphoma.	Autosomal recessive, chromosome 1q [214500]
DiGeorge syndrome: thymus hypoplasia.	Hypertelorism, mongoloid eye slant, short philtrum, ear malformation, hypoplastic or absent parathyroid, aortic arch anomalies, tetralogy of Fallot, ventricular septal defect, hypocalcemia, seizures.	Autosomal dominant, chromosome 22q11.2 [188400]
Wiskott-Aldrich syndrome: cytoskeleton defect causes T cell degenerataion.	Onset by age 6 months of eczema, petechiae, bloody diarrhea, lymph adenopathy, hepatosplenomegaly, splenomegaly, malignant reticuloendotheliosis.	X-linked, chromosome Xp11.22 [301700]

- Atopic allergic asthma and rhinitis is associated with a mutation of the beta chain of IgE receptor gene on 11q13, causing high affinity,
  - when the allele is maternally-derived.

2. Components of development include:
   - proliferation,
   - differentiation and
   - morphogenesis

- Differentiation occurs mostly in fetal life when there is a
  committment of each cell to a specific type of morphology and function, with
  - suppresssion of genes for other functions.

- After differentiation, gene expression is often timed by
  - developmental switches which produce orderly changes in function, or
  - developmental curves such as the switch from fetal to adult hemoglobins.

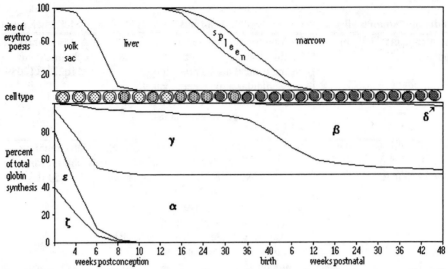

As the site of erythropoesis changes from yolk sac to liver and spleen then to marrow, the cells which synthesize globin differentiate from large primitive erythroblasts to cells of the normoblast series, and genes of globin chains are switched off and on in an orderly sequence.

- Agents that cause developmental switches, and the
  - timing mechanisms that control them, are usually
  - products of other genes.

- Mechanisms of unfortunate anatomic development include
  - malformation: intrinsically abnormal,
  - disruption: initially normal but altered during development, and
  - deformation: abnormality induced after completion of normal development.

- Categories of anatomic developmental disorders include:
  - syndrome: pattern of abnormalities in different systems due to a single cause,
  - sequence: cascade of abnormalities which may involve multiple related systems
    - but is initiated by a single cause in a single system
  - association: recurrent pattern of abnormalities of uncertain relationship

- Control of anatomic development is polygenic; hence,
  - most cases of unfortunate development represent the
  - lower end of the normal curve.

- Less frequent causes of unfortunate anatomic development are
  - chromosomal aberration and
  - teratogenic agents.

- In-vitro fertilization studies indicate that up to
  - 70% of embryos fail to implant and, when the cause can be established,
  - most of them have chromosomal aberrations.

- Studies of spontaneous abortuses indicate that
    - chromosome aberrations which frequently kill embryos early in gestation are:
        - Chromosome 16 trisomy,
        - Chromosome X monosomy and
        - Triploidy.

- Both maternal and paternal genomes are required for normal fetal differentiation.

- Duplication of the male pronucleus with
    - loss of the female pronucleus results in
    - all genes being homozygous paternal, producing a
        - hydatidiform mole instead of a fetus, with a
        - potential of development of choriocarcinoma.

- Duplication of male pronucleus without loss of female pronucleus is a form of
    - triploidy which results in a
        - partial hydatiform mole with some fetal differentiation.

3. Teratogens are agents which cause abnormal development of fetal form or function.
    - The derivation of the word implies that
        - fantasy is an intrinsic human reaction to teratogenic disorders.

τερασ (teras) = marvel, prodigy, monster
MONSTRUM = warning sign

- Factors in teratogenesis
    - Strength of agent: defects after exposure range from 3% (cytomegalovirus) to 65% (toxoplasmosis in 3rd trimester).
    - Developmental stage of exposed fetus:
        - refractory or not reachable at certain ages while very sensitive at other ages.
    - Dose of agent:
        - difficult to evaluate because significance is determined by
            - pharmacogenetic genotype of fetus
            - pharmacogenetic genotype of mother

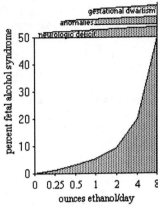

Factors to convert intake to ounces of ethanol. Liquor: 0.4. Beer: 0.04. Wine: 0.2. Wine coolers: 0.05.

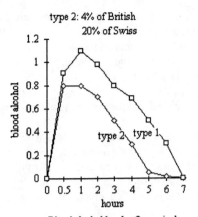

Blood alcohol levels after a single dose of 0.7 g/kg. Women with type 1 expose the fetus to higher levels.

- Recognition of teratogens involves
  - gestalt visualization of malformation patterns,
  - analysis of clustering of similar defects in fetuses exposed to the same agent,
  - animal studies (limited by species specificity).

- Teratogens can cause characteristic syndromes but most affected fetuses have only
  - poor growth and
  - poor neurological development, which continue after birth and lead to
    - short stature
    - mental subnormality and
    - abnormal neurological "soft" signs.

- Characteristic abnormalities associated with the more frequent teratogens:
  - Alcohol: blepharophimosis, faint philtrum, mental retardation
  - Cocaine: neural tube, heart and limb malformations occurring together
  - Cytomegalovirus: microcephaly, chorioretinitis, hearing defect
  - Retinoic acid: microtia, cleft palate, brain malformation.

CLUSTER ANALYSIS   A worked example that typifies some real times, places and situations from: Davis FN, Barton DE. Two space-time interaction tests for epidemicity. Brit J Prev Soc Med 1966;20:40-48.

The method:

Space Time ↓ →	Adjacent	Non-adjacent	Totals
Adjacent	X	Nt - X	Nt
Non-adjacent	Ns - X	N - Ns - Nt + X	N - Nt
Totals	Ns	N - Ns	N

Nt: adjacencies in time

Ns: adjacencies in space

N: all possible pairings

X: adjacencies in time and space, a Poisson distribution with first moment $= \mu = NsNt/N$

$$prob(X \leq \alpha) = p = \sum_{0}^{\alpha} \frac{e^{-\mu} \mu^{X}}{X!}$$

Example: Area 90 x 45 miles

Incidence of disease under study: **1:25,000**

Time interval of study 10 years

Time adjacency arbitrarily defined as 60 days

Space adjacency arbitrarily defined as 1/2 mile

96 cases were found. Some had multiple adjacencies, e.g., case 6 may have been adjacent to both case 7 and case 8. Total adjacencies were as follows:

Space Time ↓ →	Adjacent	Non-adjacent	Totals
Adjacent	5	147	152
Non-adjacent	20	4388	4408
Totals	25	4535	4560

μ = 152 x 25/4560 = 0.833

From a Poisson distribution with this μ , p = 0.0014 that chance alone would result in 5 of 96 cases being adjacent under the defined adjacency conditions, indicating clustering significant at that level of p. That means that subsequent research would be merited to identify agents to which clustered cases shared exposure during susceptible stages.

Observe the large part played in the calculations by the count of the non-adjacencies. That is the part omitted in many studies so no probability statement can be made from those studies.

The following table, which compares the probabilities for several possible values of X, may be used for "thumb-nail"evaluation of significance of clusters of cases of a disease when the disease is of similar incidence to the one in the example and the cases occur with similar adjacencies in a similar area (the size of a typical county in the USA). Many "outbreaks" fulfill those criteria.

X	1	2	3	4	5	6	7
prob	0.3622	0.1509	0.0419	0.0087	0.0014	0.0002	0.0000

CURRENTLY CHARACTERIZED HUMAN TERATOGENS
Medications

Direct effects (same as postnatal)	Teratogenic effects
Dependency-inducing drugs	(continued)
• withdrawal	**Cocaine**
Hormones & Antihormones	• limb, heart & neural tube defects
• endocrine effects: developmental in fetus.	**Fluconazole**
Streptomycin, daraprim, quinine	• craniofacial and skeletal anomalies
• deafness	**Hydantoins**
Tetracyclines	• wide face, nail & fingertip hypoplasia
• dental malformation	**Lithium**
Obstetric drugs	• Ebstein anomaly of heart
• fetus more sensitive	**Methyl mercury**
Delayed Effects	• deafness, blindness, paralysis
Diethylstilbesterol	**Penicillamine**
• genital metaplasia	• skin hyperelastosis
Teratogenic effects	**Smoking**
(poor fetal growth & development are common)	• low birth weight
Alcohol	**Trimethadione**
• blepharophimosis, faint philtrum	• V-shaped brows, dental & palatal anomaly
Aminopterin	**Thalidomide**
• dwarfism, hypoplastic cranium	• phocomelia, heart malformation, deafness
Anticoagulants	**Valproic acid**
• stippled epiphyses, hypoplastic nose	• brachycephaly, microstomia, spina bifida
Carbamepazine	**Vitamin A cogeners** (retinoic acid)
• upslanting eyes, short nose, nail hypoplasia	• microtia, clefts, brain anomalies

Infections

Maternal Infections (defects result from focal thrombotic vascular occlusions in fetus)	Fetal Infections (low birth weight, vision & hearing defect, mental retardation are common)
Purulent infections	**Cytomegalovirus**
Viral infections	**Rubella**
Amnionitis	**Syphilis**
	Toxoplasmosis
	Varicella

Maternal Disorders

Diabetes mellitus	**Myasthenia gravis**
• conotruncal defects, caudal regression	• newborn myasthenia
Hypertension	**Myotonic dystrophy**
• low birth weight, microcephaly, PDA	• arthrogryposis, mental retardation
Hyperthermia	**Phenylketonuria**
• arthrogryposis, low birth weight, neural tube defect	• microcephaly, dwarfism, prominent mid-face
Malnutrition	**Twinning**
• low birth weight	• disruption, sirenomelia, exstrophy of cloaca

CURRENTLY CHARACTERIZED HUMAN TERATOGENS (continued)
Hazardous Procedures & Trauma

Maternal Trauma, Surgical Complications	Direct Fetal Trauma
(defects result from cessation of cerebral blood flow in fetus)	**Hypertonic intravenous contrast material** • focal thrombotic vascular occlusions
Maternal hypotension **Maternal hypoxia**	**X-ray** (high dose - therapeutic or catastrophic) • microcephaly, eye & genital malformation

Radiation Hazards

All types have similar effects but the potential for mutagenesis or teratogenesis depends on the amount of energy transferred to the dividing cell or to the embryonic tissues respectively. X-ray is the form of radiation which has been studied most extensively.

Average yearly population X-ray exposure (1974)

Sources	Millirads to total body
Cosmic & terrestrial	110
Diagnostic	50
Atomic tests	8
Research & Therapy	2
Occupational	1
Nuclear power plants	1
Radiologists	0.6
Nuclear therapists	0.6

Exposure from maternal diagnostic X-rays (millirads)

Study (1972)	Average dose to early fetus
Skull series	4
Cervical spine	2
Arm	1
Leg	1
Shoulder	1
Chest	
X-ray	8
photofluorography	8
fluoroscopy	70
Thoracic spine	9
Upper GI without fluoroscopy	360
with fluoroscopy	560
Barium enema without fluoroscopy	440
with fluoroscopy	800
Cholecystogram	200
IVP or retrograde pyelogram	400
Abdomen	290
Lumbar spine	275
Pelvis	40
Hips	300

Exposure from maternal diagnostic radio-isotope studies (millirads)

Study (1972)	Total fetal	Fetal thyroid
Iodine thyroid scan	15	5000
Rose bengal	19	5000
Renal hippuran	6	100
Technetium brain scan	100	0
Technetium liver scan	30	0
Chromium placentography	4	4

Radiation Facts

X-ray as a mutagen: 50,000 millirads acute exposure is the amount estimated (from animal studies) to double the human mutation rate. To date, no single case of human disease has been proven to be due to mutation caused by X-ray, nor has there been any increase in diseases proven to be due to mutation caused by X-ray in any group of people exposed to X-ray.

X-ray as a teratogen: acute exposure of the fetus between the 3rd and 16th week of gestation in amounts above 200,000 millirads causes a syndrome characterized by cataract, pigmentary retinopathy, microphthalmos, microcephaly, mental retardation, genital hypoplasia, and short stature.

X-ray as a carcinogen: an unclear subject. Amounts over 1,000,000 millirads acute prenatal or postnatal exposure can clearly cause thyroid or bone cancer. Exceedingly poorly done studies are said by their authors to show some tendency toward leukemia with exposures as low as 1,000 millirads in utero. These studies totally lack appropriate controls and fail to consider known confounding factors. In one famous study, the data were re-examined and it was found that unexposed sibs had an even higher leukemia rate than the study subjects. It appears that these studies represent modern witch-hunts in the truest sense.

X-ray as a legal hazard: based on a combination of animal data and "logic," the National Council on Radiation Protection and Measurements (NCRPM) in 1977 issued the confusing statement that a fetal dose of less than 10,000 millirads probably did not cause congenital malformation but might have a significant teratogenic effect. These are essentially identical effects. The poor comprehension occurred because no medical geneticist was then, or is now, on the NCRPM.

- The American Colleges of OB-GYN and Radiology and the American Academy of Pediatrics noted that the NCRPM's hypothetical rate of anomalies due to low-level X-ray (.005) was less than their natural rate (.03) and issued the following statements
  - Interruption of pregnancy is never justified because of the radiation risk to the fetus from diagnostic X-ray.
  - Diagnostic X-ray during pregnancy should not be postponed except when it is not related to the patient's present illness.
  - All diagnostic X-rays should utilize the lowest possible dose which will produce the required diagnostic information whether the patient is pregnant or not.
  - The pregnant patient should be informed of the actual risks of the X-ray procedure and this should be recorded in her chart.

Additional references:

Aleck KA, Bartley DL. Fluconazole teratogenesis: A multiple malformation embryopathy resembling Antley-Bixler syndrome. Am J Hum Genet 1196;59 (Supplement):A37.

Brent RL, Gorson RO: Radiation exposure in pregnancy. Current Problems in Radiology 1972.

Cattanach BM, Kirk M. Differential activity of maternally and paternally derived chromosome regions in mice. Nature 1985;315:496-8.

Dekaban AS. Abnormalities in children exposed to X-radiation during various stages of gestation: Tentative timetable of radiation injury to the human fetus, part 1. J of Nucl Med 1968;9:471-477.

Jacobson JL, Jacobson SW, Sokol RJ, et al. Teratogenic effects of alcohol on infant development. Alcoholism:Clinical and Experimental Research 1993;177:174-183.

Jones KL. The fetal alcohol syndrome. Growth:Genetics & Hormones 1988;4:1-3.

Korthauer U, Graf D, Mages HW, et al. Defective expression of T-cell CD40 ligand causes X-linked immunodeficiency with hyper-IgM. Nature 1993;361:539-541.

Nebert DW, Bigelow SW. Genetic control of drug metabolism: Relationship to birth defects. Seminars in Perinatology 1982;6:105-115.

Larsen RJ. A statistical test for measuring unimodal clustering. Biometrics 1973;29:301-309.

Patten BM. *Human Embryology*. New York: McGraw-Hill, 1968.

Plachot M, DeGrouchy J, Cohen J, et al. Chromosome abnormalities of the fertilized human egg. Reproduction, Nutrition and Developpement. 1990;Supplement 1:83-88.

Sandford AJ, Shirakawa T, Moffatt MF, et al. Localisation of atopy and beta subunit of high-affinity IgE receptor (Fc epsilon RI) on chromosome 11q. Lancet 1993;341:332-334.

Spranger J, Benirschke K, Hall JG, et al. Errors of morphogenesis: Concepts and terms. Recommendations of an international working group. J Pediatr 1992;100:160-165.

Smith DW. Alcohol effects on the fetus. In: Schwarz RH, Yaffe SJ (editors). *Drug and Chemical Risks to the Fetus and Newborn*. New York: Liss, 1980.

Shyur S-D, Hill HR. Recent advances in the genetics of the primary immunodeficiency syndromes. J Pediatr 1996;129:8-24.

Van Allen MI, Smith DW, Shepard TH. Twin reversed arterial perfusion (TRAP) sequence: A study of 14 twin pregnancies with acardius. Seminars in Perinatology 1983;7:285-93, 1983.

Vetrie D, Vorechovsky I, Sideras P, et al The gene involved in X-linked agammaglobulinemia is a member of the src family of protein-tyrosine kinases. Nature 1993;361:226-233.

Von Wartburg JP, Schurch PM. Atypical human liver alcohol dehydrogenase. Ann NY Acad Sci 1968;151:936-946, 1968.

Weatherall DJ, Clegg JB. *The Thalassemia Syndromes*, 3rd Edition. Oxford: Blackwell, 1981.

Wilson JG. *Environment and Birth Defects*. New York: Academic Press, 1973.

ωνωμαλοσ: irregular, uneven. Sanford, 1569: *Whiche thinges because they haue neither measure, nor rule, are called anomals.* Browne, 1646: Deviation from the natural order.

Definitions

1. An anomaly is a feature that may be either unexpected, or
    *   patently abnormal.

*   Objective anomalies are defined by absence, excess or abnormal size, while
    *   subjective anomalies are defined by gestalt and are subject to question.

Normal Variation

2. Expected ("normal") variation in other mammals stems primarily from
    *   maternal effects, the contribution the mother makes to the phenotype over and above that which results from genes that she contributes to the zygote:
        *   Transcription of maternally-derived active mRNA's.
        *   Nutrition via the egg or post-natal supplies of food.
        *   Placental or breast-milk transmitted pathogens and antibodies.
        *   Imitative behavior, interaction with sibs.
    *   Cytoplasmic inheritance - see *Tenets of Genetics.*
    *   Imprinting also favors maternal resemblance.
    *   Humans are presumed to be similar.
    *   Metric traits are acquired through polygenic inheritance -
        *   see the chapter, *Segregation and Polygenic Inheritance* for human data.

*   Maternal effects account for about 1/3 of an individual's normal characteristics;
    *   resemblance to father, only about 2%:
        *   Striking examples probably represent rare Mendelian normal genes.
    *   Rare maternal Mendelian normal genes would be difficult to distinguish from maternal effects unless they hold up over several generations.

*   Most known human nuclear genes are those of abnormal Mendelian traits,
    *   normal Mendelian traits having received so little study that they may not be recognized
        *   and are liable to be thought instead to represent genetic diseases
        *   or parts of syndromes. See Appendix 1 for a list.

Abnormal Variation

3. Except when patently abnormal, a finding cannot be said to be an anomaly until
    *   proven not to exist in the normal parents of the proband,
        *   an obvious conundrum being a mild parental case of a disorder.

*   So-called "minor anomalies" such as low-set ears or high-arched palate are often
    *   not anomalies in the strict sense because they are, in most cases,
        *   not associated with any disease and are
        *   found in normal parents; however, they are also frequent
    *   concomitants of major anomalies in syndromes so are valuable bellwethers
        *   when not found in normal parents.

Major Congential Anomalies

4. Cleft lip results from
    - failure of union of lateral nasal, medial nasal and maxillary mesodermal processes which
        - should be completed by the 45th day of gestation;
        - extension into the palate occurs in 75% of cases.

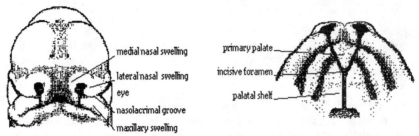

Formation of the Lip   **Formation of the Palate**

- Cleft palate results from
    - failure of union of the palatal shelves of the maxillary mesodermal processes which
        - should be completed by the 36th day of gestation;
        - partial union results in submucous cleft palate or high-arched palate.

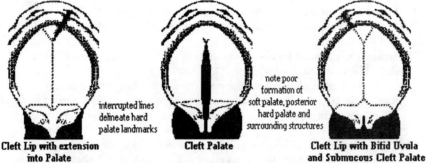

Cleft Lip with extension   **Cleft Palate**   **Cleft Lip with Bifid Uvula**
into Palate   **and Submucous Cleft Palate**

Cleft lip and cleft palate are different traits but cleft lip often extends into the primary palate and, when very severe, can disorder hard palate formation. True combinations as illustrated on the right are more typical of syndromes which entail generalized disturbance of development.

- Isolated clefts are inherited as threshhold polygenic traits (risk to 1st degree relatives: 2%).

- Bilateral clefts result from more severe developmental failure and have a
    - greater genetic risk (risk to 1st degree relatives: 6%).

- Associated defects are found in syndromal association in
  - 12% of patients with cleft lip and in
  - 40% of patients with cleft palate;
  - about 200 syndromes are associated with clefts, the
  - genetic risk depending on the mechanism of inheritance of the syndrome.

- Causes of cleft-associated syndromes, in order of occurrence, are
  - other multifactorial traits,
  - chromosome disorders,
  - single gene disorders, and
  - teratogens (very rare).

EXAMPLES OF SYNDROMES ASSOCIATED WITH CLEFT LIP

Syndrome	Findings	Etiology
Holoprosencephaly	Microcephaly, hypertelorism, scoliosis	Polygenic
Chromosome 13 trisomy	Microphthalmos, polydactyly, scalp defect	Chromosomal
Chromosome 4p-	Microcephaly, prominent glabella, dwarfsim	Chromosomal
Lip pit syndrome	Dimples, cysts or sinuses of lower lip	Autosomal dominant
Orofaciodigital syndrome I	Hyperplastic frenulae, sparse hair, cleft tongue, synbrachydactyly	Autosomal dominant, male lethal
Popliteal pterygium syndrome	Popliteal pterygium, lip pits, genital malformation, syndactyly	Autosomal dominant
Hydantoin syndrome	Gestational dwarfism, short nose, small nails, hip dislocation	Teratogenic

EXAMPLES OF SYNDROMES ASSOCIATED WITH CLEFT PALATE

Syndrome	Findings	Etiology
Pierre Robin syndrome	Micrognathia, glossoptosis, swallowing dysfunction	Polygenic
Chromosome 5p-	Gestational dwarfism, microcephaly, cat-like cry, hypertelorism	Chromosomal
Otopalatodigital syndrome I	Pugilistic face, thick skull with absent sinuses, deafness, multiple small angular bone malformations	X-linked dominant
Stickler syndrome	Severe myopia, deafness, micrognathia, joint laxity, spondyloepiphyseal dysplasia	Autosomal dominant
Treacher Collins syndrome	Downward-slanting palpebral fissures, lower lid coloboma, micrognathia, deafness, small dysplastic ears	Autosomal dominant
Retinoic acid syndrome	Microtia, hypertelorism, heart and brain malformations	Teratogenic

5.   Isolated heart malformations are inherited as threshhold polygenic traits.

- Genetic risks of isolated heart malformations are determined by
    - developmental mechanism of malformation and by
    - maternal inheritance (risk to 1st degree relatives: 14%).

- More severe developmental abnormalities result in
    - greater numbers of lesions of developmentally related heart structures and
    - greater genetic risks.

- Heart malformation results from abnormalities of about 6 developmental mechanisms.

    Lateralization defects: Risk to 1st degree relatives = 4%.
    - right atrial isomerism (includes endocardial cushion defect, transposition and
        aberrant pulmonary venous return, all of variable severity)
    - left atrial isomerism (Includes endocardial cushion defect, double-outlet right venticle and
        aberrant pulmonary venous return, all of variable severity)

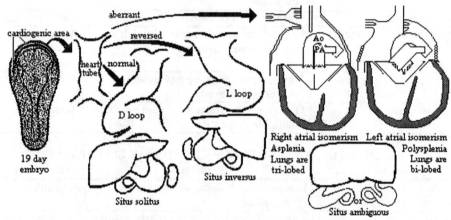

CARDIAC LATERALIZATION DEFECTS ALSO INVOLVE LUNGS AND ABDOMINAL VISCERA.

    Abnormal migration of cells of ectomesenchymal tissue: Risk to 1st degree relatives = 2%.
    - truncus arteriosus
    - transposition of great vessels
    - tetralogy of Fallot
    - ventricular septal defect type I

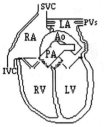 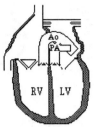 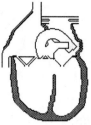 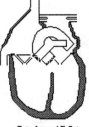 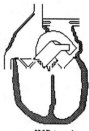

| Diagram of normal heart | Transposition | Truncus arteriosus | Tetralogy of Fallot | VSD type 1 |

CONOTRUNCAL DEFECTS RESULT FROM MIGRATION OF INSUFFICIENT NUMBERS OF MESENCHYMAL CELLS FROM BRANCHIAL ARCHES AND OCCIPITAL NEURAL CREST TO ALLOW COMPLETION OF MORPHOGENESIS. In transposition, the pulmonary artery supports peripheral circulation through a patent ductus arteriosus. In truncus arteriosus, the heart functions as 3 chambers. In tetralogy, the pulmonic valve and PA are poorly formed, causing relative pulmonic stenosis and elevating RV pressure, and displacing the ventricular septum so that is is below the aortic valve ("overriding aorta"). Type 1 VSD is also called supracristal or subarterial. It may destabilize the aortic valve ring allowing aortic insufficiency due to valve leaflet prolapse.

Abnormal embryonic hemodynamics (fetal flow): Risk to 1st degree relatives = 10%.
- aorta coarctation
- bicuspid aortic valve
- hypoplastic left heart
- pulmonic stenosis
- ventricular septal defect type II

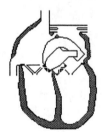 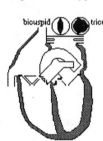 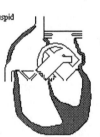 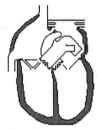 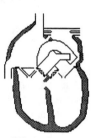

| Pulmonic stenosis | Bicuspid aortic valve | Hypoplastic left heart | Coarctation of aorta | VSD type 2 |

FETAL FLOW LESIONS RESULT FROM FAILURE OF HEMODYNAMIC STRESS TO SHAPE DEVELOPING STRUCTURES. In pulmonic stenosis, the involvement is mainly of the valve itself and there is post-stenotic dilitation of the pulmonic artery. Elevated RA pressure forces open the foramen ovale. A bicuspid aortic valve opens less wide than a normal tricuspid aortic valve, producing relative aortic stenosis, elevating LV and LA pressures. With a hypoplastic left heart, the pulmonic artery supports peripheral circulation through a patent ductus arteriosus. A preductal coartcation is illustrated, circulation to the upper body from the aorta while the pulmonary artery supports the lower body through a patent ductus arteriosus. Type 2 VSD is also called membranous VSD because that area of the septum forms from fibrous outgrowth of surrounding structures, eventually smoothed and flattened into a membrane.

Abnormal extracellular matrix determination. Risk to 1st degree relatives = 2%.
- atrioventricular canal
- ventricular septal defect type III

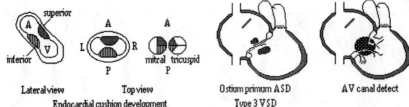

Lateral view   Top view   Ostium primum ASD   AV canal defect
Endocardial cushion development   Type 3 VSD

ATRIOVENTRICULAR CANAL DEFECTS RESULT FROM FAILURE OF ELABORATION IN THE
ENDOCARDIAL CUSHIONS OF GLYCOSAMINOGLYCANS IN AMOUNTS SUFFICIENT TO ALLOW BRIDGING
OF THE ATRIOVENTRICULAR ORIFICE. The endocardial cushion contributes to formation of the septal
leaflets of the mitral and tricuspid valves and both insufficiency and stenosis of those valves may
accompany endocardial cushion defects. Incomplete formation of the atrial septum in the area of the
foramen primum, Type 3 VSD, or a combination of both may result from defective endocardial
cushion development. Worse development leads to AV canal defect.

Abnormality of programmed cellular death (apoptosis): Risk to 1st degree relatives = 2%.
- Ebstein anomaly
- ventricular septal defect type IV

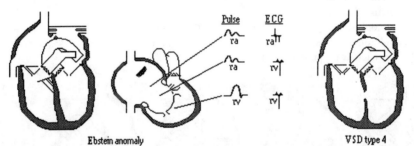

Ebstein anomaly   VSD type 4

ABERRATION OF PROGRAMMED CELL DEATH (APOPTOSIS) RESULTS IN TRABECULAR SEPTUM
ANOMALIES. In Ebstein anomaly, the basal insertion of the tricuspid septal leaflet is displaced
downward into the sinus portion of the RV, extending the RA domain into it and "atrializing" that
part of the chamber. Tricuspid insufficiency dilates the RA and forces open the foramen ovale.
Excessive apoptosis leads to type 4 VSD, also called "muscular" VSD.

Disordered targeted growth: Risk to 1st degree relatives = 2%.
- atrial septal defects
- single atrium
- anomalous pulmonary venous return

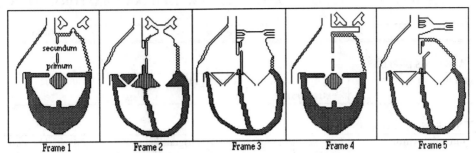

| Frame 1 | Frame 2 | Frame 3 | Frame 4 | Frame 5 |

TARGETED GROWTH IN AND AROUND THE ATRIA.

- In frame 1, the septum primum grows in from the wall of the common atrium but begins to fenestrate before it reaches the endocardial cushion, forming the foramen secundum. If it does not reach the endocardial cushion, it leaves a primum ASD. Failure of ingrowth forms a single atrium.
- In frame 2, the septum secundum grows inward beside the septum primum. Inadequate growth of its upper limb, or inadequate growth of the septum primum can form a secundum ASD.
- Frame 3 shows completed growth of both, with the septum primum forming the valve of the foramen ovale, usually kept closed by equal atrial pressures.
- In frame 1, a common pulmonary vein grows outward from the LA to meet the coalescing pulmonary venous capillaries.
- In frame 2, smooth venous wall tissue extends downward into the atrium, replacing the primitive rough atrial wall.
- In frame 3, the common pulmonary vein and branches have been absorbed into the LA, smoothing all of its lining except for the auricle.
- In frame 4, aberrant growth places the left brachiocephalic vein in the path of the pulmonary venous capillaries resulting in total anomalous pulmonary venous return into the RA as diagrammed in frame 5. The LA remains small and rough. Elevated RA pressure forces open the foramen ovale providing support to the peripheral circulation.

- In approximately 25% of patients the heart malformations is part of a syndrome as indicated by associated extracardiac malformations,
  - the genetic risk depending on the mechanism of inheritance of the syndrome.

- Approximately 12% of patients with heart malformations have chromosome aberrations.

EXAMPLES OF SYNDROMES ASSOCIATED WITH HEART MALFORMATION

	Associated findings	Etiology
APOTOSIS DEFECTS		
Fetal lithium syndrome	Polyhydramnios, non-toxic goiter, extrapyramidal disorder	Teratogenic
CONOTRUNCAL DEFECTS		
Genitopalatocardiac syndrome	Low set ears, cleft palate, micrognathia, cystic kidneys, hypospadias, XY gonadal dysgenesis	Autosomal recessive
Koussef syndrome	Low set ears, short neck, unilateral renal agenesis, sacral meningomyelocoele	Autosomal recessive
CATCH-22	Telecanthus, blepharophimosis, cleft palate, T cell deficit	Chromosome 22q11.2 microdeletion
Goldenhar syndrome	Preauricular tags, conjunctival dermoid, vertebral malformation	Polygenic
Fetal diabetes syndrome	Neural tube defect, caudal regression	Teratogenic
EXTRACELLULAR MATRIX DEFECTS		
Down syndrome	Hypotonia, brachycephaly, low nasal bridge	Chromosome 21 trisomy
FETAL FLOW DEFECTS		
Noonan syndrome	Webbed neck, sternum deformities, cryptorchidism	Autosomal dominant
Ellis-Van Creveld syndrome	Dwarfism, polydactyly, hyperplastic frenulae	Autosomal recessive
Williams syndrome	Stellate iris, patulous lips, malar hypoplasia, poor growth and development	Chromosome 7q11.23 microdeletion
Fetal rubella syndrome	Gestational dwarfism, deafness, cataracts	Teratogenic
LATERALIZATION DEFECTS		
Ivemark syndrome	Asplenia, polysplenia, situs inversus, abnormal lung lobulation	Polygenic
TARGETED GROWTH DEFECTS		
Cat eye syndrome	Preauricular tags, iris coloboma, anal atresia	Chromosome 22q duplication

6.   Non-symptomatic or sporadic hydrocephalus may be
- isolated or
- syndrome-associated

- Excessive head circumference is the most accurate indicator of hydrocephalus.
  - See Appendix 1 for norms.

- Isolated hydrocephalus may be caused by one or more of:
  - obstruction to circulation of CSF (most common)
  - interference with CSF absorption
  - excessive secretion of CSF

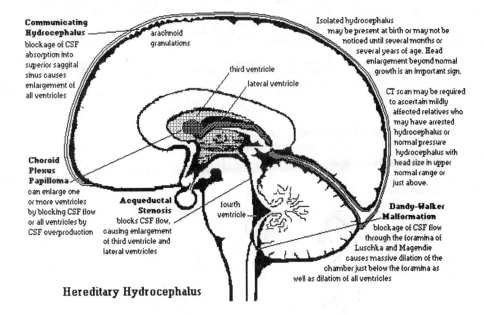

Communicating Hydrocephalus blockage of CSF absorption into superior saggital sinus causes enlargement of all ventricles

arachnoid granulations

third ventricle

lateral ventricle

Isolated hydrocephalus may be present at birth or may not be noticed until several months or several years of age. Head enlargement beyond normal growth is an important sign.

CT scan may be required to ascertain mildly affected relatives who may have arrested hydrocephalus or normal pressure hydrocephalus with head size in upper normal range or just above.

Choroid Plexus Papilloma can enlarge one or more ventricles by blocking CSF flow or all ventricles by CSF overproduction

Acqueductal Stenosis blocks CSF flow, causing enlargement of third ventricle and lateral ventricles

fourth ventricle

Dandy-Walker Malformation blockage of CSF flow through the foramina of Luschka and Magendie causes massive dilation of the chamber just below the foramina as well as dilation of all ventricles

Hereditary Hydrocephalus

- Isolated hydrocephalus is usually inherited as a threshhold polygenic trait
  - with approximately 2% risk of occurrence in subsequent sibs.

- Isolated hydrocephalus due to stenosis of the acqueduct of Sylvius
  - is also usually polygenic
    - but the risk of occurrence in subsequent sibs is 4.5%.

- Rare cases of hydrocephalus due to stenosis of the acqueduct of Sylvius are
  - X-linked and they can be differentiated from other types only if
    - genealogy shows X-linked pattern of cases.

- The most common syndrome associated with hydrocephalus is
  - neural tube defect but many cases are associated with other syndromes, the
    - genetic risk depending on the mechanism of inheritance of the syndrome.

EXAMPLES OF SYNDROMES ASSOCIATED WITH HYDROCEPHALUS

Syndrome	Findings	Etiology
Acrodysostosis	Brachycephaly, small nose, multiple small angular bone malformations	Polygenic
Triploidy	Gestational dwarfism, microphthalmia, septal heart malformations, syndactyly, micropenis	Chromosomal
Albers-Schonberg syndrome	Thick brittle bones, progressive deafness and blindness, marrow compression	Autosomal recessive
Warburg syndrome	Agyria, microphthalmia	Autosomal recessive
Fetal warfarin syndrome	Gestational dwarfism, short nose, stippled epiphyses	Teratogenic

7. Neural tube defects result from
    - failure of closure of the neural tube which
      - should be completed by the 28th day of gestation.

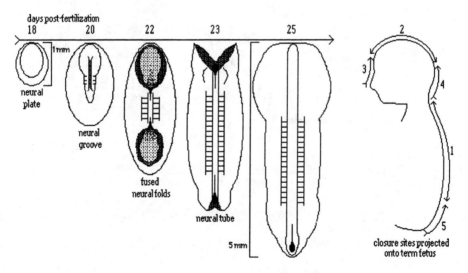

Early Development of the Nervous System

Neurulation becomes evident in the third week of gestation. The neural plate has differentiated from ectoderm of the embryonic disk. Its lateral edges then elevate to form the neural folds which approximate and form the neural tube. Fusion of closure site 1 continues cephalad toward the cranial neuropore and caudad toward the caudal neuropore. Closure at site 2 is also bidirectional, while at sites 3, 4 and 5, it is unidirectional. Cephalad closure is complete in the 25th day and caudad closure in the 27th day.

- Failure of cephalad closure results in
    - anencephaly,
    - encephalocoele and
    - Arnold-Chiari malformation

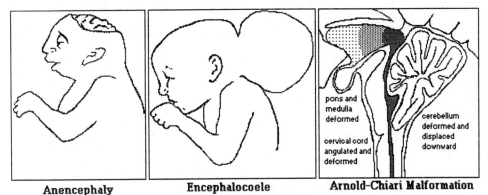

| **Anencephaly** | **Encephalocoele** | **Arnold-Chiari Malformation** |

Anencephaly is usually fatal to the newborn. Encephalocoele and Arnold-Chiari malformation vary in severity but most patients have severe global neurological impairment

- Failure of caudal closure results in
    - spina bifida and
    - meningomyelocoele

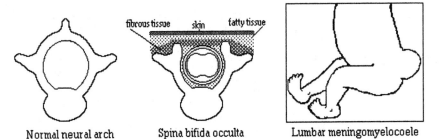

Normal neural arch   Spina bifida occulta   Lumbar meningomyelocoele

Patients with spina bifida occulta are usually asymptomatic but have the same genetic risks as patients with other neural tube defects. Patients with meningomyelocoele are usually neurologically impaired below the level of the defect (notice the neurogenic club feet in the illustration), and may also have dysplasia in other parts of the neural tube; most develop hydrocephalus.

More complicated neural tube defects involve multiple closure sites. For instance, **faciocraniorachischisis** stems from failure in sites 1, 2, 3 and 4. **Iniencephaly** entails craniorachischisis due to failure in sites 1,2, and 4, with added failure of development of mesenchymal tissues; rudimentary cervical vertebrae cause absent neck and severe retroflexion of the head, with both anterior and posterior protrusion of neural tissue. The defects may be skin-covered or visible as iniencephaly apertus. Some complicated neural tube defects breed true.

- Isolated neural tube defects comprise a
  - threshhold polygenic trait (risk to first degree relatives: 4%).

- Some cases of neural tube defects occur as part of syndromes,
  - the genetic risk depending on the mechanism of inheritance of the syndrome.
  - Occult folate dependency of various types is sufficiently common as a factor in syndromic neural tube defects to warrant supplementation during pregnancy.

EXAMPLES OF SYNDROMES ASSOCIATED WITH NEURAL TUBE DEFECTS

Syndrome	Findings	Etiology
Goldenhar syndrome	Hemifacial microsomia, preauricular tags, epibulbar dermoid, microtia, hemivertebrae	Polygenic
Chromosome 18 trisomy	Gestational dwarfism, prominent occiput, small ears, small face, short sternum, overlap of index finger onto middle finger and little finger onto ring finger, contractures of hips and fingers, septal heart malformations	Chromosomal
Meckel syndrome	Microcephaly, microphthalmia, cleft palate, polycystic kidneys, hepatic cysts, genital hypoplasia	Autosomal recessive
Fetal valproate syndrome	Fetal flow heart malformations, telecanthus, short nose, small mouth, long fingers	Teratogenic

Multiple Congential Anomalies

8. The term, multiple congenital anomalies, refers to syndromes that are
    *   evident at birth, and are characterized by
    *   primary involvement of more than one body system.

*   Syndromes of multiple congenital anomalies
    *   are much more likely to have simple etiology than are
        *   single major malformations.

Etiologies	Estimated percentages	
Polygenic	50	Mostly unfortunate family resemblance
Monogenic	19	True syndromes
Chromosomal	15	
Teratogenic	16	

*   Features of true syndromes have a common physiological basis
    *   though it is known for only a few syndromes.

9. Multiple congenital anomalies are most often due to polygenic inheritance of
    *   unfortunate family resemblance but positive evidence of this
        can usually be accumulated only through extensive evaluation and
    *   critical data may be unavailable in instances of small sibships, adoption and
        non-paternity (latter usually estimated as at least 15%).

*   The initial step in evaluation is to catalogue all of the patient's anomalies.
    *   This must be followed by evaluation of parents and normal sibs,
        the object being to identify features not associated with any malfunction.
    *   Routinely, this discloses that all of the anomalies exist in relatives,
        the patient being different in only number and severity.

*   Mathematical aspects of polygenic inheritance imply the mid-parent mean as
    *   the expectation in progeny for metric traits.
    *   Careful evaluation may disclose this,
        abnormalities of the parents having been previously ignored or overlooked.

*   Progeny worse than parents may be due to
    *   the expected spread of observations about the midparent mean but
    *   more specific etiologies must be excluded:
        *   Mitochondrial genes,
        *   Nuclear genes,
        *   Chromosome aberrations,
        *   Teratogens.
    *   Critical data required for exclusion are often unavailable: The rate of
        non-paternity favors exclusion because it is much more frequent than any other
        etiology, the unacknowledged father accounting for the actual mid-parent mean.

10. Mendelian inheritance of a syndrome is a time-honored indication
    - of monogenic etiology due to nuclear genes but is a
        - relatively infrequent observation.

- Our ability to exclude mitochondrial genes and nuclear genes at present is
    - limited to specific examples of syndromes that are recognizable *a priori*, and to
    - cases with definite Mendelian inheritance,
        - but some multiple anomaly cases with elusive diagnoses are no doubt due to those mechanisms and relatives should be counseled about that possibility,
        - especially when partial manifestation is found in relatives.

11. Some chromosome aberrations cause characteristic syndromes but there are a large number of random chromosome mutations that occur at basal frequencies
    - and cause multiple congenital anomalies; at least half of such cases stem
    - from a balanced rearrangement in a parent which may also exist
    - in other relatives.

- Chromosome analysis by high resolution technnique is required for all cases of multiple congenital anomalies that are not ascribable to a syndrome, and,
    - in familial cases with ostensibly normal chromosomes, should also be done on the parents of the patient.

12. Teratogens actually enter the body of the pregnant woman and act directly on the fetus or its support mechanisms to prevent normal development, often
    - causing syndromes that are specific to the agent and its time of entry, i.e., the gestational history and the patient's features are usually typical.

- Gestation history may suggest teratogen etiology of some syndromes; however,
    - false positive information is obtained with great frequency due to
        - societal paranoia about teratogens;
    - false negative information is also frequent and is usually due to either
        - ignorance or
        - denial.

    Hence, teratogen exposure data are acceptable only when verified and quantitated.

- Rare cases of anomalies could be caused by maternal intoxication by new agents in spite of the current rigorous pre-market testing programs but
    - worldwide surveillance over the past 40 years makes it unlikely that existing drugs and chemicals might have an undiscovered teratogenic effect.

- Cases thought to be due to mysterious teratogens have instead been either
    - known syndromes of other etiologies or
    - found *a priori* to lack the criteria for teratogenic etiology.

- Popular misconceptions causing inappropriate suspicion of teratogenic etiology:
  - Misdeeds of the father.
  - Exposure of the father to teratogens.
  - Proximity of mother to teratogens with minimal or no contact.
  - Exposure to noxious agents that are not teratogens.

- Stories of geographic distributions of cases of anomalies
  - related to proximity to mysterious environmental agents
  - have uniformly been proven to be hoaxes.

Diagnosis of Multiple Congenital Anomalies

13. Physical diagnosis and laboratory diagnosis allow recognition of
    - a few syndromes based on pathognomic findings; however,
    - genealogical study is usually also required because:
      - Many known syndromes are genetically heterogenous.
      - Many patients have syndromes not previously reported.

- Syndromes for which genealogical evaluation discloses negative results
  - may be due to mutation; however,
    - mutagens are not known to cause human sydromes;
  - rather, all cases are thought to stem from spontaneous mutation,
    - chromosome mutation being related to maternal age and
    - single gene mutation related to paternal age.

14. To be useful in recognition of syndromes, objective physical data must be collected
    - in quantity and quality to which most physicians are not accustomed,
      - and compared to extensive sets of norms.

- Gestalt evaluation of physical abnormalities requires
  - extensive experience from observation of known cases or
  - extensive photographic or descriptive literature (Appendix 3),
  - and may require photographic technique for recording findings.

15. Many syndromes require laboratory evaluation for
    - diagnosis or confirmation of diagnosis.
    - Intercurrent conditions are also not uncommon because of
      - shared genetic etiologic factors such as consanguinity.

- Chromosome analysis should be done if
  - findings are consistent with a known chromosomal syndrome or
  - findings are not consistent with a syndrome due to some other cause.

- Some syndromes have specific laboratory abnormalities;
  - appropriate choice of tests depends on prior recognition of the syndrome.
  - Screening tests for certain metabolites should be done in all other cases:
    - blood:
      - amino acids by TLC or HPLC
      - very long chain fatty acids
    - urine:
      - amino acids by TLC or HPLC
      - organic acids by TLC or GC/MS
      - sugars by TLC
      - GAG (mucopolysaccharide) quantitation & TLC
      - oligosaccharides by TLC
  - In the first year of life, the following should be added:
    - blood: titers on patient and mother for
      - cytomegalovirus
      - rubella
      - syphilis
      - toxoplasmosis
      - varicella

Additional References:

Allen WR, Skidmore JA, Stewart F, et al. Effects of fetal genotype and uterine environment on placental development in equids. J Reproduct Fert 1993;98:55-60.

Buyse ML (editor). *Birth Defects Encyclopedia*. Cambridge, MA: Blackwell Scientific, 1990.

DeGrouchy J, Turleau C. *Clinical Atlas of Human Chromosomes*, 2nd edition. New York: Wiley, 1984.

Hall JG, Froster-Iskenius UG, Allanson JE. *Handbook of Normal Physical Measurements*. New York: Oxford, 1989.

Hu JR, Nakasima A, Takahama Y. Heritability of dental arch dimensions in humans. J Craniofac Gen Developmen Biol 1991;11:165-9.

Jones KL. *Smith's Recognizable Patterns of Human Malformation*. Philadelphia: Saunders, 1988.

McKusick VA. *Mendelian Inheritance in Man. Catalogs of Autosomal Dominant, Autosomal Recessive, and X-linked phenotypes*, 9th Edition. Baltimore: The Johns Hopkins Press, 1990.

Carter CO. Multifactorial Genetic Disease. In McKusick VA, Claiborne R (editors). *Medical Genetics*. New York: Hospital Practice Publishers, 1973.

Emery AEH. *Methodology in Medical Genetics. An Introduction to Statistical Methods*. New York: Churchill Livingstone, 1986.

Fraser-Roberts JA. Multifactorial inheritance in relation to normal and abnormal human traits. Brit Med Bull 1961;17:241-246.

Hamill PVV. NCHS growth charts, 1976. Monthly Vital Statistics Report 1976;25 (3).

Lande R, Price T. Genetic correlations and maternal effect coefficients obtained from offspring-parent regression. Genetics 1989;122:915-22.

Lucock MD, Wild J, Schorah CJ, et al. The methylfolate axis in neural tube defects: in vitro characterisation and clinical investigation. Biochem Med Metabol Biol 1994;52:101-14.

Mitchell LE, Duffy DL, Duffy P, et al. Genetic effects on variation in red-blood-cell folate in adults: Implications for the familial aggregation of neural tube defects. Am J Hum Genet 1997;60:433-8.

Nadas AS, Fyler DC. *Pediatric Cardiology*, 3rd Edition. Philadelphia: Saunders, 1972.

Nora JJ, Fraser FC. *Medical Genetics. Principles and Practice*, 3rd Edition. Philadelphia: Lea & Febiger, 1989.

Perloff JK. *The Clinical Recognition of Congenital Heart Disease*. Philadelphia: Saunders, 1978.Pierpont MEM, Moller JH. *Genetics of Cardivascular Diseases*. Boston: Martinus Nijhoff Publishing, 1987.

Romero R, Pilu G, Jeanty P, et al. *Prenatal Diagnosis of Congenital Anomalies*. Norwalk, CT: Appleton & Lange, 1988.

Sadler TW.*Langman's Medical Embryology*. Baltimore: Williams & Wilkins, 1990.

Toriello HV, Higgins JV. Occurrence of neural tube defects among first, second and third degree relatives of probands: Results of a United States study. Am J Med Genet 1983;15:601-606.

Tyson KRT. Congenital heart disease in infants. Clinical Symposia 1975;27 (3), CIBA Pharmaceutical Corporation.

Van Allen MI, Kalousek DK, Chernoff GF, et al. Evidence for multi-site closure of the neural tube in humans. Am J Med Genet 1993;47:726-743.

- Normal size is best defined as the mid-parent mean.
  - This is well-defined for height but probably applies to weight also.

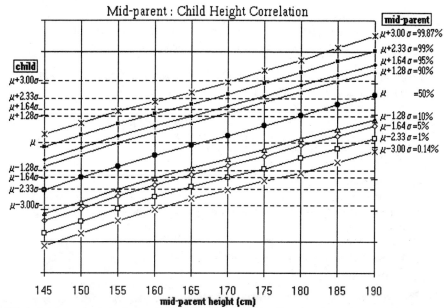

Find child's height standard deviation (σ) on left axis, trace horizontal line to intersect with vertical representing mid-parent height, follow mid-parent scale to read σ for child's expected height: A child's height σ of μ-1.64 would be mean (μ) of expected height if mid-parent height were 150 cm.

1. Tall stature is defined as height greater than
   - 2 standard deviations above the mean for age (≈ 97th percentile).

- Isolated tall stature is usually polygenic.
  - A major gene for stature is on the Y chromosome at Yq12,
    - effecting faster growth, slower maturation and larger tooth size.

- At least 50 syndromes are associated with tall stature.
  - Syndromes of fibrillin and collagen deficiency (see chapter on Genetic Erudita) should be suspected in persons who appear to have isolated tall stature, because signs of those
    - syndromes may not be evident except to medical evaluation.

EXAMPLES OF SYNDROME-ASSOCIATED TALL STATURE

Syndrome	Associated findings	Etiology
Acromegaloid syndrome	Prognathism; large hands & feet; corneal leukoma; soft skin; cutis verticis gyrata	Autosomal dominant
Chromosome XYY syndrome	Prominent glabella, long ears, large teeth, abrupt behavior, poor coordination.	Chromosomal
Multiple endocrine neoplasia I	Peptic ulcer disease; endocrine hyperplasia or tumors (pituitary, parathyorid, pancreas)	Autosomal dominant

2.   Short stature is defined as height less than
- 2 standard deviations below the mean for age (≈ 3rd percentile).

- Isolated short stature (no other abnormalities) is usually "constitutional" or polygenic
  - and is accounted for by the expected spread of children's statures of
    - several centimeters about the midparent mean.

- Constitutional short stature is the most likely diagnosis if children
  - short children are born to short parents with short relatives
    - so diagnosis requires genealogical data
  - but mid-parent height percentile (x) is the most potent genetic risk factor:
    - The mean height of future progeny is (50-x)/2 below the population mean,
    - and approximately (50-x) X 1.06383 will be below the third percentile.

- Regression toward mean is expected so
  - stature percentile less than that of the shorter parent is unusual in
  - constitutional short stature and must always be a diagnosis of exclusion.

- The growth hormone axis is normal in constitutional short stature. Reports of
  - response to growth hormone therapy may reflect
    - undiagnosed defects of the growth hormone axis, or some patients may have an
    - undue assortment growth hormone production and reception genes.

- Deficiency of production or reception of growth hormone can produce short stature
  - as a part of several syndromes
  - or as an isolated trait,
- and this can be distinguished from constitutional short stature by
  - a typical Mendelian inheritance pattern and
  - response to growth hormone stimulation tests.

- Patients with features in addition to short stature may have either
  - an inborn error of metabolism or
  - a syndrome of which short stature is only one aspect.

- Patients who have unsuccessfully treated *disorders of amino acids, urea cycle and organic acids*, or who have unnoticed mild forms of those disorders, may have
  - short stature, often accompanied by
    - mental retardation or
    - epilepsy,
      and in cases with excessive systemic organic acids,
    - weakness or hypotonia due to carnitine depletion.

- Diagnosis in cases of short stature due to metabolic disease is difficult because most cases are unique types; however, tests for certain metabolites are practical in nearly all cases:
  - blood:
    - amino acids by TLC or HPLC
    - very long chain fatty acids
  - urine:
    - amino acids by TLC or HPLC
    - organic acids by TLC or GC/MS
    - sugars by TLC
    - GAG (mucopolysaccharide) quantitation & TLC
    - oligosaccharides by TLC

- Chromosome analysis is also required in the diagnostic evaluation of short stature.

- About 40% of cases of short stature are syndrome-associated, and the majority of genetic syndromes are associated with short stature,
  - each of the several hundred syndromes being relatively equal in rarity,
  - genetic risk depending on the mechanism of inheritance of the syndrome.

EXAMPLES OF SYNDROME-ASSOCIATED SHORT STATURE

Syndrome	Findings	Etiology
Aarskog syndrome	Hypertelorism, short nose, low-set ears, shawl scrotum, broad hands and feet	X-linked dominant
Achondroplasia	Large head, frontal bossing, flat nasal bridge, short hands and feet, lordosis	Autosomal dominant
Diastrophic dysplasia	Pinnal swelling, hitchhiker thumbs, cleft palate, club foot	Autosomal recessive
Chromosome X monosomy (Turner syndrome)	Webbed neck, shield chest, lymphedema, coarctation of aorta	Chromosomal
Fetal alcohol	Short nose, faint philtrum, mental retardation	Teratogenic

- Poor intrauterine growth and low birth weight characterize gestational short stature,
  - originating in either the fetus or fetal support mechanism, for diagnosis
  - requiring, in addition to genealogical evaluation, as a minimum,
    - careful quantitative evaluation of teratogenic agents that may have entered the pregnant woman ("exposure" history is misleading),
    - careful evaluation for effects of heat, hypertension, hypotension and trauma on the pregnant woman,
    - careful assessment of uterine and placental anatomy and function,
    - chromosome analysis,
    - titers of cytomegalovirus, rubella, syphillis, toxoplasmosis, varicella,
    - bone survey X-rays for chondrodystrophies and dysostoses.

Disproportionate Gestational Short Stature
(measurements of body parts in different percentiles)

DISORDERS	ETIOLOGIES	McKusick number	CLUES
Achondrogenesis 1B	Autosomal recess	600972	Poor ossification
Achondrogenesis IA	Autosomal recess	200600	Poor ossification
Achondrogenesis II	Autosomal recess	200610	Poor long bone ossification
Achondroplasia	Autosomal dom	100800	Lordosis
Acromesomelic dwarfism	Autosomal recess	201250	Short distal limbs & hands
Atelosteogenesis	Sporadic	108270	Rhizomelia
Camptomelic dysplasia	Autosomal recess	211970	Bowed tibiae
Cerebrocostomandibular syndrome	Autosomal dom	117650	Rib gaps, micrognathia
Chondrodysplasia punctata asymmetric	Autosomal dom X-linked dom	118650 302950	Punctate epiphyses
Chondrodysplasia punctata rhizomelic	Autosomal recess	215100	Rhizomelia
Chondroectodermal dysplasia	Autosomal recess	225500	Polydactyly
Diastrophic dysplasia	Autosomal recess	222600	Club feet, calcified pinnae
Femoral hypoplasia syndrome	Sporadic	134780	Short legs, small nose
Fibrochondrogenesis	Autosomal recess	228520	Dumbbell femora
Grebe syndrome	Autosomal recess	200700	Distal limb reductions
Hypophosphatasia	Autosomal recess	241500	Poor ossification
Jarcho-Levin syndrome	Autosomal recess	277300	Short trunk
Jeune thoracic dystrophy	Autosomal recess	208500	Short ribs
Kniest dysplasia	Autosomal dom	156550	Barrel chest, stiff joints
Mesomelic dysplasia	Autosomal recess	249700	Short distal limbs
Metatropic dysplasia	Autosomal dom Autosomal recess	156550 250600	Progressive scoliosis
Osteogenesis imperfecta II	Autosomal dom	259400	Poor ossification
Roberts SC phocomelia	Autosomal recess	269000	Limb reduction, face clefts
Short rib-polydactyly I	Autosomal recess	263530	Pulmonary hypoplasia
Short rib-polydactyly II	Autosomal recess	263520	Pulmonary hypoplasia
Spondyloepiphyseal dysplasia congenita	Auto	189300	Short trunk
Thanatophoric dwarfism	Sporadic	187600	Telephone receiver femora
Thanatophoric dwarfism cloverleaf skull	Autosomal dom	187601	Kleeblattschaedel

Proportionate Gestational Short Stature
(measurements of body parts roughly in same percentile)

DISORDERS	ETIOLOGIES	McKusick number*	CLUES
Bloom syndrome	Autosomal recess	210900	Photosensitivity
Chromosome trisomies, monosomies	Chromosomal		Malformations
Constitutional	Polygenic		Midparent height
De Lange syndrome	Sporadic	122470	Synophrys, small hands
De Sanctis-Cacchione syndrome	Autosomal recess	278800	Xeroderma pigmentosum
Dubowitz syndrome	Autosomal recess	223370	Uneven eye sockets
Fanconi syndrome	Autosomal recess	227650	Radial defect, pancytopenia
Hallerman-Strieff syndrome	Autosomal recess	234100	Small nose, bulbous head
Johanson-Blizzard syndrome	Autosomal recess	243800	Hypoplastic alae nasi
Leprechaunism	Autosomal recess	246200	Hypoglycemia
Maternal malnutrition	Starvation		Brain sparing
Mucolipidosis II	Autosomal recess	252500	Stiff joints, tight skin
Mulibrey dwarfism	Autosomal recess	253250	Pigmentary retinopathy
Placental insufficiency	Sporadic		Placenta inspection
Placental hypoperfusion	Maternal disease		Brain sparing
Pena-Shokeir syndrome	Autosomal recess	208150	Arthrogryposis
Rubenstine-Taybi syndrome	Autosomal dom	180849	Broad thumbs
Russell-Silver syndrome	Autosomal dom	180860	Triangular face
Seckel syndrome	Autosomal recess	210600	Prominent nose
Teratogens: alcohol, anticonvulsants	Fetal exposure		Malformations
TORCH agents	Infection		Malformations
Twin ateriovenous transfusion	Sporadic		Brain sparing

*McKusick VA. *Mendelian Inheritance in Man. Catalogues of Autosomal Dominant, Autosomal Recessive, and X-linked Phenotypes*, 10th edition. Baltimore: The Johns Hopkins Press, 1992.

- Malnutrition is the major non-genetic cause of short stature of postnatal onset and is signalled by less than 5th percentile value for
  - **Mid-Arm Muscle Circumference** $(((10 \times mac)-(3.14 \times tsf))/10)$
  - See Appendix 1 for norms.

- Mid-arm muscle circumference may be low but
  - triceps skin fold may be normal in: **neuropathies myopathies**;
  - triceps skin fold may be high in **kwashiokor.**

3.   Normal corpulence is probably best expressed by the conicity index.
*   It ranges in value between 1.00 and 1.73, and probably has a child:mid-parent relationship similar to height but the relationship is still being defined.
*   Conicity $= w/[0.109 \times (wt/ht)^{1/2}]$
     w = waist in meters
     wt = weight in kilograms
     ht = height in meters

*   Obesity is best defined by the body-mass index over 95th percentile, an observation which is seldom occurs in normal persons.
   *   **Body-mass Index** = weight/height^2 X 100
   *   See Appendix 1 for norms.

*   Isolated obesity is probably polygenic in most cases, but
   *   plentiful food is required for its manifestation, and this produces the impression that all obesity is exogenous.
   *   Persons with some types of obesity may be asthenic, sickly or short-lived in situations in which food is in short supply.

*   Research models have identified three major mechanisms of polygenic obesity.
   *   Combinations also occur.
   *   Careful attention to diagnostic evaluation allows better management.

*   Neurotransmitter defect.
   *   Decreasing intake is difficult.
   *   Responds to fenfluramine and intense environmental light 24 hours a day.
   *   Desired weight may be achieved safely.

*   Thermogenesis defect.
   *   Easily treated with decreased intake.
   *   Achievement of desired weight may risk malnutrition.

*   Re-esterification defect.
   *   Treatment requires behavior modification and precise control of intake.
   *   Achievement of desired weight may produce physical and mental characteristics of anorexia nervosa.

Genetic Heterogeneity of Obesity
(Weight/Height^2 > 95th Percentile)
A Tentative Classification Based on Research and Clinical Data

Social-political obesity (about 5% of obese persons)

Type	Intake	Mechanism	Research Models
Exogenous	Hyperphagia	Easy availability of wide range of attractive foods induces overeating	Cafeteria diet rat: rats on monotonous diet do not become obese

Polygenic obesity (about 90% of obese persons, equally divided among 3 types)

Type	Intake	Mechanism	Research Models
Neurotransmitter defect	Excessive carbohydrate snacks in the evening.	Carbohydrate facilitates tryptophan uptake and that increases brain serotonin, producing salubrious feelings, allowing sleep	NZO mouse KK mouse
Thermogenesis defect	Normal	Lack of normal heat response to stimulation by food or cold leads to storage of calories as fat	sand rat spiny mouse
Re-esterification defect	Hyperphagia	Triglyceride metabolism anomaly requires excessive intake to maintain normal fatty acid blood levels	Well-characterized in human subjects with this type of obesity

Formerly obese persons with re-esterification defect can stay slim only by maintaining 3/4 the normal ratio of calories:weight-height. They then have low thyroid function, leukopenia, hypotension, bradycardia, amenorrhea, cold intolerance, obsessive thoughts of food. Their fat cells are tiny but numerous.

Single gene obesity (about 5% of obese persons)

Type	Intake	Mechanism	Research Models
Syndromes	Hyperphagia	Uncertain, possibly related to poor perception of satiety	ob mouse fa rat

Obesity Syndromes	Eye	Ear	Mental retardation	Hypo-gonadism	Short stature	Diabetes	Other findings
Alstrom	R	P	?	+		+	nephropathy
Bardet-Biedl	r		+	+	+	+	polydactyly, renal malformation
Biemond II	c		+	+	+		polydactyly
Cohen	s	L	+		+		narrow hand, tapered fingers
Laurence Moon	R		+	+			spastic paraplegia
Prader-Willi			+	+	+	+	hypotonia, small hands & feet
Vasquez	m	D	+	+	+		gynecomastia

EYE: R: retinitis pigmentosa, r: pigmented retina, c: coloboma, s: strabismus, m: malformations.
EAR: D: congenital deafness, L: large, P: progressive deafness.

4. Infection, perinatal brain injury, metabolic disease, neurotoxic illness, or trauma
   - may cause symptomatic mental retardation.

- As for short stature, diagnostic evaluation of mental retardation requires testing for inborn errors, chromosome aberrations and gestational complications.

- Most (95%) mental retardation is non-symptomatic or sporadic and may be
  - isolated or
  - syndrome-associated.

- Most (70%) sporadic mental retardation is isolated (non-syndromic), with
  - polygenic inheritance and
  - genetic risk depending on
    - severity of index case
    - number of affected relatives and
    - mating type.

- IQ criteria used to define mental retardation.
  - below 71-80:   borderline
  - below 35-70:   mild
  - below 20-34:   severe
  - below 20:   profound

When mental retardation is sporadic, the risk of mental retardation in relatives of the proband is higher when IQ of proband is lower so IQ determination allows a more concrete estimation of risk.

- Mating type and number of affected relatives with sporadic mental retardation.
  - Risk of first retardate

retarded	x	retarded	40%
retarded	x	normal	12%
normal sib of retarded	x	retarded	24%
normal sib of retarded	x	normal	2.5%
normal	x	normal	0.5%

  - Risk of second retardate

retarded	x	retarded	42%
retarded	x	normal	20%
normal sib of retarded	x	retarded	?%
normal sib of retarded	x	normal	13%
normal	x	normal	6%

- Over 200 syndromes are associated with mental retardation, some of which are
  - neurologic, and some of which are
  - morphologic, the
  - genetic risk depending on the mechanism of inheritance of the syndrome.

EXAMPLES OF NEUROLOGIC SYNDROMES ASSOCIATED WITH MENTAL RETARDATION

Syndrome	Findings	Etiology
Ceroid lipofuscinosis	Seizures, myoclonic jerks, mental retardation, neuronal inclusions	Autosomal recess
Pelizaeus-Merzbacher disease	Nystagmus, jerky movements of limbs, mental retardation	X-linked recess

EXAMPLES OF MORPHOLOGIC SYNDROMES ASSOCIATED WITH MENTAL RETARDATION

Syndrome	Findings	Etiology
Chromosome 13 trisomy	Infantile spasms, microphthalmia, cleft lip/palate, heart malformation, polydactyly, scalp defect	Chromosomal
Holoprosencephaly	Bilateral cleft lip/palate, hypotelorism, mental retardation	Autosomal recess

Additional references:

Bouchard C, Perusse L. Genetic aspects of obesity. In Williams CL, Kimm SYS (editors). Childhood Obesity. Ann NY Acad Sci 1993;669:26-35.

Cronk CE, Roche AF. Race and sex specific reference data for triceps and subscapular skin folds and weight/stature[2]. Am J Clin Nutr 1982;35:347-354.

Crow JF, Kimura M. *An Introduction to Population Genetics Theory.* New York: Harper & Row, 1970.

Gurney JM, Jeliff DB. Arm anthropometry in nutritional assessment: nomogram for rapid calculation of muscle circumference and cross-sectional muscle and fat areas. Am J Clin Nutr 1973;26:912-915.

Hamill PVV. NCHS growth charts, 1976. Monthly Vital Statistics Report 1976;25 (3).

Jequier E. Energy expenditure in obesity. Clin Endoc Metab 1984;13:563-580.

Leahy AM. Nature-nurture and intelligence. Genetic Psychology Monographs 1935;17: 236-308.

Liebel RL, Hirsch J. Metabolic characterizarion of obesity. Ann Int Med 1985;103:1000-1002.

Mueller WH, Meininger JC, Liehr P, et al. Conicity: A new index of body fat distribution. What does it tell us? Am J Hum Biol 1996;8:489-96.

Outhit MC. A study of the resemblance of parents and children in general intelligence. Arch Psychol 1933;149:1-60.

Reed EW, Reed SC. *Mental Retardation: A Family Study*. Philadelphia: Saunders, 1965.

Rothwell NJ, Stock MJ. The development of obesity in animals: The role of dietary factors. Clin Endoc Metab 1984;13:437-449.

Tanner JM, Goldstein H, Whitehouse RH. Standards for children's height at ages 2-9 years allowing for height of parents. Arch Dis Childh 1970;45:755-762.

Warshaw JB. Intrauterine Growth Restriction Revisited. Growth, Genetics & Hormones 1992;8:5-8.

Wurtman JJ, Wurtman RJ. D-fenfluramine selectively decreases carbohydrate but not protein intake in obese subjects. International Journal of Obesity 1984;8 (Supplement1):79-84.

1. Infection, perinatal brain injury, metabolic disease, neurotoxic illness, trauma or tumor may cause symptomatic epilepsy.

- As for short stature and mental retardation, diagnostic evaluation of epilepsy requires testing for inborn errors, chromosome aberrations and gestational complications - see the chapter on *Stature Abnormalities, Mental Retardation.*

- Non-symptomatic or sporadic epilepsy may be
   - isolated or
   - syndrome-associated.

- Most (80%) epilepsy is sporadic, with
   - polygenic inheritance and
   - genetic risk depending on type.

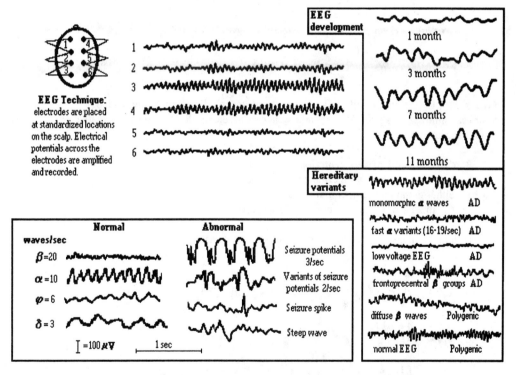

Illustrations in this section are composite drawings of informative parts of multiple electroencephalograms that are intended to point out diagnostic findings rather than to represent results obtained from actual patients.

- Grand mal epilepsy or major motor epilepsy (risk to 1st degree relatives: 6%).

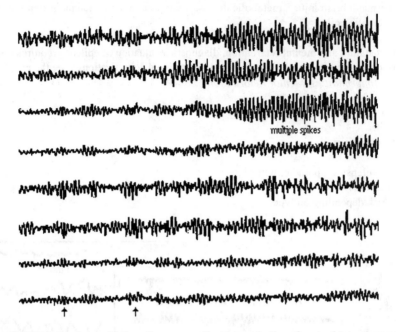

multiple spikes

Grand Mal Epilepsy: multiple spike waves. Centrencephalic refers to the tendency of wave patterns to appear simultaneously and synchronously across all electrodes as if they originated from a central point - see arrows.

- Rare cases of epilepsy are centralopathic, with
  - autosomal dominant inheritance of centrencephalic EEG and
  - either grand mal or petit mal epilepsy
    - in 25% of those who have the EEG pattern.

- Petit mal epilepsy or absence seizures (risk to 1st degree relatives: 6%).

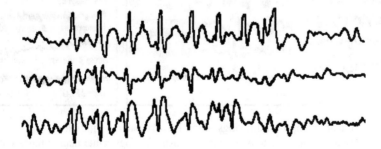

Petit Mal Epilepsy: A burst of synchronous, rhythmic 3/second spike and wave patterns accompanies a brief lapse of consciousness during which the patient remains upright but is unresponsive.

- Infantile spasms with hypsarrhythmic EEG (risk to 1st degree relatives: 6%).

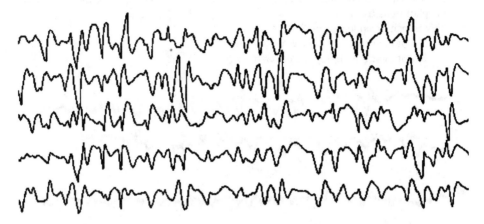

Hypsarrhythmia: Cortical high voltage random slow waves and spikes in a child with infantile spasms.

- Partial (Rolandic) epilepsy:
  - 50% of 1st degree relatives have the EEG pattern;
  - 12% have seizures (slightly higher risks to daughters of affected females).

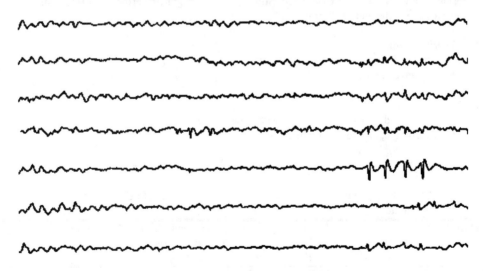

Rolandic epilepsy: A child with partial epilepsy has spikes over the Rolandic area in an inter-ictal EEG.

- Flickering light elicits seizure potentials in some persons;
  - this photosensitive EEG is also found in 40% of their 1st degree relatives.
  - Photosensitive grand mal or petit mal epilepsy occurs in a small proportion of those with the photosensitive EEG;
  - photosensitive epilepsy occurs in
    - 5% of their male 1st degree relatives and
    - 8% of their female 1st degree relatives.

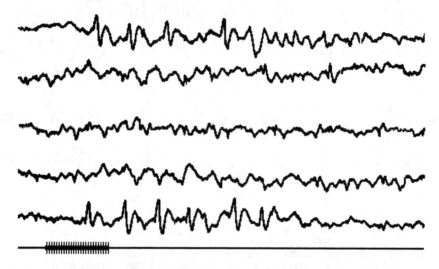

Photosensitive EEG pattern: Brief photic stimulation with light flickering at 16 Hz elicits spikes that persist beyond the end of stimulation.

- Febrile seizures:
  - 30% of 1st degree relatives have febrile seizures;
  - 4% have afebrile seizures.

- Over 130 syndromes are associated with epilepsy, some of which are
  - neurologic, and some of which are
  - morphologic, the
  - genetic risk depending on the mechanism of inheritance of the syndrome.

EXAMPLES OF NEUROLOGIC SYNDROMES ASSOCIATED WITH EPILEPSY

Syndrome	Findings	Etiology
Lafora disease	Grand mal epilepsy, myoclonus, ataxia, dementia, intracellular and extracellular Lafora bodies in brain	Autosomal recess
Hartung disease	Grand mal epilepsy, myoclonus, ataxia, dementia, diffuse atrophy of brain	Autosomal recess

EXAMPLES OF MORPHOLOGIC SYNDROMES ASSOCIATED WITH EPILEPSY

Syndrome	Findings	Etiology
Zellweger syndrome	Seizures, hypotonia, large fontanelles, high forehead, flat face, absent reflexes, poor growth	Autosomal recess
Tuberous sclerosis	Infantile spasms, adenoma sebaceum, mental retardation, white nevi, shagreen patches	Autosomal dom
Craniodiaphyseal dysplasia	Grand mal epilepsy, cranial hyperostosis dysplasia and sclerosis, cranial nerve compression, "nightstick" long bones	Autosomal recess

2. Visual impairment has a genetic cause in at least 50% of cases, and about
   - 50% of those are syndrome-associated, the
   - genetic risk depending on the mechanism of inheritance of the syndrome

EXAMPLES OF SYNDROME-ASSOCIATED BLINDNESS

Syndrome	Findings	Etiology
Albinism	Lack of pigment of skin and eyes, visual impairment, nystagmus	Autosomal recess
Chromosome 13 trisomy	Microphthalmos, polydactyly, scalp defect	Chromosomal
Galactosemia	Cataracts, hepatomegaly, mental retardation	Autosomal recess
Lowe syndrome	Congenital cataract, hypotonia, mental retardation, renal tubular dysfunction	X-linked recess
Reiger syndrome	Congenital glaucoma, iris hypoplasia, short philtrum, prognathism, hypodontia, cone-shaped teeth	Autosomal dom
Rubella syndrome	Gestational dwarfism, congenital cataract, sensorineural deafness, microcephaly, patent ductus arteriosus	Teratogenic

- Mendelian inheritance is responsible for most genetic cases of
  - visual impairment of early onset and marked severity.

- Polygenic inheritance is responsible for most genetic cases of
  - visual impairment of late onset and chronic course.

- Strabismus is the deviation of one eye from parallelism with the other and
  - causes vision loss (misuse amblyopia) in one eye which becomes
    - permanent after infancy if not treated, most cases being
  - polygenic traits with 15% genetic risk.

- Corneal dystrophy is opacification of the cornea, usually progressive, comprising
  - one congenital form (autosomal recessive)
  - nine chronic forms (2 autosomal recessive, 7 autosomal dominant).

- Cataract is opacification of the lens, 65% of cases being genetic:
  - 5 congenital forms (1 X-linked, 4 autosomal dominant) and
  - 7 chronic forms (1 X-linked, 1 autosomal recessive, 5 autosomal dominant)
  - each causing most noticeable symptoms in older persons:
    - return of ability to read without presbyopia correction lenses,
    - blurring of central vision,
    - yellowing of colors.

- Glaucoma causes progressive damage to the optic nerve through
  - elevated intraocular pressure, most often being
    - primary open-angle in type but occasionally
    - acute closed-angle, both types usually
  - polygenic traits with 12% genetic risk,
  - some congenital cases being autosomal recessive, termed buphthalmos
    - because of enlarged globes and corneal edema.

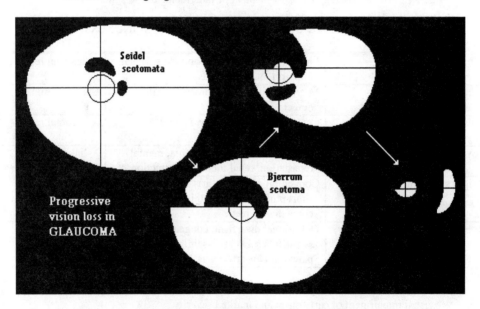

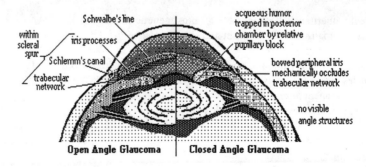

- Retinitis pigmentosa is progressive deterioration of the retina with
  - accumulation of pigment clumps peripherally, which, in most cases, is
    - so peripheral that it requires the indirect ophthalmoscope for visualization of the lesions even in advanced cases.
    - After total blindness ensues are the lesions visible to the direct ophthalmoscope.
  Causes include:
  - autosomal recessive inheritance (70%),
  - autosomal dominant inheritance (20%) or
  - X-linked inheritance (10%).

3. Deafness has a genetic cause in at least 50% of cases, and about
   - 50% of those are syndrome-associated, the
   - genetic risk depending on the mechanism of inheritance of the syndrome.

EXAMPLES OF SYNDROME-ASSOCIATED DEAFNESS

Syndrome	Findings	Etiology
Alport syndrome	Progressive sensorineural deafness, progressive nephritis	Autosomal dom
Jervell-Lange-Neilson	Congenital deafness, cardiac rhythm abnormalities, sudden death	Autosomal recess
Usher syndrome	Congenital sensorineural deafness, retinitis pigmentosa	Autosomal recess
Waardenberg syndrome	Congenital sensorineural deafness, white forelock, heterochromia irides	Autosomal dom
Cytomegalovirus	Congenital or progressive deafness, chorioretinitis, microcephaly, epilepsy	Teratogenic

- Isolated cases of congenital deafness are often polygenic traits with
  - genetic risk of 10%.

- Isolated cases of deafness may be due to Mendelian inheritance and can be
  - differentiated from polygenic cases only if
    - genealogy shows a specific inheritance pattern,
  - 50% being due to many different autosomal recessive genes
  - 30% autosomal dominant and
  - 20% X-linked.

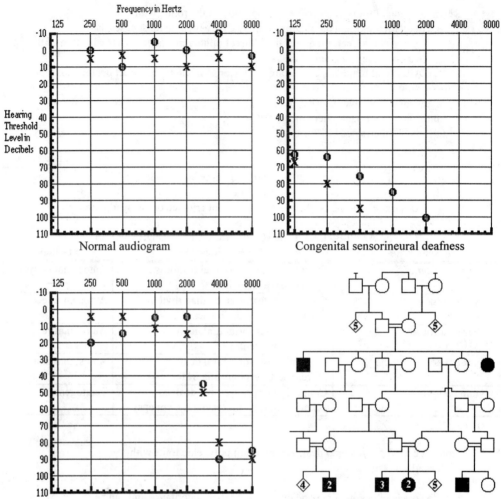

Normal audiogram

Congenital sensorineural deafness

"Noise-induced" hearing deficit, often found
among obligate heterozygotes in this family

Note the autosomal recessive inheritance pattern

An "outbreak" of deaf-mutism in Chackbay, LA
Eight cases occurred in families living near a petroleum installation over a brief span of years.
None was aware of the genealogical connections nor the consanguinity.

- Because there are many different autosomal recessive genes causing deafness,
  - mating between homozygotes produces
    - all deaf children in only 10% of cases and
    - all hearing children in 75% of cases.

- Otosclerosis is one of the more common autosomal dominant types of deafness and
  - has about 40% penetrance.

Additional references:

Cotlier E, Maumenee IH, Berman ER. *Genetic Eye Diseases. Retinitis Pigmentosa and Other Inherited Eye Disorders*. Birth Defects Original Article Series 18(6). New York: Alan R. Liss, Inc., 1982

Duke-Elder S. System of Ophthalmology. London: Kimpton, 1964.

Ford FR. *Diseases of the Nervous System in Infancy, Childhood and Adolescence*, 6th Edition. Springfield, IL:Charles C Thomas, 1973.

Fraser GR, Friedmann AI. *The Causes of Blindness in Childhood. A Study of 776 Children with Severe Visual Handicaps*. Baltimore: The Johns Hopkins Press, 1967.

Fraser GR. *The Causes of Profound Deafness in Childhood*. Baltimore: The Johns Hopkins Press, 1976.

Holmes GL. *Diagnosis and Mangement of Seizures in Children*. Philadelphia: Saunders, 1987.

Keith CG. *Genetics and Ophthalmology*. New York: Churchill Livingstone, 1978.

Lavrich JB, Nelson LB. Diagnosis and treatment of strabismus disorders. In: Nelson LB (editor). *Pediatric Ophthalmology*. Ped Cl N A 1993;40:737-752.

Nelson LB. *Pediatric Ophthalmology*. Major Problems in Clinical Pediatrics 25. Philadelphia: W.B. Saunders, 1984.

Paton D, Craig JA. Cataracts. Development, Diagnosis and Management. CIBA Symposia 1974;26(3). Summit, NJ:CIBA Pharmaceutical Co.

Paton D, Craig JA. Gluacomas. Diagnosis and Management. CIBA Symposia 1976;28(2). Summit, NJ:CIBA Pharmaceutical Co.

Raymond V. Molecular genetics of the glaucomas: Mapping of the first five "GLC" loci. Am J Hum Genet 1997;60:272-277.

Ruben RJ, De Water TR, Steel KP. Genetics of Hearing Impairment. Ann NY Acad Sci 1991;630.

van Beijsterveldt CEM, Molenaar PCM, de Geus EJC, et al. Heritability of human brain functioning as assessed by electroencephalography. Am J Hum Genet 1996;58:562-573.

1. Whether environmental or hereditary, cancers are characterized by genetic events:
    *   Chromosome aberrations in the cancer cells, occasionally constitutional,
        *   obscure in effect but possibly one vehicle of the next two characteristics.
    *   Activation of oncogenes in the cancer cells.
    *   Inactivation of tumor suppressor genes in the cancer cells.

EXAMPLES OF CHROMOSOME ABERRATIONS	TUMORS
deletion (1q)	lymphoproliferative disease
	carcinomas
trisomy (1)	lymphoproliferative disease
	carcinomas
translocation (2;8)	Burkitt lymphoma
translocation (3;8q24)	renal cell carcinoma
translocation (3;8q21)	mixed salivary gland tumor
deletion (3p)	small cell carcinoma of lung
deletion (5q)	myeloid leukemia
	colon carcinoma
monosomy (5)	myeloid leukemia
monosomy (7)	myeloid leukemia
deletion (6q)	lymphoproliferative neoplasia
translocation (6;9)	myeloid leukemia
translocation (6;14)	ovarian cystadenocarcinoma
trisomy (8)	acute myelogenous leukemia
translocation (8;21)	acute myelogenous leukemia
translocation (8;14)	Burkitt lymphoma
translocation (8;22)	Burkitt lymphoma
translocation (9;22) "Philadelphia chromosome"	chronic myelogenous leukemia
translocation (9;6)	myeloid leukemia
deletion (11p)	Wilms tumor-aniridia
translocation (11;14)	B-cell neoplasia
	acute lymphatic leukemia
	lymphomas
translocation (11;22)	Ewing sarcoma
trisomy 12	chronic lymphocytic leukemia
deletion (13q)	retinoblastoma
translocation (14;14)	B-cell neoplasia
	acute lymphatic leukemia
	lymphomas
translocation (15;17)	acute promyelocytic leukemia
deletion (20q)	preleukemia
	polycythemia vera
monosomy 22	meningioma
X monosomy (Turner)	endometrial carcinoma
trisomy X	carcinoma of breast
disomy X (Klinefelter)	mediastinal carcinoma
Y with X monosomy	gonadoblastoma

Gene, McKusick number	ONCOGENES Tumors	Gene, McKusick number	TUMOR SUPPRESSOR GENES Tumors
abl, 189980	chronic myelogenous leukemia (K562)	APC, 175100	colon cancer, stomach cancer
erbB, 190120	epidermoid carcinoma, squamous carcinoma, glioblastoma	BRCA1, 113705	breast cancer, ovarian cancer
erbB-2, 190160	adenocarcinoma of salivary gland, gastric carcinoma, mammary carcinoma	BRCA2, 600185	breast cancer
ets-1, 600541	acute monomyelocytic leukemia	CDKN2, 600160	esophageal cancer, lymphoblastic leukemia, melanoma, mesothelioma, pancreatic cancer
myb, 189990	adenocarcinoma of colon, acute myelogenous leukemia	DPC4, 600993	pancreatic cancer
myc, 190080	promyelocytic leukemia (H160), colon APUDoma (COLO320), small cell carcinoma of lung, carcinoma of breast (SKBr-3 etc), gastric adenocarcinoma	MTS1, 154280	pancreatic cancer, skin cancer
L-myc, 164850	small cell carcinoma of lung	NF-1, 162200	myeloid leukemia, pheochromocytoma
N-myc, 164850	neuroblastoma, small cell carcinoma of lung, retinoblastoma	NF-2, 162210	brain cancer
K-ras, 190070	carcinoma of lung, gastric carcinoma	p53, 191170	adrenal cancer, brain cancer, breast cancer, leukemia, lung cancer, sarcoma
N-ras, 164790	mammary carcinoma (MCF-7)	VHL, 193300	renal cancer
ret, 164761	multiple endocrine neoplasia, medullary thyroid carcinoma	WT1, 194070	Wilm's tumor

PROPORTIONS OF CANCER PATIENTS WHO HAVE A FAMILY HISTORY OF CANCER

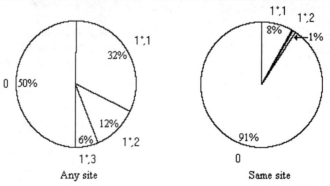

"1°,2" means, "first degree relatives, 2 in number."

- Most types of cancers occur in both environmental and hereditary forms.
- Environment is said to cause 80% of cancers but control has not produced anticipated results.
  - About 25% of hereditary cancers are thought to be Mendelian, and 75%, polygenic;
    - known environmental agents probably influence the occurrence of either very little.
    - Initiating events of hereditary cancers are obscure.

EXAMPLES OF POLYGENIC INHERITANCE OF CANCER

Type	Risk factor	Type	Risk factor
Endometrium	2.7	Prostate	1.9
Lung	3	Stomach	2.6
Melanoma	2.5	Testis	9
Ovary	3.6	Thyroid	8.2

To estimate risk to 1° relatives, multiple factor by relative's age-specific risk.

AGE-SPECIFIC RISKS OF CANCERS

Age	Endometrium	Lung male	Lung female	Melanoma male	Melanoma female	Ovary
0 to 4	0.00000030	0.00000080	0.00000060	0.00000010	0.00000010	0.00000050
5 to 9	0.00000001	0.00000030	0.00000020	0.00000010	0.00000010	0.00000060
10 to 14	0.00000010	0.00000040	0.00000030	0.00000020	0.00000020	0.00000240
15 to 19	0.00000070	0.00000080	0.00000060	0.00000150	0.00000110	0.00000420
20 to 24	0.00000250	0.00000220	0.00000110	0.00000440	0.00000330	0.00000500
25 to 29	0.00000450	0.00000510	0.00000230	0.00000840	0.00000670	0.00000720
30 to 34	0.00000750	0.00001950	0.00000740	0.00001320	0.00001010	0.00001410
35 to 39	0.00001620	0.00005670	0.00002060	0.00001740	0.00001310	0.00003430
40 to 44	0.00003220	0.00015050	0.00004720	0.00002040	0.00001570	0.00007650
45 to 49	0.00005570	0.00033430	0.00008390	0.00002440	0.00001770	0.00014050
50 to 54	0.00009520	0.00066660	0.00012500	0.00002860	0.00001920	0.00020400
55 to 59	0.00015160	0.00113210	0.00016840	0.00003180	0.00002240	0.00025570
60 to 64	0.00022180	0.00167490	0.00021080	0.00003690	0.00002600	0.00030040
65 to 69	0.00028810	0.00206520	0.00025710	0.00004320	0.00003060	0.00033730
70 to 74	0.00035650	0.00219250	0.00031870	0.00005070	0.00003660	0.00036680
75 to 84	0.00042050	0.00191280	0.00038620	0.00006770	0.00004770	0.00037270
≥ 85	0.00048200	0.00120820	0.00038740	0.00008940	0.00006720	0.00030060

AGE-SPECIFIC RISKS OF CANCERS

Age	Prostate	Stomach male	Stomach female	Testis	Thyroid male	Thyroid female
0 to 4	0.00000070	0.00000030	0.00000020	0.00000090	0.00000010	0.00000010
5 to 9	0.00000020	0.00000010	0.00000010	0.00000030	0.00000010	0.00000010
10 to 14	0.00000020	0.00000010	0.00000001	0.00000040	0.00000010	0.00000001
15 to 19	0.00000040	0.00000030	0.00000030	0.00000500	0.00000020	0.00000020
20 to 24	0.00000030	0.00000110	0.00000060	0.00001140	0.00000020	0.00000030
25 to 29	0.00000030	0.00000280	0.00000270	0.00001930	0.00000050	0.00000050
30 to 34	0.00000030	0.00000760	0.00000720	0.00001840	0.00000060	0.00000080
35 to 39	0.00000070	0.00001840	0.00001410	0.00001580	0.00000110	0.00000140
40 to 44	0.00000260	0.00003840	0.00002650	0.00001260	0.00000210	0.00000250
45 to 49	0.00000920	0.00007700	0.00004400	0.00000890	0.00000380	0.00000440
50 to 54	0.00003650	0.00014680	0.00007230	0.00000710	0.00000580	0.00000840
55 to 59	0.00011090	0.00025790	0.00011980	0.00000670	0.00001020	0.00001390
60 to 64	0.00029910	0.00044400	0.00019770	0.00000680	0.00001480	0.00002130
65 to 69	0.00066820	0.00072010	0.00031960	0.00000850	0.00001990	0.00003180
70 to 74	0.00134150	0.00106120	0.00050940	0.00001000	0.00002690	0.00004460
75 to 84	0.00285160	0.00159030	0.00086410	0.00001360	0.00003030	0.00006130
≥ 85	0.00465240	0.00189370	0.00123560	0.00001900	0.00003120	0.00006950

- Cancers appear to arise during cell division as a result of two mutations;
  - the first, called initiation, promotes somatic mutations in subsequent divisions,
    - which may be cumulative or random but which eventually
  - lead to the second, called conversion, which transforms that daughter cell
  - into a cancer cell, at rates which are variable but specific to cancer type.

- In sporadic cancers, all mutations occur during divisions of somatic cells, generally
  - requiring more time for manifestation, hence cancer at a later age,
  - than Mendelian cancers in which the first mutation is inherited;
  - the rates of cancers among relatives of sporadic cases are consistent with expectations of
    - polygenic inheritance of cancer propensity.

- Germ-line mutation can produce a gamete that has the first mutation,
  - in which case the same progression of somatic mutations may produce
  - a sporadic case of cancer but also allowing
  - genetic transmission of the mutant gene to progeny.

- The first mutation may be silent, or
  - may be detectable by genetic analysis, or
  - may produce a recognizable phenotype associated with cancer,
    - either a condition or a syndrome.

2. The effect of the initial mutation leading to tumors of infancy and childhood
   - may be to cause persistence of rests of primordial embryonal tissue.
   - Many are also associated with hamartomas or benign tumors.

- Retinoblastoma is an embryonal neoplasm of the retina,
    - signaled by a white pupillary reflex, and
    - occurring usually shortly after birth.

- Retinoblastoma is caused by homozygous malfunction of RB1, a tumor suppressor gene at
    - at chromosome 13q14 (McKusick 180200), in other tissues causative of osteogenic sarcoma, pinealoma, bladder cancer, lung cancer, among others.

- In all cases of bilateral retinoblastoma and
    - 15% of cases of unilateral retinoblastoma,
    - the patient has inherited one malfunctioning supressor gene and
    - somatic mutation of the other occurs in a retinal cell.

- In 85% of cases of unilateral retinoblastoma,
    - There is somatic mutation of both retinoblastoma genes in a retinal cell.

- Retinoblastoma is also associated with
    - several syndromes caused by aberrations involving chromosome 13q,
        - usually involving hemizygosity of the retinoblastoma gene and
        - usually accompanied by mental retardation and congenital malformations,
        - sometimes transmitted by parents who have a balanced translocation.

(also see Appendix 3, and "chromosome 13 aberrations" in *Laboratory Diagnosis: Cytogenetics*)

- Wilms tumor is an embryonal neoplasm of the kidney, derived from the
    - metanephric blastema, occurring most frequent in mid-childhood,
    - caused by homozygous malfunction of the WT1 tumor
    - at chromosome 11p13 (McKusick 194070).

- At least 33% of Wilms tumors are inherited and another
    - 3% have the same mutant gene as the inherited type which is
    - an autosomal dominant gene with 63% penetrance,
    - inherited cases being usually bilateral and earlier onset.

- Wilms tumor occurrence within a family of a sporadic case
    - conforms to the expectations of a polygenic trait with a genetic risk of 6%.

- Wilms tumor is also associated with several syndromes and the
    - genetic risk depends on the mechanism of transmission of the syndrome.

3. The breast cancer frequency of 7% is a cumulative lifetime incidence.
    - Risks to relatives of a sporadic case conform to the expectations of a polygenic trait.
    - Infrequent cases caused by single genes entail higher risks to relatives.

- As many as 4/1000 women have a mutation in the BRCA1 gene on 17q:
    - producing a cumulative lifetime incidence of breast or ovarian cancer of 85%,
    - characteristically occurring before age 50, and bilateral.
- The BRCA2 gene on 13q confers a risk mainly of breast cancer

Patient	Sister	Additional 1°	Additional 1°	% BRCA1	% BRCA2
breast cancer <age 50	breast cancer <age 50	breast cancer <age 50		40	42
breast cancer <age 50	breast cancer <age 50	ovarian cancer < age 50		82	
breast cancer <age 50	breast cancer <age 50	ovarian cancer < age 50	ovarian cancer < age 50	91	

Figures in the % columns represent the relative likelihoods of DETECTING inherited BRCA1 or BRCA2 in the patient <u>who has cancer</u> and among various relatives <u>who themselves have</u> various types of cancers. Additional 1° means a mother or another sister, who has cancer.

BREAST CANCER RISK FACTORS

Age-specific risk of breast cancer

Age	risk
0 to 4	0.00000050
5 to 9	0.00000010
10 to 14	0.00000010
15 to 19	0.00000030
20 to 24	0.00000210
25 to 29	0.00001530
30 to 34	0.00005720
35 to 39	0.00013550
40 to 44	0.00027120
45 to 49	0.00043340
50 to 54	0.00058470
55 to 59	0.00069250
60 to 64	0.00078650
65 to 69	0.00087290
70 to 74	0.00103410
75 to 84	0.00132770
≥ 85	0.00183540

Fibrocystic disease and family history

Relative who has breast cancer	Factor: patient has fibrocystic disease
none	3.4
one 1° relative	7.4

To estimate breast cancer risk, find patient's age in table at left, multiply her age-specific risk by the appropriate factor from the table above.

Number of relatives

Relative (s) with cancer	Factor
one 2° relative >age 51	1.09
one 1° relative >age 51	1.36
one 2° relative <age 50	1.63
one 1° relative <age 50	2.31
two 2° relatives >age 51	1.63
two 1° relatives >age 51	2.45
two 2° relatives <age 50	3.13
two 1° relatives <age 50	5.44
patient has BRCA1	11.56

To estimate breast cancer risk, find applicable data in column 1, read factor at left, multiply patient's age-specific risk by factor.

- Breast cancer can be a part of several syndromes and the
  - genetic risk depends on the mechanism of transmission of the syndrome.

Causative gene (McKusick number)	Proportion of breast cancers		Associated cancers
	< 50 years age	≥ 50 years age	
Androgen resistance (313700)	<1%	-	male breast only
Ataxia telangiectasia (208900)	7%	7%	leukemia
BRCA1 (113705)	5%	1%	ovary, colon, prostate
BRCA2 (600185)	?	?	male breast, prostate
hRAS (190020)	-	-	leukemia
p53 (191170)	<1%	-	sarcoma, brain

4. About 85% of colorectal cancers are associated with colon polyps.
   - Colon polyps can have either dominant or polygenic inheritance, or
   - can be part of autosomal dominant syndromes.

- Familial and sporadic nonpolyposis colorectal cancers share similar mutations.
  - About 5% are Mendelian; the remainder are sporadic.
  - Risks to relatives of a sporadic case conform to the expectations of a polygenic trait.

MENDELIAN COLON CANCER

Disorder (gene): McKusick number	Tumors	Etiology
Cancer family-Lynch I (APC | KRAS | p53 | DCC): 114500	Colorectal cancer arising from a cascade of mutations in which the p53 is transitional.	Autosomal dom chromosome 17p
Familial colorectal cancer (DCC): 120470	Colorectal cancer	Autosomal dom chromosome 18q
Non-polyposis colon cancer (PMSL1): 600258	Colon cancer, genomic instability	Autosomal dom chromosome 2q
Non-polyposis colon cancer (PMSL2): 600259	Colon cancer, genomic instability	Autosomal dom chromosome 7p
Non-polyposis colon cancer 1, cancer family-Lynch II, Muir-Torre syndrome (MSH2): 120435	Breast cancer, colon cancer, endometrial cancer, ovarian cancer, soft tissue sarcomas, sebaceous skin tumors, keratoacanthoma, genomic instability	Autosomal dom chromosome 2p
Non-polyposis colon cancer 2 (MLH1): 120436	Colon cancer, genomic instability	Autosomal dom chromosome 3p
Familial adenomatous polyposis, Turcot syndrome, Gardner syndrome (APC): 175100	Epidermoid cysts, cutaneous fibromas, osteomas, supernumerary teeth, duodenal polyps, duodenal cancer, colon polyps, colon carcinoma, glioma, astrocytoma	Autosomal dom chromosome 5q
Familial juvenile polyposis: 174900	Intestinal polyposis onset in childhood, colon cancer in fourth decade	Autosomal dom

5. Cancer occurs as part of many different syndromes and the
   - genetic risk depends on the mechanism of transmission of the syndrome.

EXAMPLES OF SYNDROMIC CANCER

Syndrome, synonyms (gene): McKusick number	Findings	Etiology
Basal cell nevus syndrome (NBCCS): 109400	Calcified falx cerebri, telecanthus, odontogenic cysts of jaw, rib anomalies, vertebral anomalies, palmar pits, multiple basal cell nevi	Autosomal dom chromosome 9q22.3
Beckwith-Wiedeman (BWS): 130650	Macrosomia, macroglossia, organomegaly, omphalocoele, Wilms tumor	Autosomal dom chromosome 11p15
Cowden syndrome: 158350	Multiple hamartomas of skin and mucous membranes, fibroadenomatous enlargement of breasts, breast cancer	Autosomal dom
Denys-Drash syndrome (WT1): 194070	Pseudohermaphroditism, progressive nephropathy, Wilms tumor.	Autosomal dom chromosome 11p
Familial atypical mole melanoma, dysplastic nevus syndrome (CMM1): 155600	Fair complexion, freckles, mutiple reddish brown irregular 5 to 15 mm nevi on upper trunk and limbs, melanoma around age 45.	Autosomal dom chromosome 1p
Li-Fraumeni syndrome (p53): 191170	Breast cancer, medulloblastoma, leukemia, adenocarcinoma of lung, rhabdomyosarcoma, adrenocortical carcinoma	Autosomal dom chromosome 17p
Multiple endocrine neoplasia III (MENIIB): 162300	Mucosal neuromas, patulous lips, marfanoid habitus, prognathism, megacolon, pheo-chromocytoma, medullary carcinoma of thyroid	Autosomal dom chromosome 10q11.2
Peutz-Jeghers syndrome (PJS): 175200	Melanin spots of lips, buccal mucosa, digits; intestinal polyposis; polyps of respiratory tree and urinary tract; breast cancer; pancreatic cancer	Autosomal dom
von Hippel-Lindau syndrome (VHL): 193300	Cerebellar hemangioblastoma, retinal angioma, renal cell carcinoma, pancreatic carcinoma, pheochromocytoma	Autosomal dom chromosome 3p26
WAGR syndrome (WT1): 194070	Aniridia, hypogenitalism, mental retardation, Wilms tumor	Autosomal dom chromosome 11p

(also see Appendix 3, and "Meiotic Instability Syndromes" in *Laboratory Diagnosis: Cytogenetics*)

5. Diabetes mellitus is a group of disorders characterized by
   * chronic hyperglycemia with
   * heterogenous pathogeneses;
      * many different pathological processes culminate as diabetes.

* Most cases are either
   * insulin dependent (IDDM) with juvenile onset or
   * non-insulin dependent (NIDDM) with adult onset,
   * a small number being non-insulin dependent with juvenile onset (MODY),
      * maturity onset diabetes of the young.

	IDDM	NIDDM
Clinical	Thin, ketosis-prone, insulin required for survival	Frequently obese, responsive to diet or oral hypoglycemics, ketosis resistant
Onset	Childhood, early adulthood Fall and winter Acute or subacute Inflammatory cells in islets	Over 30 years of age Not seasonal Usually slow onset No islet inflammation
Family	Increased IDDM	Increased NIDDM
Twins	<50% concordance in monozygotic twins	Nearly 100% concordance in monozygotic twins
Insulin levels	Low to absent	Variable
Insulin response to glucose	Flat	Variable
Autoimmune disease association	Yes	No
Islet cell antibodies	Yes	No
HLA asssociation	Yes	No
Pathogenesis	Viral infections, beta-cell toxins, autoimmunity	Insulin resistance, premature aging of beta cells

HLA Typing and Frequency of IDDM

HLA Phenotype	IDDM	HLA Genotype	IDDM
DR1	1:1000	DR3/DR3	1:125
DR2	1:2500	DR3/DRX	1:500
DR3	1:185	DR4/DR4	1:147
DR4	1:208	DR4/DRX	1:476
DR5	1:2500	DR3/DR4	1:42
DR6	1:1429	DRX/DRX	1:5565
DR7	1:1250		
DR8	1:556		
DR9	1:345		

HLA DR3 or DR4 Haploypes and IDDM

Characteristic	DR3	DR4
Islet cell antibody production	Low or absent	High
Islet cell antibodies	Persistent	Disappear after diagnosis
Antipancreatic immunity	Increased	No increase
Autoimmune endocrinopathies	More frequent	Less frequent
Onset	Variable, initially may be NIDDM	Young
Parental transmission	Mother or father	Father
Residual b-cell function	High (short term after diagnosis)	Low
Proliferative retinopathy	No increase	Frequent

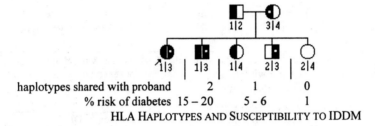

haplotypes shared with proband   2   1   0

% risk of diabetes   15 – 20   5 - 6   1

HLA HAPLOTYPES AND SUSCEPTIBILITY TO IDDM

- Occurrence of IDDM or NIDDM within a family
  - usually conforms to the expectations of a polygenic trait.

	Risk to sibs	Risk to offspring
IDDM	5-20%	2-5%
NIDDM		
Overt disease	5-10%	5-10%
Glucose intolerance	15-25%	15-25%

- MODY is often inherited as an autosomal dominant trait.

- Diabetes mellitus occurs as part of over 25 different syndromes and the
  - genetic risk depends on the mechanism of transmission of the syndrome.

EXAMPLES OF SYNDROME-ASSOCIATED DIABETES MELLITUS

Syndrome	Findings	Etiology
Alstrom syndrome	Retinitis pigmentosa with early loss of central vision, nerve deafness, obesity	Autosomal recess
Prader-Willi syndrome	Hypotonia, hypogenitalism, obesity, mental retardation	Autosomal recess
Familial lipodystrophy	Symmetrical loss of fat of the limbs and lower trunk, phlebectasia	Autosomal dom
Insulin resistant acanthosis nigricans	Acanthosis nigricans, hirsutism, polycystic ovaries	Autosomal dom

6. Blood pressure is a continuous polygenic trait.
    - Absolute definition of hypertension: 2σ above mean. Associated with
      - cardiomegaly, encephalopathy, nephropathy, and retinopathy at any age.
    - Past age 50 years, rates of complications increase in proportion to diastolic pressures over 90 mm so this constitutes another definition of hypertension.

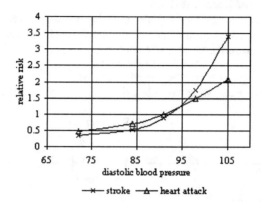

HYPERTENSION COMPLICATIONS IN OLDER ADULTS

	Birth	1 year	Until age 18		Mid 40's – mid 70's
systolic	75mm±20	95mm±15	Female: +3mm/Y ±20	Male: +4mm/Y ±20	+5mm/Y ±15
diastolic	45mm±15	55mm±15	+3mm/Y ±15	+3mm/Y ±15	+5mm/Y ±10

BLOOD PRESSURE AGE-SPECIFIC NORMS ($\mu \pm 2\sigma$). Also see Appendix 1 for graphic charts.

DIET	high calorie, high salt, low calcium , low potassium
DRUGS	alcohol, amphetamines, caffeine, cigarette smoking, corticosteroids, cyclosporin, imipramine, lead, mercury, methotrexate, methylphenidate, oral contraceptives. sympathomimetics
DISEASES	adrenocortical disorders, hyperthyroidism, hyperparathyroidism, coarctation of aorta, renal parenchymal diseases, renal vascular diseases, Wilms tumor, pheochromocytoma, neuroblastoma spectrum tumors, aldosterone-secreting tumor, juxtaglomerular renin-secreting tumor, increased intracranial pressure, head injury, cerebrovascular accident, Guillain-Barre syndrome, spinal cord injury, posterior fossa lesions, chronic upper airway obstruction, traction, burns, pregnancy, intravascular volume overload, pain, anxiety, stress

MAJOR ENVIRONMENTAL FACTORS THAT CAUSE HYPERTENSION

- A cause cannot be defined in most cases of hypertension, so it is called "essential".
  - When a cause can be defined, it is called secondary hypertension.

- Pathogenesis of essential hypertension may involve at least 2 mechanisms:
  - Sodium-lithium countertransport defect: results in accumulation of sodium in cells.
  - Abnormal neuroendocrine response.
    - Poorly understood but a rat model has defective receptors for catecholamines that promote vasodilation through agonist-related c-AMP production.
    - Angiotensin variations may also contirbute.

- Essential hypertension risk to 1st degree relatives $\cong$ 5%
  - This is approximately what would be expected on the basis of the absolute definition.

Types of Hypertension

	Newborn	Childhood	Adult
Essential hypertension	57%	72%	93%
Secondary hypertension	43%	28%	7%
% Renal parenchymal disease	39	34	36
% Renovascular disease	35	17	21
% Coarctation of aorta	9	35	-
% Oral contraceptives	-	-	34
% Endocrine disease	-	7	6
% Other	17	7	3

- Regression toward mean occurs so blood pressure in a percentile higher than that of the highest parental percentile is unexpected and makes secondary hypertension likely.

- Secondary hypertension occurs as part of over 100 syndromes and the
  - genetic risk depends on the mechanism of transmission of the syndrome.

Syndrome	Findings	Etiology
Polycystic kidney	Bilateral multiple renal cysts, progressive renal dysfunction, portal hypertension, hepatic cysts	Autosomal dom
Fibromuscular dysplasia	Occlusive thickening of renal artery wall. May be either female-limited or a part of neurofibromatosis	Autosomal dom
Williams syndrome	Infantile hypercalcemia, supravalvular aortic stenosis, peripheral pulmonic artery stenosis, elfin face, stellate iris, short stature	Autosomal dom
Pheochromocytoma	Paroxysmal hypertension, episodes of sweating and palpitations, VMA in urine.	Autosomal dom
Adrenogenital syndrome III	Virilization, hyponatremia	Autosomal recess

EXAMPLES OF SYNDROME-ASSOCIATED HYPERTENSION

Additional references:

Cancer

Aaltonen LA, Peltomaki P, Leach FS, et al. Clues to the pathogenesis of familial colorectal cancer. Science 1993;260:812-816.

Biesecker BB, Boehnke M, Calzone K, et al. Genetic counseling for families with inherited susceptibility to breast and ovarian cancer. JAMA 1993;296:1970-1974.

Claus EB, Risch N, Thompson WD. Genetic analysis of breast cancer in the Cancer and Steroid Hormone Study. Am J Hum Genet 1991;48:232-242.

Dupont WD, Page DL. Risk factors for breast disease in women with proliferative breast disease. NE J Med 1985;312:146-151.

Easton DF. The inherited component of cancer. Brit Med J 1994;50:527-35.

Easton DF, Ford D, Bishop DT. Breast and ovarian cancer incidence in BRCA-1 mutation carriers. Am J Hum Genet 1995;56:265-271.

Feuer EJ, Wun L-M, Boring, CC, et al. The lifetime risk of developing breast cancer. Jour Natl Cancer Inst 1993;85:892-897.

Helman LJ, Thiele CJ. New insights into the causes of cancer. Pediatric Clinics of North America 1991;38 (2):201-221.

King MC. Genetic and epidemiological analysis of cancer in families: Breast cancer as an example. In Bodmer WF (editor). *Inheritance of Susceptibility to Cancer in Man*. New York: Oxford, 1982.

King MC, Lee GM, Spinner NB, et al. Genetic epidemiology. Annu Rev Public Health 1984;5:1-52.

King MC, Rowell S, Love SM. Inherited breast and ovarian cancer. What are the risks, What are the choices? JAMA 1993;269:1975-1980.

Kundson AG. Hereditary cancer, oncogenes and antioncogenes. Cancer Research 1985;45:1437-1443.

London SJ, Connolly JL, Schnitt SJ, et al. A prospective study of benign breast disease and the risk of breast cancer. JAMA 1992; 267:941-944.

Lynch HT, Brodkey FD, Lynch P, et al. Familial risk and cancer control. JAMA 1976;236:582-4.

Lynch HT, Follett KL, Lynch PM, et al. Family history in an oncology clinic. Implications for cancer genetics. JAMA 1979;242:1268-72.

Lynch HT, Hirayama T (editors). *Genetic Epidemiology of Cancer*. Boca Raton, FL: CRC Press, 1989.

Mason TJ, McKay FW, Hoover R, et al. Atlas of Cancer Mortality for U.S. Counties: 1950-1969. DHEW Publication No. (NIH) 75-780. Washington DC: US Department of Health, Education, and Welfare, 1975.

McKusick VA. *Mendelian Inheritance in Man. Catalogues of Autosomal Dominant, Autosomal Recessive, and X-linked Phenotypes*, 10th edition. Baltimore: The Johns Hopkins Press, 1992.

Peltomaki P, Aaltonen LA, Sistonen P, et al. Genetic mapping of a locus predisposing to human colorectal cancer. Science 1993;260:810-812.

Purtilo DT, Paquin L, Gindhart T. Genetics of neoplasia. Impact of ecogenetics on oncogenesis. Am J Pathol 1978; 91:609-687.

Schneider NR, Chaganti SR, German J, et al. Familial predisposition to cancer and age at onset of disease in randomly selected cancer patients. Am J Hum Genet 1983;35:454-67.

Schottenfeld D, Fraumeni JF. Cancer Epidemiology and Prevention. WB Saunders, Philadelphia, PA: WB Saunders, 1982.

Shattuck-Eidens D, McClure M, Simard J. A collaborative study of 80 mutations in the BRCA1 breast and ovarian cancer susceptibility gene. JAMA 1995;273:535-41.

Skolnick MH, Cannon-Albright LA, Goldgar DE et al (1990): Inheritance of proliferative breast disease in breast cancer kindreds. Science 1990;250:1715-1720.

Slattery ML, Kerber RA. A comprehensive evaluation of family history and breast cancer risk. JAMA 1993;270:1563-1568.

Stanbridge EJ. Human tumor suppressor genes. Ann Rev Genet 1990;24:615-657.

Taylor JA. Epidemiologic evidence of genetic susceptibility to cancer. In: Spatz L, Bloom AD, Paul NW (editors). *Detection of Cancer Predisposition: Laboratory Approaches. Monograph 3*. White Plains, NY: March of Dimes Birth Defects Foundation, 1990:113-127.

Thibodeau SN, Bren G, Schaid D. Microsatellite instability in cancer of the proximal colon. Science 1993;260: 816-819.

Vandenbroucke JP. Is "The Causes of Cancer" a miasma theory for the end of the twentieth century? Int J Epidemiol 1988;17:708-9.

Wooster R, Neuhausen SL, Mangion J, et al. Localization of a breast cancer susceptibility gene, BRCA2, to chromosome 13q12-13. Science 1994;265:2088-2090.

Young JL, Percy CL, Asire AJ. Surveillance, Epidemiology and End Results: Incidence and Mortality Data, 1973 - 77. National Cancer Institute Monograph 57. NIH Publication No. 81-2330. Bethesda, MD: US Department of Health and Human Services, 1981.

Diabetes

Hollingsworth DR, Resnik R (editors). *Medical Counseling Before Pregnancy*. New York: Churchill Livingstone, 1988.

Hypertension

Feld LG, Spingate, JE. *Hypertension in Children*. Current Problems in Pediatrics 1988;18:6. Year Book Medical Publishers, Chicago.

Filer LJ, Lauer RM (editors). *Children's Blood Pressure*. Report of the 88th Ross Conference on Pediatric Research. Columbus, OH: Ross Laboratories, 1985.

Jeunemaitre X, Soubrier F, Kotelevtsev YV, et al. Molecular basis of human hypertension: role of angiotensinogen. Cell 1992;71:7-20.

Lauer RM, Burns TL, Clarke WR. Assessing children's blood pressure - considerations of age and body size. The Muscatine Study. Pediatrics 1985;75:1081-1090.

Lieberman E. Hypertension in Childhood and Adolescence. CIBA Symposia 1978;30(3). CIBA Pharmaceutical Co, Summit, NJ.

Wilkins RW, Hollander W, Chobanian AV. *Evaluation of Hypertensive Patients.* CIBA Symposia 1972;24(2). CIBA Pharmaceutical Co, Summit, NJ.

Williams RR, Dadone MM, Hunt SC, et al. The genetic epidemiology of hypertension: A review of past studies and current results for 948 persons in 48 Utah pedigrees. In: Rao DC, Elston RC, Kuller LH, et al (editors). *Genetic Epidemiology of Coronary Heart Disease. Past, Present and Future.* New York: Alan R Liss, 1984.

1.   Atherosclerosis is related to hypercholesterolemia which is often familial.
   •   The most common form is polygenic, in which correlation of total cholesterol level among relatives without dyslipoproteinemia is 0.25.
      •   Heritability of total cholesterol level is 65% (environmental component 35%).
      •   Heart attacks occur after 50 years of age.
      •   Men with levels over 245 mg/dl account for 50% of coronary artery disease deaths,
         •   while men with levels below 145 mg/dl account for 5%.

Cholesterol Levels in British Males

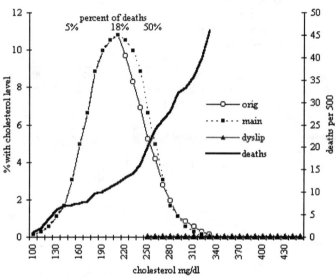

Data from Martin MJ, Hulley SB, Browner WS, Kuller LH, Wentworth D. Serum cholesterol, blood pressure and mortality: implications from a cohort of 361662 men. *Lancet* 1986;2:933-936. Deaths are graphed by the line with circle symbols, the cholesterol data from the original study. Two other lines resolve the cholesterol data into 2 curves. The first resolved curve ("main") represents the polygenic distribution of cholesterol levels in the population. The other ("dyslip") represents the distribution of dyslipoproteinemia heterozygotes, the most common of which is familial hypercholesterolemia. The homozygote frequency of .000001 contributes little.

   •   See Appendix 1 for blood lipid norms.

   •   Separate from the environmental component of polygenic hypercholesterolemia, there are
      •   many environmental factors that contribute to coronary artery disease disease through
      •   elevation of cholesterol or depression of HDL cholesterol.

   •   Control of environmental factors can lower cholesterol by 10% to 20%,
      •   with corresponding decreases in population frequency of coronary artery deaths,
         •   and possibly decreasing some individuals risks.

Environmental Factors in Coronary Heart Disease

Elevated Cholesterol		Depressed HDL Cholesterol	
Diet	high cholesterol	Diet	polyunsaturated:saturated fats < 1:1
Drugs	beta adrenergic antagonists, oral contraceptives, corticosteroids, hydrochlorthiazides	Drugs	androgens, progestins, probucol, propranolol, pyrazinamide, sulfonylureas
Diseases	anorexia nervosa, congenital biliary atresia, diabetes mellitus, dysglobulinemia, acute hepatitis, idiopathic hypercalcemia, hypopituitarism, hypothyroidism, Klinefelter syndrome, systemic lupus erythematosis, nephrosis, obesity, porphyria, pregnancy, progeria, renal transplant, storage diseases, uremia, Werner syndrome.	Diseases	azotemia, diabetes mellitus, hyperthyroidism, hypothyroidism, immunoglobulin disorders, malnutrition, myeloproliferative disorders, obesity, Wolman disease

Modified from Lee J, Burns TL. Genetic dyslipoproteinemias associated with coronary atherosclerosis. In: Pierpont MEM, Moller JH (editors). *The Genetics of Cardiovascular Disease.* Boston, MA: Martinus Nijhoff Publishing, 1986:161-191.

- HDL cholesterol level is inversely related to death rate from coronary heart disease.
  - It is also polygenic.
    - Correlation for first degree relatives is 0.20.

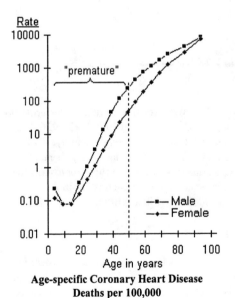

Age-specific Coronary Heart Disease Deaths per 100,000

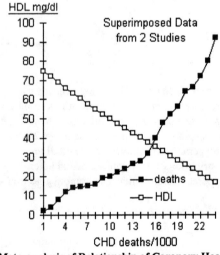

Meta-analysis of Relationship of Coronary Heart Disease Deaths to HDL Cholesterol

- About 0.5% of the population has one of the dyslipoproteinemias, which are more specific defects of lipid level regulation that can be differentiated by lipid profiles,
  - manifested by premature coronary artery disease,
  - accounting for nearly 10% of coronary heart disease deaths.

Lipoprotein Determinations		Lipoprotein Profiles		
Tests				Elevated components:
Fasting	1. Total cholesterol	Types	1	Chylomicrons
	2. Total triglyceride		2a	LDL
	3. HDL cholesterol		2	LDL+VLDL
	4. Chylomicrons		b	
Calc	LDL cholesterol= total cholesterol -		3	b-VLDL
	((triglyceride/5)+HDL cholesterol)		4	VLDL
	VLDL cholesterol = triglyceride/5		5	Chylomicrons+VLDL

Modified from Lee J, Burns TL. Genetic dyslipoproteinemias associated with coronary atherosclerosis. In: Pierpont MEM, Moller JH (editors). *The Genetics of Cardiovascular Disease.* Boston, MA: Martinus Nijhoff Publishing, 1986:161-191.

Dyslipoproteinemias

Disorder, synonyms: features (all cause premature coronary artery disease)	McKusick number*	Profile	Cholest	Triglyc
Apolipoprotein E defect, broad-beta disease, dysbetalipoproteinemia: xanthomas (planar, tendon, tuberous, tuberoeruptive), peripheral vascular disease.	107741	3	elevated	elevated
Analphalipoproteinemia, Tangier disease: large orange tonsils, neuropathy, weakness, lymphadenopathy, hypersplenism.	205400	low HDL-C, abnormal LDL and chylomicrons	low	normal
Combined hyperlipidemia	144250	2a**, 2b**, 4, 5 (rare)	elevated	elevated
Familial hypercholesterolemia, LDL receptor defect: corneal arcus, xanthelasma, xanthomas (tendon in heterozygotes, tendon and planar in homozygotes).	143890	2a**, 2b (rare)**	elevated	normal
Familial hypercholesterolemia B: xanthomas (tendon in heterozygotes, tendon and planar in homozygotes), corneal arcus, xanthelasma	144010	abnormal LDL	elevated	normal
Familial hypertriglyceridemia: abnormal glucose tolerance, atheroeruptive xanthoma	145750	4, 5 (rare)	normal	elevated
Hyperlipoproteinemia II, hyperbetalipoproteinemia: corneal arcus, xanthomas (tendon and tuberous).	144400	2a** 2b**	elevated elevated	normal elevated
Hyperlipoproteinemia IV: abnormal glucose tolerance, atheroeruptive xanthoma	144600	4	normal	elevated
Hyperlipoproteinemia V	144650	5 low LDL and HDL	normal	elevated

Data from Lee J, Burns TL. Genetic dyslipoproteinemias associated with coronary atherosclerosis. In: Pierpont MEM, Moller JH (editors). *The Genetics of Cardiovascular Disease*. Boston, MA: Martinus Nijhoff Publishing, 1986:161-191.

* McKusick VA. *Mendelian Inheritance in Man. Catalogues of Autosomal Dominant, Autosomal Recessive, and X-linked Phenotypes*, 11th edition. Baltimore: The Johns Hopkins Press, 1995.

**Note: profile 2a, and rarely, 2b, also characterizes the common polygenic type of hypercholesterolemia which is many times more prevalent than the dyslipoproteinemias.

2. Alzheimer disease, bipolar affective disorder, schizophrenia, and alcoholism may be confused at times in some cases due to
    * clinical variability,
    * diagnostic inaccuracy, and
    * genetic heterogeneity.

* Alzheimer disease progresses over 5 to 10 years; 75% are dead by 10 years after onset.
    * Initial features:
        * Changes in mood and loss of judgement, spatial orientation and memory. Depression, collapse of social relationships. Diagnosis can be made at this point.
        * Benign, childlike state. Patient follows the caretaker closely, cooperating to the level of his ability. Speech and communication deteriorate.
    * Intermediate features:
        * Episodic bouts of irritability. Patient becomes irrascible, anxious, uncooperative and physically active. Communication is lost. Disrupted sleep and night wandering.
    * Advanced features:
        * Apathy: loss of response to most stimuli, incontinence.
        * Terminal disease: patient shrivels. Seizures, deglutition abnormalities, infections.

Criteria of Alzheimer disease

A. Criteria of POSSIBLE Alzheimer disease:
    1. An Alzheimer-like dementia syndrome with variations of onset, presentation or clinical course, in the absence of other neurologic, psychiatric, or systemic disorder sufficient to cause dementia.
    2. An Alzheimer-like dementia syndrome in the presence of a second systemic or brain disorder sufficient to produce dementia but not thought to be the cause of the dementia.
    3. A single, gradually progressive severe cognitive defect in the absence of other identifiable cause
B. Criteria of PROBABLE Alzheimer disease:
    1. Dementia established by clinical examination and documented by the Mini-Mental Test, Blessed Dementia Scale or similar examination and confirmed by neuropsychological testing.
    2. Deficits in 2 or more areas of cognition.
    3. Progessive worsening of memory and other cognitive functions.
    4. No disturbance of consciousness.
    5. Onset between ages 40 years and 90 years.
    6. Absence of systemic disorders or other brain diseases that in and of themselves could account for the progressive deficits of memory and cognition.
C. Clinical features supporting a diagnosis of PROBABLE Alzheimer disease:
    1. Progressive deterioration of specific cognitive functions such as language (aphasia), motor skills (apraxia), and perception (agnosia).
    2. Impaired activities of daily living and altered patterns of behavior.
    3. Family history of similar disorder, particularly if confirmed neuropathologically.
    4. Laboratory results:
        * normal cerebrospinal fluid by standard techniques.
        * normal EEG pattern or nonspecific changes such as increased slow-wave activity.
        * cerebral atrophy on CT with progression documented by serial observation.

Criteria of Alzheimer disease(contuinued)

D. Other clinical features consistent with a diagnosis of PROBABLE Alzheimer disease, after exclusion of other causes of dementia:
1. Plateaus in the progression of the illness.
2. Associated symptoms of depression, insomnia, incontinence, delusions, illusions, hallucinations, sexual disorders, weight loss, catastrophic verbal, emotional or physical outbursts.
3. Other neurological abnormalities in some patients, especially with more advanced disease, including motor signs such as increased muscle tone, myoclonus, or gait disorder.
4. Seizures in advanced disease.
5. CT normal for age.
E. Clinical features which make unlikely a diagnosis of PROBABLE Alzheimer disease:
1. Sudden, apoplectic onset.
2. Focal neurological findings such as hemiparesis, sensory loss, visual field defects, or incoordination early in the course of the illness.
3. Seizures or gait disturbances at the onset or very early in the course of the illness.
F. Criteria of DEFINITE Alzheimer disease:
1. Clinical criteria of probable Alzheimer disease PLUS:
2. Histopathological evidence of Alzheimer disease from biopsy or autopsy.
G. Classification of Alzheimer disease should specify features that may differentiate subtypes:
1. Familial occurrence.
2. Onset before age 65 years.
3. Chromosome 21 trisomy in patient.
4. Coexistence of other relevant conditions such as Parkinson disease.

Pathological changes of Alzheimer disease:
- Plaques and neurofibrillary tangles in hippocampus amygdala, neocortex and basal forebrain nuclei.
- Loss of neurons in hippocampus and amygdala.
- Loss of temporal and mid-frontal large neurons.
- Decreased activity of acetylcholinesterase and choline acetyltransferase in cortex.

Similar changes of lesser degree are part of normal aging.

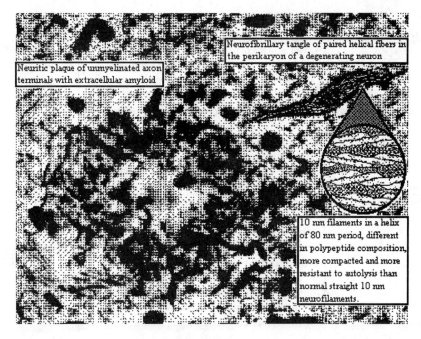

Neuritic plaque of unmyelinated axon terminals with extracellular amyloid

Neurofibrillary tangle of paired helical fibers in the perikaryon of a degenerating neuron

10 nm filaments in a helix of 80 nm period, different in polypeptide composition, more compacted and more resistant to autolysis than normal straight 10 nm neurofilaments.

PATHOLOGICAL CHANGES OF ALZHEIMER DISEASE

TYPES OF ALZHEIMER DISEASE

Type	Gene: locus	Inheritance: McKusick number*
AD1: Early onset	Amyloid precursor: Chromosome 21q21.3	Autosomal dominant: 104300:104760
AD2: Late onset	Apolipoprotein E4: Chromosome 19q	Autosomal dominant: 104310:107741
AD3: Early onset	S182 (presenilin-1): Chromosome 14q24.3	Autosomal dominant: 104311
AD4: Early onset	STM2 (presenilin-2): Chromosome 1q31	Autosomal dominant: 600759

* McKusick VA. *Mendelian Inheritance in Man. Catalogues of Autosomal Dominant, Autosomal Recessive, and X-linked Phenotypes*, 11th edition. Baltimore: The Johns Hopkins Press, 1995.

- Careful genealogical evaluations [Breitner JCS, Silverman J, Mohs RC, et al] have provided data consistent with autosomal dominant inheritance of Alzheimer disease.
  - Controversy about possible non-genetic cases may stem from:
    - Inadequate genealogical evaluation:
      - Penetrance is incomplete until at least age 87 years;
      - non-paternity leads to erroneous genealogy data in 15% of cases.
    - Inadequate diagnostic evaluation:
      - Non-genetic conditions similar to Alzheimer disease include
        - deficiencies for folic acid and vitamin B12,
        - hypothyroidism,
        - neurosyphilis.

Disorders clinically similar to Alzheimer disease

Disorder	Differentiating features	McKusick number
Cerebroarterial amyloidosis	Onset in fifth decade of migraine headaches, progressive intellectual deterioration and memory loss, cerebral and cerebellar hemorrhages.	104760 (allele of AD1)
Cruetzfeldt-Jacob disease	Rapid course (average=8 months), status spongiosus of brain.	123400
Lewy body dementia	Paralysis agitans, eosinophilic ovoid cytoplasmic inclusions (Lewy bodies) in degenerating neurons in substantia nigra, asymmetric focal cerebral atrophy.	127750
Multi-infarct dementia	Onset in third decade of migraine headaches and seizures, followed by bipolar affective disorder, attacks of focal subcortical ischemia, pseudobulbar palsy.	125310
Pick disease	Frontal atrophy prior to symptoms, temporal lobar atrophy, argyophilic cytoplasmic inclusions (Pick bodies) in degenerating neurons, ballooned neurons (Pick cells).	172700
Unclassified encephalopathy	Diffuse nerve cell degeneration and glial proliferation in brain without other recognizable features.	Heterogeneous

Research Diagnostic Criteria of bipolar affective disorder

Manic Disorder	Major Depressive Disorder
A. One or more periods of persistent elevated, expansive, or irritable mood not due to substance use.	A. One or more periods of persistent dysphoric/ irritable mood or pervasive loss of interest or pleasure.
B. At least 3 of the following is mood is elevated or expansive, at least 4 if only irritable:	B. At least 5 of the following:
1. More active than usual.	1. Poor appetite/weight loss or increased appetite/weight gain.
2. More talkative than usual.	2. Insomnia or hypersomnia.
3. Flight of ideas or racing thoughts.	3. Loss of energy.
4. Grandiosity.	4. Psychomotor agitation or retardation.
5. Decreased need for sleep.	5. Loss of interest or pleasure in usual activities.
6. Distractibility	6. Feelings of self-reproach or inappropriate guilt.
7. Poor judgement (e.g., buying sprees, foolish investments.	7. Diminished ability to think or concentrate.
	8. Recurrent thoughts of death or suicide.
C. At least 1 of the following:	C. Duration of dysphoric features at least 1 week.
1. Meaningful conversation is impossible.	
2. Serious social or occupational impairment.	
3. Hospitalization.	
D. Duration of manic features at least 1 week (shorter if hospitalized).	D. Sought or was referred for help, took medication, or had impaired functioning.
E. No psychotic symptoms suggestive of schizophrenia.	E. No psychotic symptoms suggestive of schizophrenia.
	F. Does not meet criteria for schizophrenia, residual subtype.

Family data about bipolar affective disorder:

Bipolar:

Inheritance: Polygenic (also, oligogenes apparently on chromosomes 5q, 6, 13, 15, 18q, and Xq)

	Population	MZ twins reared together or apart	DZ twins	Other first degree relatives
Risk %:	1	70	20	bipolar: 6 unipolar: 8

Unipolar (major depressive disorder only):
Inheritance: Polygenic

	Population	MZ twins reared together or apart	DZ twins	Other first degree relatives
Risk %:	male: 3 female: 7	50	20	bipolar: 1 unipolar: 6

Research Diagnostic Criteria of schizophrenia

A. During an active phase of the illness (may or may not now be present) at least 2 of the following are required for a definite diagnosis, or 1 for a probable diagnosis:
   1. Thought broadcasting, insertion, or thought withdrawal.
   2. Delusions of being controlled (or influenced), other bizarre or multiple delusions.
   3. Delusions having a somatic, grandiose, religious, or nilhilistic content, or other delusions without themes of persecution or jealousy, lasting for at least 1 week.
   4. Delusions of any type if accompanied by hallucinations of any type for at least 1 week.
   5. Auditory hallucinations in which either a voice keeps up a running commentary on the patient's behavior or thoughts as they occur, or 2 or more voices converse with each other.
   6. Non-affective verbal hallucinations spoken to the patient.
   7. Hallucinations of any type throughout the day for several days or intermittently for at least 1 month.
   8. Definite instances of marked formal thought disorder accompanied by either blunted or inappropriate affect, delusions, or hallucinations of any type, or grossly disorganized behavior.

B. Signs of the illness have lasted at least 2 weeks from the onset of a noticeable change in the patient's usual condition (current signs of the condition may not now meet criterion A and may be residual symptoms only, such as extreme social withdrawal, blunted or inappropriate affect, mild formal thought disorder, or unusual thoughts or perceptual experiences).

C. At no time during the active period (delusions, hallucinations, marked formal thought disorder, bizarre behavior, etc.) of illness being considered did the patient meet the full criteria for either probable or definite manic or depressive syndrome to such a degree that it was a *prominent* part of the illness.

Family data about schizophrenia

Inheritance: Polygenic (also, oligogenes apparently on chromosomes 5q11.2 6p23, 19p13, 22q11)

% risk of	Population	MZ twins	DZ twins	Sibs	One parent affected	Both parents affected
schizophrenia	1	40	10	10	16	34
schizoid	3	40	9	9	32	32

Syndrome	Associated findings	Etiology
DiGeorge syndrome	Hypertelorism, mongoloid eye slant, short philtrum, ear malformation, hypoplastic or absent parathyroid, conotruncal heart malformation, hypocalcemia, seizures.	Autosomal dom
Hashimoto struma	Autoimmune thyroiditis	Autosomal dom
Saethre-Chotzen syndrome	Craniosynostosis, flat face, long nose, asymmetric shallow orbits, long ears, cleft palate, syndactyly	Autosomal dom
Urogenital adysplasia	Wide-set eyes; flat face; receding chin; large ears; pulmonary hypoplasia; vaginal, uterine & fallopian anomalies; hypertension	Autosomal dom
Muscular dystrophy	Weakness, hypotonia, cardiomyopathy, calf enlargement, cardiomyopathy, obstirpation	X-linked recessive

EXAMPLES OF SYNDROME-ASSOCIATED SCHIZOPHRENIA

Diagnostic criteria for alcohol dependence (type 1 alcoholism)

A. Criteria of alcohol abuse (see below) plus either
B. Tolerance:
1. Need for markedly increased amounts of alcohol to achieve the desired effect.
2. Markedly diminished effect with regular use of the same amount.
C. Withdrawal:
1. Symptoms ("shakes" or malaise relieved by alcohol) after cessation or reduction of drinking.

Diagnostic criteria for alcohol abuse (type 2 alcoholism)

A. Pattern of pathological alcohol use:
1. Need for daily use of alcohol for normal functioning.
2. Inability to cut down or stop drinking.
3. Repeated efforts to control or reduce drinking by temporary abstinence or restriction of drinking by time of day.
4. Binges (continuously intoxicated for at least 2 days).
5. Occasional volume consumption (750 ml spirits or equivalent during one drinking session).
6. Amnesic periods (blackouts) for events occurring while intoxicated.
7. Knowingly drinking in spite of a serious physical illness exacerbated by alcohol.
8. Drinking of non-beverage alcohol.
B. Impairment of social or occupational functioning due to alcohol use:
1. Violence while intoxicated.
2. Absence from work.
3. Loss of job.
4. Legal difficulties: arrest for intoxicated behavior, traffic accidents while intoxicated.
5. Arguments or difficulties with family or friends because of excessive alcohol use.
C. Duration of disturbance of at least 1 month.

- Types of alcoholism breed true within families:
  - Type 1
    - onset after 25 years age
    - both sexes; if female, usually transmitted from mother
    - more dependent on environment for manifestation
  - Type 2
    - onset before 25 years age
    - mostly in males
    - almost always father to son transmission

Family data about alcoholism

Mode of inheritance: Polygenic. Type 2 has stronger heritability.

	MZ twins reared together or apart	DZ twins	Other first degree relatives
Risk %:	40	20	15

- Wernicke encephalopathy (ataxia, apathy, confusion, drowsiness, oculomotor apraxia) may occur in some chronic alcoholics and may advance into Korsakoff psychosis (amnesia, inability to acquire new memory). Predisposing factors include:
  - Central European ethnicity.
  - Nutritional inadequacy, especially of thiamin.
  - Variant transketolase (chromosomes 3p14.3 [TKT1], Xq28 [TKT2]).

Additional references:

Beighton PH, Lindenberg R (1971): Alzheimer's disease in multiple members of a family. In: Bergsma D (editor). *The Second Conference on the Clinical Delineation of Birth Defects. Part VI. Nervous System*. Birth Defects Original Article Series 1971;7(1).

Breitner JCS, Silverman J, Mohs RC, et al. Familial aggregation in Alzheimer's disease: comparison of risk among relatives of early-onset and late-onset cases, and among male and female relatives in successive generations. Neurology 1988;38:207-212.

Gershon ES. Genetics of the affective disorders. Hospital Practice, 1979; March Issue, 117-122.

Goedde HW, Agarwal DP (editors). *Alcoholism. Biomedical and Genetic Aspects*. New York: Pergamon Press, 1989.

Gordon DJ, Knoke J, Probstfield JL, et al. High density lipoprotein cholesterol and coronary heart disease in hypercholesterolemic men: The Lipid Research Clinics Coronary Primary Prevention Trial. Circulation 1986;74:1217-1225.

Kety SS, Rowland LP, Sidman RL, et al. *Genetics of Neurological and Psychiatric Disorders*. Research Publications: Association for Research in Nervous and Mental Disease. Volume 60. New York: Raven Press, 1983.

Lee J, Burns TL. Genetic dyslipoproteinemias associated with coronary atherosclerosis. In Pierpont ME, Moller JH, (editors). *Genetics of Cardiovascular Disease*. Boston: Martinus Nijhoff Publishing, 1986.

Martin MJ, Hulley SB, Browner WS,et al. Serum cholesterol, blood pressure and mortality: implications from a cohort of 361662 men. Lancet 1986;2:933-936.

Mason TJ, Fraumeni JF, Hoover R, et al. *An Atlas of Mortality from Selected Diseases*. NIH Publication No. 81-2397. Washington, DC: US Department of Health and Human Services, 1981.

Stern C. Chapter 27. Heredity and Environment: III. Behavior Genetics. In: *Principles of Human Genetics*, 3rd Edition. San Francisco: WH Freeman, 1973.

Tsaung MT, Faraone SV. *The Genetics of Mood Disorders*. Baltimore: The Johns Hopkins Press, 1990.

Vandenberg SG, Singer SM, Pauls DL. *The Heredity of Behavior Disorders in Adults and Children*. New York: Plenum Medical Book Company, 1986.

TABLE 1. FREQUENCIES OF GENETIC DISEASES

Category	Disease	Cases per 100,000		
Congenital anomalies	Heart malformation		800	
	Hypospadias		540	
	Pyloric stenosis		300	
	Hydrocephalus		200	
	Omphalocoele		160	
	Chromosome 21 trisomy		150	
	Cleft lip/palate		100	
	Neural tube defects		100	
	Albinism			6
Connective tissue disorders	Ankylosing spondylitis		50	
	Marfan syndrome			7
	Osteogenesis imperfecta			4
	Ehlers-Danlos syndrome			1
Hematologic	Sickle cell anemia		30	
	Thalassemia		10	
	Hemophilia			4
Inborn errors	Phenylketonuria			7
Neuromuscular	Alcoholism	2700		
	Affective disorders	2000		
	Alzheimer disease	2000		
	Mental retardation	2000		
	Epilepsy	1000		
	Shizophrenia	1000		
	Parkinson disease		100	
	Multiple sclerosis		30	
	Duchenne muscular dystrophy		10	
	Mytonic dystrophy			7
	Werdnig-Hoffman disease			4
	Ataxia-telangiectasia			2
	Amyotrophic lateral sclerosis			1
	Becker muscular dystrophy			1
Organ disorders	Hypertension	16000		
	Diabetes	5000		
	Psoriasis	2000		
	Deafness	1200		
	Short stature	1000		
	Blindness		700	
	Familial hypercholesterolemia		500	
	Ichthyosis		400	
	Alpha-1 antitrypsin deficiency		100	
	Cystic fibrosis		18	
	Wilson disease			3

TABLE 1. FREQUENCIES OF GENETIC DISEASES (CONTINUED)

Category	Disease	Cases per 100,000		
Tumors	Breast cancer	7000		
	Neurofibromatosis		30	
	Familial polyposis		13	
	Gardner syndrome			6
	Wilms			6
	Retinoblastoma			6
	Tuberous sclerosis			2

Data with modifications from: Berini RY, Kahn E. *Clinical Genetics Handbook.* Oradell NJ: Medical Economics Books, 1986.

- Table 1 lists the genetic disease frequencies for which reliable data are available.
  - Divide any of the frequencies by 5 for an estimate of the number of patients
    - that a primary care physician is likely to encounter during a practice lifetime.

- The more common diseases are more illustrative of the epidemiology of genetic diseases,
  - but the rarer diseases are concentrated in Medical Genetics clinics,
    - and their management exemplifies this medical specialty.

- Etiological clarity may be inversely proportional to frequency.
  - Rarer diseases tend to stand out, and their
  - genetic factors are usually simpler,
    - making them worthwhile vehicles for study.

"Significant" Rare Genetic Diseases

Autosomal dominant	Autosomal recessive	X-linked	Mitochondrial
Ehlers-Danlos syndrome familial hypercholesterolemia Huntington disease Marfan syndrome myotonic dystrophy neurofibromatosis osteogenesis imperfecta	cystic fibrosis Hurler syndrome phenylketonuria sickle cell disease thalassemia	Duchenne muscular dystrophy fragile X syndrome hemophilia	Leber optic atrophy MELAS MERRF

1. Ehlers-Danlos syndrome is recognizable from descriptions as far back as 1668 but
   - development of the concept dates to the 1891 description in Russian by Tschernogubow,
     - followed by a description in Danish by Ehlers in 1901,
       - and in French by Danlos in 1908, all describing stretchy skin.
   - Subsequent imprecise descriptions resulted in several different tissue integrity disorders
     - being called Ehlers-Danlos syndrome, at least one without stretchy skin.
     - illustrating one source of genetic heterogeneity.

- Additional physical characteristics of the Ehlers-Danlos phenotype include:
  - Skin fragility: scars stretch and become papyraceous.
  - Vascular fragility: easy bruisability and internal hemorrhages.
  - Tissue fragility: hernias, aneurysms.
  - Mitral prolapse is common.
  - Fragile fetal membranes of an affected fetus may lead to premature birth.
  - There is variability in the number of features and in the ages when they manifest.

- Genes for most types of Ehlers-Danlos syndrome have not been identified.
  - Mutations of several types in collagen genes can cause some types:
  - COL1A1 (chromosome 17q21),
  - COL1A2 (chromosome 7q21), and
  - COL3A1 (chromosome 2q31).

Disorders that have been called Ehlers-Danlos Syndrome

Type	Skin elasticity	Skin fragility	Skin bruisability	Joint fragility	Other	Seg	MIM
I Gravis	+++	+++	++	+++	Occasional arterial & intestinal ruptures	AD	130000
II A. Mitis B. Recessive	++	++	+	++	Like I but milder COL1A2 null alleles	AD	130010
III Familial hypermobility	++	+	+	+++	Arthritis	AD AR?	130020 208050
IV Arterial	-	+++	+++	+	Acrogeria, ruptures of arteries, intestines, uterus. Pneumothorax. COL3A1 mutations	AD AD? AR? AR? AR?	130050 120180 201200 225350 225360
V? X-linked	++	+(+)	+	+		XR	305200
VI Ocular	++	++	++	+++	Microcornea, rupture of eye, hypotonia, osteoporosis, kyphoscoliosis. Deficiency of lysyl hydroxylase due to LOH mutation.	AR AD? AR?	225400 153454 229200
VII A & B. Arthrochalasis multiplex congenita C. Dermatosparaxis	++	+(+)	+	+++	Congenital luxations, short stature COL1A1 exon 6 loss deletes N-proteinase cleavage site Soft skin, umbilical hernia N-proteinase lack	AD AD? AR? AR?	130060 120160 225410 225410
VIII	+	++	++	++	Periodontal disease	AD	130080

Disorders that have been called Ehlers-Danlos Syndrome (continued)

Type	Skin elasticity	fragility	bruisability	Joint fragility	Other	Seg	MIM
IX X-linked cutis laxa Occipital horn syndrome	+/-	+	-	+	Lax skin, osteoporosis bladder diverticula, occipital exostoses. Menke syndrome allele: defect in copper utilization.	XR	304150
X	+	+	+	++	Petechiae, platelet dysfunction, striae Abnormal fibronectin	AR	225310
Etc 1	+++	+++	+++	+++	Progeroid face, short stature, hypotonia, mental retardation, loose joints, lax skin	AD	130010
Etc 2	++	++	++	+	Kyphoscoliosis, aortic dissecting aneurysm, hernias, myxomatous heart valve disease	AD	130090
Etc 3	+++			+++	Lop ears, loose joints, hernias, luxations	AR	225320

Modified from: Steinmann B, Royce PM, Superti-Furga A. The Ehlers-Danlos syndrome. In Steinmann B, Royce PM, Editors. *Connective Tissue and Its Heritable Disorders. Molecular, Genetic and Medical Aspects.* New York: Wiley Liss, 1993. p 360.

2.   The most common dyslipoproteinemia is familial hypercholesterolemia, which is
  • due to mutations of several types in the low-density lipoprotein receptor (LDL) gene locus, at chromosome 19p13.2, a 45 kb gene with a 5.3 kb mRNA transcript and a protein product of 860 amino acids length.
  • Effects of the mutations range from failure to produce a protein product to failure of one of the steps in the functioning of the LDL receptor.
    • Heterozygote frequency is 0.2%. Their features include:
      • Tendon xanthomas after age 20 years.
      • Cholesterol levels ranging from 250 to 450 mg/dl.
      • First heart attack before age 50 years.
    • Approximately equal numbers of homozygotes and compound heterozygotes account for severe cases, with a total frequency of 0.000001. Their features include:
      • Cutaneous xanthomas, either congenital or by age 4 years.
      • Cholesterol levels over 500 mg/dl
      • First heart attack between ages 5 years and 30 years.
  • Lipoprotein profiles 2a (elevated LDL) or 2b (elevated LDL and VLDL) are typical.
    • However, only 5% of patients with those profiles have familial hypercholesterolemia;
      • 95% have the more common polygenic hypercholesterolemia.

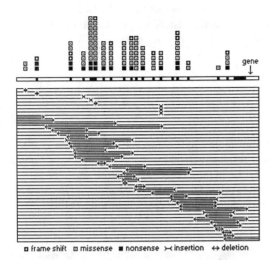

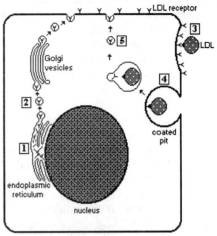

Mutations in the LDL receptor gene. Exons are in black. Positions of point mutations are indicated by symbols above the gene. Each open bar below the gene represents an outline of the gene; positions of deletions and insertions are indicated in the bars.

Classification of LDL receptor mutations. Class 1: null alleles. Class 2: transport defective alleles. Class 3: binding-defective alleles. Class 4: internalization-defective alleles. Class 5: recycling-defective alleles.

3. Huntington disease begins with scattered neuron death in the caudate nucleus, demonstrable presymptomatically first by PET scan and later by MRI.
   - It spreads slowly through the basal ganglia, then to the third and fifth cortical layers.
   - Clinical manifestations are progressive chorea and dementia. Either may appear first.
     - Prodromal behavioral and psychological symptoms may precede them.
     - The disease culminates in a rigid, bedridden state after an average of 17 years.
       - Death is usually due to either cardiac arrest or pneumonia.

- The most frequent age of onset of Huntington disease is 35 years but may be at any age.
  - Cases within a family usually have onset at a similar age.
  - Transmission from an affected father may result in earlier onset and greater severity.

- Variations in the clinical picture of Huntington disease are familial.
  - Early onset variety.
  - Rigid variety.
  - Chorea without dementia.
  - African variety: rarer but more severe.

- The disease is due to focal meiotic instability in the huntingtin gene at chromosome 4p16.3. There is normally a segment of from 11 to 36 copies of CAG (repeats) in the 5' end.
  - Copy numbers of CAG greater than 37 cause the disease.
    - Increases or decreases in copies of CAG may occur at that site in gametes of persons with the Huntington disease gene, up to 120.
    - Greater numbers of copies cause earlier onset and greater severity.
    - Earlier onset in succeeding generations is termed, anticipation.

4. The clinical triad of arachnodactyly, ectopia lentis, aortic dilatation typifies Marfan syndrome, but unfolding of the full picture may require time, and severity ranges from
    - neonatal lethality to
    - single signs such as
        - isolated ectopia lentis,
        - isolated aortic aneurysm,
        - unusual tallness.

- Mutations in the fibrillin gene (FBN1) at chromosome 15q21 cause Marfan syndrome.
    - Missense mutations which alter a cysteine residue: typical cases.
        - These entail reduced deposition of fibrillin in the extracellular matrix.
            - Severity of cardiovascular features is related to degree of reduction
    - Premature termination codons in the central region: typical cases, neonatal lethality.
    - Exon skipping: milder cases.
    - MRNA instability: milder cases.

- Disorders clinically similar to Marfan syndrome include
    - Contractural arachnodactyly, also a fibrillin deficiency, but caused by
        - mutations in the FBN2 gene at chromosome 5q23.
    - Marfan-like connective tissue disorder: no fibrillin deficiency.
    - Syndromes with collagen abnormalities.
    - Chance concurrences: Mitral prolapse population frequency is 6%, tallness is 3%.

Differential Diagnosis of Marfan Syndrome

Achard syndrome	Fragilitas oculi	Myotonic dystrophy
Ankylosing spondylitis[2]	Homocystinuria[1,3]	Nemaline myopathy
Camptodactyly B	Klinefelter syndrome	Osteogenesis imperfecta[2]
Chromosome 8 trisomy	Lujan-Fryns syndrome[1]	Pseudoxanthoma elasticum
Cobalamin C defect[1]	Marfanoid craniosynostosis[1]	Reiter syndrome[2]
Cobalamin D defect[1]	Marfanoid cutis laxa[1]	Relapsing polychondritis[2]
Contractural arachnodactyly	Marfanoid hypermobility	Snyder-Robinson syndrome[1]
Ehlers-Danlos syndrome[2,3]	Marfanoid mental retardation[1]	Stickler syndrome[3]
Erdheim cystic medial necrosis[2]	Marfanoid microcephaly nephritis[1]	Syphilitic aortitis[2]
Familial bicuspid aortic valve[2]	Marfanoid retinal detachment	Weill-Marchesani syndrome[3]
Familial ectopia lentis[3]	Mitral prolapse syndrome[2]	
Fragile X syndrome	Multiple endocrine adenomatosis III	

[1]neuropsychiatric symptoms [2]cardiovascular symptoms [3]ocular symptoms
Modified from Pyeritz RE, Murphy EA, McKusick VA. Clinical variability in the Marfan syndrome(s). Birth Defects Original Article Series 1979;XV(5B):155-178. See also McKusick VA. *Mendelian Inheritance in Man. Catalogues of Autosomal Dominant, Autosomal Recessive, and X-linked Phenotypes*, 11th edition. Baltimore: The Johns Hopkins Press, 1995.

THE PHENOTYPE OF THE MARFAN SYNDROME

Objective observations:

Metric trait	Parameter	Normals	Marfan syndrome
Long limbs	U/L ratio	White: Mean 1.1 birth .. 0.90 age 12Y	All below Mean, 2/3 below -2 s.d.
		White: -2 s.d 1.0 birth .. 0.85 age 12Y	
		Black: Mean 1.0 birth .. 0.85 age 14Y	
		Black: -2 s.d 0.95 birth .. 0.75 age 14Y	
	Hand/height	< 0.11	> 0.11
	Foot/height	< 0.15	> 0.15
Arachnodactyly	Middle finger/palm	< 1.5	> 1.5

Subjective observations:

Face: Long and narrow, giving children an appearance of soberness and wiseness.

Skeletal: Ligamentous laxity causes loose-jointedness.

Dislocated hips may be present at birth. Protrusio acetabuli is present in most adults.

Arthritis and spondylitis are frequent in older cases.

With growth, some develop fifth finger camptodactyly, elongation of great toe, tallness.

Ocular: Blue sclerae are found in some cases.

Ectopia lentis is easily observed in 50% of adult cases. If examined by slit lamp in maximum mydriasis, redundant suspensory ligaments of lens are present in nearly all cases, and ectopia lentis can be found in 80% of adult cases.

Myopia is present in most cases and may be accompanied by keratoconus or megalocornea.

Cardiac: Aortic dilitation is clinically obvious at birth in some cases and may be found by an experienced echocardiographer in many other cases. Nearly all cases have it by age 10 years.

Severe cases also have dilitation of the pulmonary artery and dissecting aneurysm of the pulmonary artery has been described.

Aortic dilitation begins in the aortic root. There may be saccular enlargements of the valve cusps which drag on the coronary ostia causing angina.

The anterior leaflet of the mitral valve is contiguous with the aortic root and it begins to prolapse into the left atrium while aortic root dilitation progresses. This causes a click which is audible to experienced observers under optimal conditions by age 10. In some cases, it is present at birth.

Mitral insufficiency follows; in severe cases, it is present at birth, causing a soft, late systolic apical murmur a bit lower in intensity than the transmitted background noise of most hospitals.

Catastrophic progression of cardiovascular disease can occur at any age. Most cases develop some degree of aortic insufficiency during puberty. Women frequently develop dissecting aortic aneurysm during or just after pregnancy. Aneurysm may occur in either sex with age. The sudden development of a musical or buzzing murmur is a valuable early sign. Rarely, babies die rapidly of malfunction of all heart valves. This may occur suddenly in adults in rare cases. However, spotty valve involvement and irregular progression is the rule. Average age at death is 32 years, most occurring after age 20, 90% due to aortic disease.

Other: Underdevelopment of muscles and subcutaneous fat.

Hernias.

Cystic disease of the lungs.

Modified from Thurmon TF. *Medical Genetics Primer*. Shreveport, LA: LSU School of Medicine Bookstore, 1995.

5. Myotonic dystrophy is due to focal meiotic instability in the myotonin-protein kinase gene at chromosome 19p13.2. There are normally from 5 to 35 copies of CTG (repeats) in the 3' end.
    *   Copy numbers of CTG greater than 50 cause a disease characterized by
        *   myotonia, muscle wasting and cataracts, usually becoming apparent
        *   sometime in the third or fourth decade of life but occasionally in the second.

    *   Decreases in copies of CTG may occur at that site in gametes, or increases up to 3000.
        *   Greater numbers of copies cause earlier onset and greater severity.
        *   Anticipation is observed in families with this disease.
        *   Transmission from the mother may result in the neonatal form, characterized by
            *   hypotonia, psychomotor retardation and facial diplegia, which may be fatal.
            *   Survivors develop myotonia around 10 years, then follow the course of the adult form.

    *   Types of malignant hyperthermia may exhibit symptoms similar to myotonic dystrophy,
        *   such as myopathy and hypertonicity.
            *   Laboratory proof of myotonic dystrophy makes malignant hyperthermia less likely.

6. Type I neurofibromatosis (von Recklinghausen disease) is typically a progressive disorder.
    *   Cafe-au-lait spots may be present at birth or may appear during infancy or childhood.
        *   The spots increase in size and number with age.
    *   Dermal neurofibromas may appear at any time but typically after age 10 years.
        *   They may also occur in other organs and body parts.
        *   The tumors increase in size and number with age.
    *   Axillary freckling and Lisch nodules of the iris increase in frequency with age.
    *   Other common features include macrocephaly, short stature and developmental disorder.
    *   Many tumors occur with increased frequency in neurofibromatosis, including
        *   pheochromocytoma, optic glioma, acoustic neuroma, meningioma, and others.
        *   Some are malignant.

    *   Neurofibromatosis is caused by mutations ranging from point mutations to megabase deletions in the NF1 gene at chromosome 17q11.2, a 350 kb gene with a 12 kb mRNA and 59 exons
        *   which result in absence or dysfunction of its 2818 amino acid product, neurofibromin,
            *   the normal function of which is to down-regulate the p21-ras oncogene.

    *   Type II neurofibromatosis has mainly an etymological relationship to Type I.
        *   It is also called NF2 but the gene designation is SCH, a tumor suppressor gene
            *   at chromosome 22q12.2, the product of which is called merlin or schwannomin.

    *   The disease produced by mutations in SCH is also called bilateral acoustic neurinoma.
        *   Typical features include neurological tumors at any age but usually around age 22 years:
            *   Bilateral eighth cranial nerve schwannomas,
                *   also called neuromas, neurinomas, neurofibromas.
            *   Meningiomas of the brain.
            *   Schwannomas of the dorsal roots of the spinal cord.

- Typical eighth nerve tumor symptoms include tinnitus, deafness, blindness.
  Other features of type II neurofibromatosis include:
  - Circumscribed, slightly raised, roughened skin areas often pigmented and hairy.
  - Scattered cafe-au-lait spots, usually less than 6.
  - Neuropathy, sometimes with spherical subcutaneous tumors on peripheral nerves.

Disorders that have been called Osteogenesis Imperfecta
(all are characterized by fractures from minimal trauma)

Type	blue sclerae	deafness	dentinogenesis imperfecta	short stature	Other	Seg	MIM
I Tarda	+++	++	+/-	+/-	Null allele of COL1A1, or structural mutation in either COL1A1 or COL1A2	AD	166200 166220 166230 166240 166260
II Congenita. Perinatal lethal.	++	+/-	+/-	++++	Frequently lethal. Poor skull mineralization, congenital fractures. Rearrangements in COL1A1 or COL1A2	AD AR	166210 259400 259410 259440 259450
III Progressive deforming	+	++	++	++++	Recurrent fractures, progressive deformity sclerae lighten with age. Point mutations in COL1A1 or COL1A2. Frameshift mutation in COL1A2	AD AR	none 259420 259440
IV Normal sclerae	-	+/-	++	+/-	Point mutation or small deletion in COL1A2, rarely in COL1A1.	AD	166220

Modified from: Byers PH. Osteogenesis imperfecta. In Steinmann B, Royce PM (editors). *Connective Tissue and Its Heritable Disorders. Molecular, Genetic and Medical Aspects.* New York: Wiley Liss, 1993:317.

7. Osteogenesis imperfecta is a collection of diseases due to mutations in collagen genes
   - COL1A1 and COL1A2, the same genes that are associated with
     - some types of Ehlers-Danlos syndrome.
   - The central feature is fragility of bones, which, in the most severe form,
     - osteogenesis imperfecta congenita, occur in the fetus.
   - Fractures in the other forms may occur at any age, including the newborn.
     - When noticed incidentally, fractures may raise suspicion of child abuse.

- Each phenotypic category of osteogenesis imperfecta
  - may be caused by several different genetic abnormalities.
  - There is also unexplained variability in expression of the phenotype
    - in patients with the same genetic abnormality.

- Other features of osteogenesis imperfecta stem from the generalized defects of collagen:
  - Hearing loss appears to be due to innumerable microfractures in the auditory apparatus,
    - and is potentially preventable.
  - Sclerae are thin, fragile, and translucent, and have a blue hue which is exaggerated by
    - underlying dark choroid
  - Teeth may also be translucent, which is termed, opalescent dentin.
    - Dentinogenesis imperfecta may result if the dental tissue defect is severe.

8. Cystic fibrosis may be apparent in the newborn as meconeum ileus, but usually shows up as
   - chronic malabsorption sometime in the first year of life.
   - Lung infections follow, and gradually become chronic and destructive,
     - eventually culminating in death due to pulmonary failure.
   - Heat intolerance and infertility are also observed.

- Cystic fibrosis is caused by homozygosity or compound heterozygosity for mutations in the
  - gene for the cystic fibrosis transmembrane receptor (CFTR) at chromosome 7q31.2, an ATP-binding transporter protein comprised of 5 domains: 2 membrane-spanning domains (MSD) which constitute the chloride channel pore, 1 R domain which opens the channel, and 2 nucleotide binding domains (NBD) which interact with ATP.
    - Mutations in CFTR cause defective chloride transport in the apical membrane of epithelial cells of sweat glands, airways, pancreas and intestine, rendering it more or less impermeable to the chloride ion, leading to insufficient, thickened, inspissated exocrine secretions:
      - Class 1 (null alleles): defective protein synthesis.
      - Class 2: defective protein processing.
      - Class 3: defective regulation of channel.
      - Class 4: defective conduction through channel (milder phenotypes).
    - 70% of mutant genes in Europeans is accounted for by DF508, a Class 2 mutation which deletes a CTT that should code for phenylalanine in exon 10 of the first NBD.
    - Over 400 other mutations are known, and there is no general test for all of them

9. Hurler syndrome is a progressive disorder. It may not be noticed at birth, or
   - the affected baby may seem particularly plump and healthy-looking.
   - Abnormalities usually appear in the first year: poor weight gain (failure to thrive),
     - poor development or coarsening of features.
       - All are usually present by age 2 years.

- Gargoylism is an effete synonym which refers to the somatic changes.
  - The eyes slowly grow to bulge, the face widens, the jaw thickens,
    - and a perpetual grimace develops.
  - Joint sockets fill in, joint movements become awkward and range of motion is limited.
  - Growth is stunted and the body assumes a gnarled habitus with protuberant abdomen,
    - due in part to hepatosplenomegaly
  - Corneal dystrophy leads to poor vision. Progressive sensorineural deafness occurs.
  - Heart failure occurs due to compromise of valve function.
  - The disease is eventually fatal in early adulthood.

- Hurler syndrome is caused by homozygosity or compound heterozygosity for mutations
  - in the alpha-L-iduronidase gene near the huntingtin gene at chromosome 4p16.3.
    - Alpha-L-iduronidase participates in degradation of intracellular mucopolysaccharide as part of the normal mechanisms that refresh cell components.
  - The gene comprises 14 exons that span 19 kb, with a 13 kb intron between introns 1 & 2.
  - Many different types of mutations have been identified but half are accounted for by two common alleles (Trp402→ter, Gln70→ter) and one minor allele (Pro533→Arg).

  - Clinically important mutations cause poor or absent function of alpha-L-iduronidase.
    - Mucopolysaccharides and chemical by-products accumulate in lysosomes until they compromise cell integrity, then spillage occurs, and, eventually, cell death.

10. Most cases of phenylketonuria are caused by compound heterozygosity for mutations at the phenylalanine hydroxylase locus at chromosome 12q22. Some cases are homozygotes.
    - The gene comprises 13 exons spanning 90kb, and has over 70 RFLP hsplotypes. Over 100 different mutations are known (missense, nonsense, insertions, deletions).
    - Each ethnic group has a characteristic array of mutations and associated haplotypes for which phenotypes vary in clinical severity.
    - A few of the more severe cases are accounted for by mutations in the
      - dihydrobiopterin reductase locus at chromosome 4p15.1,
      - GTP cyclohydrolase locus, possibly at chromosome 14q11,
      - 6-pyruvoyl-tetrahydropterin synthetase locus at chromosome 11q23.3,
      - and other yet unidentified loci.

- Mild cases of phenylalanine hydroxylase deficiency (blood phenylalanine always below 1000μM [N=58±15] on normal diet) account for about 1/3 of cases of hyperphenylalaninemia. They may be asymptomatic, but most probably have different degrees of progressive cognitive disorder.

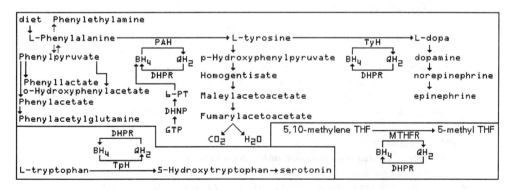

Metabolic pathways related to hyperphenylalaninemias. PAH: phenylalanine hydroxylase. QH_2: quininoid dihydrobiopterin. BH_4: tetrahydrobiopterin. DHPR: dihydrobiopterin reductase. 6-PT: 6-pyruvoyltetrahydropterin. DHNP: dihydroneopterin triphosphate. GTP: guanosine triphosphate. TyH: tyrosine hydroxylase. TpH: tryptophan hydroxylase. THF: tetrahydrofolate. MTHFR: methylene tetrahydrofolate reductase.

- Clinical picture of classic phenylketonuria (phenylalanine intake produces symptoms):
  - Most are asymptomatic in first year, few ever diagnosed without laboratory screening; 25% have eczema and some have a musty odor and depigmentation.
  - Thereafter, a progressive neuroencephalopathy occurs. Some never walk or talk. Many have seizures. Most have hyperactive, agitated and aggressive behavior.
  - Other common findings are tremor, microcephaly, prominent maxilla with widened interdental spaces and enamel hypoplasia, decalcification of long bones, poor growth.
  - Severe older cases may develop *Schneidersitz*, a sitting posture with incessant rhythmic movements of arms.

- Clinical picture of dihydrobiopterin reductase (DHPR) defect.
  - Low birth weight, poor growth and development, and other symptoms of DOPA and serotonin deficiency: poor feeding, choking, seizures. Biopterin is a co-factor in the paths from tyrosine to DOPA, typtophan to serotonin, and folate to activated folate. Symptoms occur without phenylalanine intake.

- Clinical picture of dihydrobiopterin synthesis defect: deficiency of either GTP cyclohydrolase or 6-pyruvoyl-tetrahydropterin synthetase.
  - More profound deficit of biopterin. Additional symptoms include spasticity, drooling, athetosis, myoclonus. Symptoms occur without phenylalanine intake.

11. The sickle mutation changes the sixth codon from GAG to GTC (Glu6→Val) in the
    - hemoglobin beta locus chain at chromosome 11p15.5.
      - It deletes a MstII recognition site, causing a longer fragment to be diagnostic.
    - A Glu6→Lys in the same codon causes hemoglobin C.

- Sickle cell disease is classified as an autosomal recessive disorder but there has been
  - controversy as to whether heterozygotes are truly free of disease.
    - They are identifiable by their relative resistance to malaria.

- Hemolytic anemia is a characteristic feature of sickle cell anemia.
  - It becomes evident toward the first year of life after fetal hemoglobin has dwindled.
  - Transfer of oxygen from red blood cells in peripheral vasculature to tissue
    - polymerizes sickle hemoglobin into long strands which
      - deform the erythrocyte into the sickle shape.
  - Some sickled cells circulating through the spleen snag there and lyse.

- Painful episodes called sickle cell crises begin shortly after the hemolytic anemia.
  - Tangles of sickled cells embolize small blood vessels,
    - causing ischemia randomly throughout the body.
  - Resulting damage to the brain and other vital organs eventually debilitates
    - and, finally, kills the patient in early adulthood.

- Coexisting with either heterozygosity or homozygosity for the sickle cell mutation
  - may be varying numbers of copies of genes for
    - alpha thalassemia, beta thalassemia, and hemoglobin C, reported in most cases
      - to produce phenotypes less severe than pure sickle cell homozygosity.

- Heterozygosity for hemoglobin D or hemoglobin O-Arab (alpha locus), combined with
  - heterozygosity for the sickle cell mutation is termed, double heterozygosity.
    - It produces a disease picture like homozygosity for the sickle cell mutation

- DNA polymorphisms in the hemoglobin beta gene that are non-randomly associated with the
  - sickle cell mutation link bearers of the sickle cell mutation to one of five family groups:
    - equatorial, eastern and southern Africa Bantu,
    - Atlantic west Africa Senegal,
    - central west Africa Benin,
    - central Africa Cameroon Eton,
    - Saudi Arabia-India.

12. Thalassemia has been present for thousands of years but was first differentiated from the
    - background of human suffering in 1925 by Cooley and Lee.
    - Whipple and Lee coined the name from θαλασσα, the Greek word for sea, because studies of the genetic demography of the disease suggested to them that it had been spread by Greek colonization of the Mediterranean.

- Mutations of many types in the loci for hemoglobin chains, including beta, delta (also at chromosome 11p15.5), delta-beta fusions, and alpha (chromosome 16p13.3),
  - cause inadequate or absent synthesis of hemoglobin, which is the basis of the disease,
  - anemia that is unresponsive to iron therapy.
  - The most severe varieties do not allow adequate synthesis of fetal hemoglobin,
    - and manifest as hydrops fetalis.
  - Most other types begin in the first year of life when fetal hemoglobin dwindles,
    - and rapidly develop into their final forms.

- In the severe forms of postnatal onset thalassemia, compensatory mechanisms switch in and
  - hematopoetic tissues hypertrophy, resulting in bony deformities and hepatosplenomegaly.
  - Growth is stunted and secondary sexual characteristics fail to develop.
  - Infertility and leg ulcers are later signs.
  Milder forms may cause only chronic anemia.

- Careful and detailed nosology allows some order in categorization.
  - The most basic groupings are into the forms involving primarily the alpha chain
    - and those involving primarily the beta chain.
  - Another variety is called delta beta thalassemia.
  - The complex hemoglobin molecule provides many other possible sites of disorder and
    - most have been found to exist, albeit rare.

Thalassemia Examples

Disease	Clinical	Laboratory	Genetic	Parents	
Homozygous α thalassemia	hydrops fetalis	A 0 A_2 0 F 0 Bart's 85% Portland 15%	all four α genes inactive	—/αα	—/αα
Hemoglobin H disease	thalassemia intermedia	A 75% H 25% Bart's 25% (cord)	three α genes inactive	—/αα	–α /αα
Heterozygous α thalassemia	thalassemia minor	Bart's 15% (cord)	two α genes inactive	—/αα .... –α /αα	αα /αα .... –α /αα
Silent	none	Bart's 1% (cord)	one α gene inactive	–α /αα	αα /αα
Homozygous $β^0$ thalassemia	thalassemia major	A 0 A_2 5% F 95%	both β genes inactive	$β^0/β$	$β^0/β$
Homozygous $β^+$ thalassemia	thalassemia major	A 25% A_2 5% F 60%	mutations in both β genes	$β^+/β$	$β^+/β$
Heterozygous $β^0$ thalassemia	thalassemia minor	A 90 A_2 5% F 5%	one β gene inactive	$β^0/β$	β/β
Heterozygous $β^+$ thalassemia	thalassemia minor	A 25% A_2 5% F 60%	mutations in one β gene	$β^+/β$	β/β
Homozygous δβ thalassemia	thalassemia intermedia	A 0 A_2 0% F 100%	both δ and β genes inactive	$δβ^0/β$	$δβ^0/β$
Heterozygous δβ thalassemia	thalassemia minor	A 80% A_2 5% F 15%	one δ and β gene inactive	$δβ^0/β$	β/β

13. Muscular dystrophy is an X-linked disorder.
    - Females who have the gene are usually heterozygous,
        - while males are hemizygous.

- Most forms are due to various mutations in the 2.3 mb DMD gene at chromosome Xp21,
    - which produces an mRNA transcript of 14 kb; space for a vast repetoire of mutations. Many types have been observed. See the LDL receptor illustration for examples of types.
    - The type of mutation correlates with disease severity but there is
        - poor correlation with amount of gene involved.

- Duchenne muscular dystrophy is the most severe variety and is characterized by
  - absence of the 3685 amino acid gene product, dystrophin.
  - Progressive muscle weakness begins before three years of age,
    - and peaks before 12 years of age.
  - Creatine phosphokinase levels over 10,000 IU/ml are common.
  - Fatty hypertrophy of calves occurs sometimes.
  - Mental retardation and cardiomyopathy are frequently observed,
  - Survival beyond the third decade is rare.

- Becker muscular dystrophy is a milder variety and is characterized by
  - dystrophin that is abnormal in either size or quantity.
  - Creatine phosphokinase levels over 1,000 IU/ml are observed during childhood,
    - but then tail off.
  - Fatty hypertrophy of calves is common.
  - Survival is prolonged but patients usually cannot walk after 40 years of age.

- Different promoter genes of the DMD gene operate in brain, heart, and muscle.
  - Deletion of the brain promoter can cause X-linked mental retardation.
  - Deletion of the heart promoter can cause X-linked dilated cardiomyopathy.

14. Cell culture for chromosome analysis done under conditions of thymidine deprivation reveals fragile site heteromorphisms where chromosome arms may fracture, most associated with no perceptible phenotypic abnormality, but the *fragile X syndrome* is associated with
  - excessive frequency of fractures at the fragile site on Xq27:
    - familial mental retardation (mainly in males) or subnormality (mainly in females),
    - long face with large ears and prominent jaw,
    - high-pitched jocular speech in males, shyness in females,
    - hypermobile joints, especially in fingers,
    - macroorchidism in males.

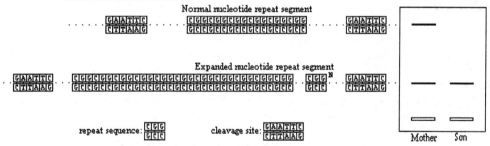

Electrophoresis and probe visualization of DNA fragments from the FMR-1 locus. The restriction enzyme cleaves at sites that bracket the FMR-1 gene. The mother has a normal repeat sequence on one X chromosome and an expanded one on the other, so she has two bands; one containing the normal segment which is smaller and moves faster in the electrophoresis gel, and one containing the expanded segment which is larger and moves slower. Each son receives only one X chromosome from his mother. In this case, it happened to be the one with the expanded segment, causing fragile X syndrome.

- Meiotic instability of short tandem repeats on the X chromosome causes the fragility.
  - Fragile X syndrome results when greater than 150 CGG repeats occur at the 5' end of the FMR-1 gene on Xq (mean=30 [range=5-51]), accompanied by
    - methylation of an adjacent CpG island (multiple repeats of 5'-CG-3'),
      - which shuts down gene function.
  - Females are less uniformly affected than males.
  - Unaffected carriers ("premutation") having over 57 repeats, estimated to be
    - approximately 0.2% - 0.8% of females, do not methylate the CpG island, but
    - have a tendency toward amplification of repeats during meiosis, which results in expression of the phenotype in their children.
  - Rarely, men with the gene fail to methylate the CpG island (Normal Transmitting Males), and do not express the phenotype, nor do their daughters who receive the gene from that father, but subsequent transmission of the gene by a daughter can result in expression.

15. Hemophilia is a category of X-linked disease in which
    - many forms of bleeding disorders are included.
      - Most types are caused by mutations in FVIII, a 186kb gene on the X chromosome
        - near the tip (Xq28), which produces a 9 kb mRNA transcript.
        - Point mutations account for 95% of cases, and deletions, 5%.
      - Hemophilia A, the best known type of hemophilia is due to deficiency of the 2332
        - amino acid protein product, factor VIII, which, with factor IX normally functions to activate factor X in the coagulation chain reaction.
      - Severity depends on the degree to which the mutation inactivates factor VIII.
        - Mild 10-30 U/dl [N≥35], moderate 2-10 U/dl, severe <2 U/dl (50% of patients)

    - Hemophilia A may cause bleeding from the umbilical cord or circumcision in the newborn
      - but usually becomes apparent as excessive bruises in the toddler.
    - Minor trauma causes bleeding from mucous membranes.
    - Internal bleeding may also occur.
    - Painful bleeding into joints increases in frequency with age
      - and often results in degenerative joint disease.
    - Bleeding from surgical or dental procedures can be fatal in the undiagnosed patient.
    - The eventual cause of death in most cases is intracranial hemorrhage.

  - Standard bleeding and clotting times are usually within normal limits.
    - The best initial test is the activated partial thromboplastin time.
      - If it is prolonged, the next appropriate test is a factor VIII level.
    - Hemophilia B may be so clinically similar that a factor IX level
      - should be done if the factor VIII is normal.
    - If factor VIII and factor IX both are normal,
      - still rarer factor deficiencies may be at fault.

  - Factor IX deficiency (hemophilia B or Christmas disease) is caused by
    - one of a number of mutations in FIX, a 34 kb gene at chromosome Xq27.1,
      - that produces factor IX, a 415 amino acid protein.

- Von Willebrand disease is a much more common variety of factor VIII deficiency.
  - It is usually a much milder bleeding disorder with autosomal dominant transmission,
    - and rarely causes joint disease. It is caused by one of several mutations
  - in the 180 kb vWF gene at chromosome 12p13.3.
    - The FVIII gene is normal.
  - The product of the vWF gene is von Willebrand factor, a 2813 amino acid protein
    - that binds to factor VIII and stabilizes it in blood, and is
    - required for survival of factor VIII in vivo.
  - This protein is also required for platelet aggregation
    - so the standard bleeding time is prolonged.

16. Leber hereditary optic atrophy (LHON) typically begins between 12 and 30 years of age, with
    - blurring and color fading in the center of the visual field. This progresses to
    - marked deficiency of visual acuity over about 4 months. Examination discloses
    - tortuosity of the retinal vessels and telangiectasia around the optic nerve is seen.
    - Cardiac conduction defects are frequently observed.

  - At least 12 different mutations in the mitochondrial genome are causative. LHON occurs in
    - 85% of males and 20% of females who harbor one of these mutations

  - Most patients have a G to A point mutation at mitochondrial locus 11778 (NADHd4),
    - which impairs its function in oxydative phosphorylation.
    - 20% of cases have a G to A point mutation at mitochondrial locus 3460 (NADHd1).
    - In a few cases, a T to C point mutation at mitochondrial locus 4160 (NADHd1) causes LHON in association with a complex neurological disorder.
    - A number of other mutations have also been found.
      - Some cases have several mutations in the same or different mitochondrial genomes.
    - Age of onset, progression time and residual vision are highly variable.
      - Identification of the mutation, or mutations, involved can clarify this to a degree.

17. Mitochondrial myopathy, encephalopathy, lactic acidosis, and stroke-like episodes (MELAS)
    - typically begins around 10 years of age with an acute episode of vomiting and a
      - tonic-clonic or atonic seizure during which a moderate elevation of
        - blood lactate is discovered.
      - It usually clears with supportive therapy and anticonvulsants but tends to recur.
    - Actual strokes and paralysis occur in severe cases, and there may be
    - vision loss ranging from hemianopsia to cortical blindness.
    - Hearing loss also occurs, and
    - progressive dementia is observed in some cases.
    - Some have ragged red fibers on muscle biopsy.

  - Children with MELAS are often said to be normal prior to its onset
    - but accurate evaluation may disclose pre-existing
      - muscle weakness, learning problems, and poor growth.

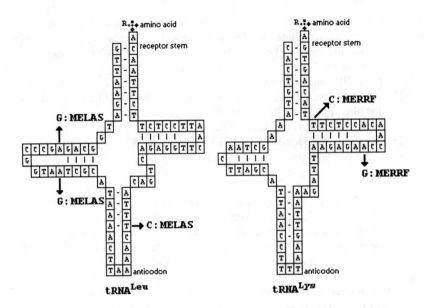

Mutations in mitochondrial transfer RNA that produce MELAS or MERRF

- Most patients have an A to G point mutation at mitochondrial locus 3243 (tRNA-leu (UUR)).
  - A few have a T to C mutation at locus 3271, or A to G mutation at locus 3252.
    - There are numerous cases with unidentified mutations.

18. Myoclonic epilepsy associated with ragged red fibers (MERRF)
    - typically begins around 10 years of age with an seizure in which there is
      - involuntary muscle jerking (myoclonus).
    - The patient is often ataxic afterwards.
    - In more severe cases, there are frequent myoclonic seizures,
      - and the weakness and ataxia progress to a bed-ridden state.
    - Some patients have hearing loss, nephropathy and dilated cardiomyopathy.

    - Lactic acidosis is often discovered during diagnostic evaluation
      - as are ragged red muscle fibers. The muscle biopsy abnormality is often segmental,
        - which is consistent with the mitochondrial genetic drift tendency.

    - Children with MERFF are often said to be normal prior to its onset
      - but accurate evaluation may disclose pre-existing
        - muscle weakness, learning problems, and poor growth.

    - Most patients have an A to G mutation at mitochondrial locus 8344 (tRNA-lys (MTTK)).
      - A few have a T to C mutation at locus 8356.
      - Various other tRNA mutations may produce a more severe form,
        - lethal infantile mitochondrial myopathy (LIMM).

Additional references:

Ainsworth PJ, Rodenhiser DI, Costa MT. Identification and characterization of sporadic and inherited mutations in exon 31 of the neurofibromatosis (NF1) gene. Hum Genet 1993;91:151-56.

Andrew SE, Goldberg YP, Kremer B, et al. The relationship between trinucleotide (CAG) repeat length and clinical features of Huntington's disease. Nature Genet. 1993; 4:398-403.

Bernstam VA. *Handbook of Gene Level Diagnostics in Clinical Practice*. Boca Raton, FL: CRC Press, 1992:385-94.

Boileau C, Jondeau G, Babron M-C, et al. Autosomal dominant Marfan-like connective-tissue disorder with aortic dilation and skeletal anomalies not linked to the fibrillin gene. Am J Hum Genet 1993;53:46-54.

Byers PH. Disorders of collagen biosynthesis and structure. In: Scriver CR, Beaudet AL, Sly WS, et al (editors). *The Metabolic and Molecular Bases of Inherited Disease. 7ᵗʰ Edition*. New York: McGraw-Hill, 1995:4029-4077.

Cooley TB, Lee P. A series of cases of splenomegaly in children with anemia and peculiar bone changes. Trans Am Pediat Soc 1925;37:29.

Dietz HC. Marfan syndrome caused by a recurrent de novo missense mutation in the fibrillin gene. Nature 1991;352:337-9.

Dougherty FE, Ernst SG, Aprille JR. Familial recurrence of atypical symptoms in an extended pedigree with the syndrome of mitochondrial encephalopathy, lactic acidosis, and stroke-like episodes. J Pediatr 1994;125:758-61.

Eisensmith RC, Woo SLC. Molecular basis of phenylketonuria and related hyperphenylalaninemias: mutations and polymorphisms in the human phenylalanine hydroxylase gene. Hum. Mutat. 1992;1:13-23.

Emery AEH. *Oxford Monographs on Medical Genetics No 15. Duchenne Muscular Dystrophy*. Oxford: Oxford University Press,1987.

Folstein SE, Abbott MH, Franz ML,et al. Phenotypic heterogeneity in Huntington disease. J Neurogenet 1984;1:175-184.

Folstein SE, Chase GA, Wahl WE, et al. Huntington disease in Maryland: clinical aspects of racial variation. Am J Hum Genet 1987;41:168-179.

Folstein SE, Phillips JA, Meyers DA, et al. Huntington's disease: two families with differing clinical features show linkage to the G8 probe. Science 1985;229:776-779.

Fullerton SM, Harding RM, Boyce AJ, et al. The origin of the sickle cell mutation in human populations: Insights from the study of DNA sequence polymorphism at the beta-globin locus. Am J Hum Biol 1995;7:123.

Harper PS. Myotonic dystrophy and other autosomal muscular dystrophies. In: Scriver CR, Beaudet AL, Sly WS, et al (editors). *The Metabolic and Molecular Bases of Inherited Disease. 7ᵗʰ Edition*. New York: McGraw-Hill, 1995:4227-51.

Lee B, Godfrey M, Vitale E, et al. Linkage of Marfan syndrome and a phenotypically related disorder to two different fibrillin genes. Nature 1991;352:330-4.

Loesch DZ, Hay DA. Clinical features and reproductive patterns in fragile X female heterozygotes. J Med Genet 1988;25:407-14.

Mandel JL, Hagerman R, Froster U, et al. Fifth International Workshop on the Fragile X and X-Linked Mental Retardation. Am J Med Genet 1992;43:5-27.

McKusick VA. *Heritable Disorders of Connective Tissue*. New York: Mosby, 1972.

Muntoni F, Cau M, Ganau A, et al. Deletion of the dystrophin muscle-promoter region associated with X-linked dilated cardiomyopathy. N Engl J Med 1993;329:921-5.

Nagel RL, Fleming AF. Genetic epidemiology of the beta-s gene. Baillieres Clin Hematol 1992;5:331-65.

Nelson DL, Eichler E, King JE, et al. Characterization of the FMR-1 gene at the FRAXA locus of man. Abstract 186. Am J Hum Genet 1992;51 (Supplement):A49.

Neufeld EF, Muenzer J. The mucopolysaccharidoses. In: Scriver CR, Beaudet AL, Sly WS, et al (editors). *The Metabolic and Molecular Bases of Inherited Disease. 7th Edition*. New York: McGraw-Hill, 1995:2465-2494.

Nussbaum RL, Ledbetter DH. The fragile X syndrome. In: Scriver CR, Beaudet AL, Sly WS, et al (editors). *The Metabolic and Molecular Bases of Inherited Disease. 7th Edition*. New York: McGraw-Hill, 1995:795-810.

Newman NJ. Leber's hereditary optic neuropathy: New genetic considerations. Arch Neurol 1993;50:540-48.

Orkin SH. Disorders of hemoglobin synthesis: The thalassemias. In: Stamatoyannopoulos G, Nienhuis AW, Leder P, et al (editors). *The Molecular Basis of Blood Diseases*. Philadelphia PA: W. B. Saunders, 1987:106-126.

Pyeritz RE. The Marfan syndrome. American Family Physician 1986;34:1-12.

Riccardi VM, Eichner JE. *Neurofibromatosis: Phenotype, Natural History and Pathogenesis*. Baltimore, MD: Johns Hopkins Univ Press, 1986.

Sadler JE, Davie EW. Hemophilia A, hemophilia B, and von Willebrand's disease. In: Stamatoyannopoulos G, Nienhuis AW, Leder P, et al. *The Molecular Basis of Blood Diseases*. Philadelphia PA: W. B. Saunders, 1987:575-630.

Scriver CR, Kaufman S, Eisensmith RC, Woo SLC. The hyperphenylalaninemias. In: Scriver CR, Beaudet AL, Sly WS, et al (editors). *The Metabolic and Molecular Bases of Inherited Disease. 7th Edition*. New York: McGraw-Hill, 1995:1015-1075.

Schechter AN, Noguchi CT, Rodgers GP. Sickle cell disease. In: Stamatoyannopoulos G, Nienhuis AW, Leder P, et al (editors). *The Molecular Basis of Blood Diseases*. Philadelphia PA: W. B. Saunders, 1987:179-218.

Shoffner JM, Wallace DC. Oxidative phosphorylation diseases. In: Scriver CR, Beaudet AL, Sly WS, et al (editors). *The Metabolic and Molecular Bases of Inherited Disease. 7th Edition*. New York: McGraw-Hill, 1995:1535-1609.

Snow K, Doud LK, Hagerman R, et al. Analysis of a CGG repeat at the FMR-1 locus in Fragile X families and in the general population. Abstract 185. Am J Hum Genet 1992;51 (Supplement):A49.

Welsh MJ, Tsui L-C, Boat TF, et al. Cystic fibrosis. In: Scriver CR, Beaudet AL, Sly WS, et al (editors). *The Metabolic and Molecular Bases of Inherited Disease. 7th Edition*. New York: McGraw-Hill, 1995:3799-3876.

Wertelecki W, Rouleau GA, Superneau DW, et al. Neurofibromatosis 2: clinical and DNA linkage studies of a large kindred. N Engl J Med 1988;319:278-83.

Whipple GH, Bradford WL. Mediterranean disease-thalassemia (erythroblastic anemia of Cooley). J Pediatr 1936;9:279.

PHARMACOKINETICS

1.   Pharmacokinetic genetic variations include
    * polygenic control of distribution, and
    * polymorphisms.

    * Population distribution parameters for most drugs are Gaussian.
        * Within a normal population, ranges are sufficient that
            * toxicity may result among the few persons at one extreme of the curve, and
            * inadequate therapeutic effect among the few persons in the other extreme.

Examples of Heritability of Drug Distribution

Drug	Dose	Parameter	Range	h^2
Antipyrine	18 mg/kg po once	plasma half-life	5.1 - 16.7 hr	0.99
Phenylbutazone	6 mg/kg po once	plasma half-life	1.2 - 7.3 days	0.99
Dicumarol	4 mg/kg po once	plasma half-life	7.0 - 74.0 hr	0.98
Halothane	3.4 mg iv once	excretion/24 hr	2.4 - 11.4 %	0.63
Ethanol	1.2 ml/kg once	absorption/hr	0.40 - 2.24 mg/ml	0.57
	1.2 ml/kg once	clearance/hr	0.073 -0.255 mg/ml	0.41
Diphenylhydantoin	100 mg iv once	serum half life	7.7 - 25.5 hr	0.85
Lithium	600 mg /da x 7	plasma level	0.16 - 0.38 mEg/l	0.86
Amobarbital	125 mg iv once	clearance	16.0 - 67.2 ml/min	0.83
Nortriptyline	0.6 mg/kg/da x 8	plasma level	8 - 78 ng/ml	
Sodium salicylate	40 mg/kg iv once	decay slope	0.64 - 1.02 mg/dl/hr	0.86
Aspirin	65 mg/kg/da x 3	plasma level	11.9 - 36.4 mg/dl	0.98
	65 mg/kg/da x 3	excretion rate	0.84 - 1.91 mg/kg/hr	0.89

Data from Vogel F, Motulsky AG (1986)

* Pharmacogenetic polymorphisms predate the drugs and probably function for other purposes though few such purposes are known. Forces thought to maintain the polymorphisms are
    * genetic drift and selection.
        * Malaria selects for G6PD deficiency which protects against it.
        * Selection by other diseases, environmental agents and dietary factors is possible.

* Plasma pseudocholinesterase rapidly degrades the surgical paralytic, succinyldicholine, to its inactive form, succinylmonocholine, over about 10 minutes after a single iv dose.
    * Three well-known alleles have less activity that the common allele (E^u_1),
        * based on the reaction rate with the substrate benzoylcholine:
        Fluoride resistant (E^f_1): Slightly decreased activity. Frequency 1.2% in caucasians.
        Atypical (E^a_1): Moderately decreased activity. Frequency 3.4% in caucasians.
        Silent (E^s_1): Absent activity. Frequency 0.5% in Caucasians, 1.5% in Eskimos.
        * Homozygotes or compound heterozygotes experience prolonged paralysis.
    * Other alleles may be detected if succinyldicholine is used as the substrate.

Pseudocholinesterase Phenotypes

Phenotype	Caucasian frequency	Dibucaine inhibition	Fluoride inhibition	Succinyldicholine sensitivity
E^u_1/E^u_1	0.95	0.80	0.59	normal
E^u_1/E^a_1	0.035	0.62	0.48	+
E^u_1/E^f_1	0.012	0.74	0.50	+
E^u_1/E^s_1	0.005	0.80	0.59	?
E^a_1/E^f_1	0.0004	0.49	0.33	+++
E^a_1/E^a_1	0.0003	0.22	0.27	+++
E^a_1/E^s_1	0.00009	0.22	0.27	+++
E^f_1/E^f_1	0.00003	0.66	0.35	++
E^f_1/E^s_1	0.00003	0.67	0.43	++
E^s_1/E^s_1	0.000005	1.00	1.00	++++

- Hepatic N-acetyltransferase participates in drug metabolism by acetylation.
  - Homozygosity for a common allele (Ac^s) causes poor acetylation ("slow inactivation"),
    - which can result in adverse effects from excessive blood levels of drugs..
  - Normal acetylation ("rapid inactivation") results from
    - homozygosity or heterozygosity from the other allele (Ac^R).

N-acetyltransferase "Slow Inactivator" Polymorphism

Ethnic group	Phenotype frequency	Drugs affected	Reported adverse effects
Ashkenizim	0.71	Dapsone	methemoglobinemia
Africans	0.55	Diphenylhydantoin	ataxia, nystagmus
Europeans	0.49	Hydralizine	hypotension
Siamese	0.42	Isoniazid	polyneuritis
Chinese	0.15	Nitrazepam	ataxia, nausea
Japanese	0.12	Phenelzine	vertigo
Eskimos	0.14	Procainamide	lupus erythematosis
		Sulfadimizine	methemoglobinemia
		Sulfapyridine	methemoglobinemia

- Many hepatic cytochromes P-450 participate in metabolism of many drugs.
  - There are at least 12 families containing at least 17 subfamilies,
    - most of which are clusters of tightly linked genes.
  - Better defined polymorphisms include:

Family	Polymorphism	Ethnic group frequency				
		Africa	Arab	Europe	China	Japan
CYP1A2	Phenacetin O-deethylase defect: methemoglobinemia from phenacetin.			5%		
CYP2C	Mephenytoin hydroxylation defect: ataxia, nausea, lethargy from mesantoin or diphenylhydantoin.			5%	5%	23%
CYP2D	Debrisoquine hydroxylation defect: see table.	6%	1%	9%	30%	rare

Cytochrome P-450 CYP2D "Poor Metabolizer" Polymorphism

Drugs	Adverse effects	Drugs	Adverse effects
Alprenolol	bradycardia, hypotension	Nifedipine	hypotension, dizziness, weakness
Amitriptyline	postural hypotension	Nortriptyline	postural hypotension
Bufuralol	bradycardia, hypotension	Penicillamine	proteinuria, thrombocytopenia
Captopril	agranulocytosis	Perhexilene	peripheral neuropathy, agranulocytosis
Debrisoquine	hypotension	Phenformin	lactic acidosis
Desipramine	hypotension, stupor	Propafenone	somnolence, cardiac arrhythmias
Encainide	inactive	Propranolol	bradycardia, hypotension
Guanoxan	hypotension	Sparteine	cardiac depression, uterine contraction
Metiamide	agranulocytosis	Timolol	bradycardia, hypotension
Metoprolol	bradycardia, hypotension		

- Ethanol intolerance is mediated through a polymorphism of acetaldehyde dehydrogenase 2.
  - It is a factor in alcoholism.
    - Alcohol dehydrogenase polymorphism affects level and half-life of ethanol,
      - but does not correlate with alcoholism.

Acetaldehyde dehydrogenase (ALDH2) Polymorphism

Ethnic Group	Proportion
Japanese	44
Chinese	32
Native South Americans	42
Native North Americans	3
Europeans	0

Data from Japanese Studies

	ALDH2 Profile	
	Deficient	Normal
Healthy	44	56
Alcoholics	2	98

Levels after ethanol dose

	Acetaldehyde	Alcohol
Normal	2.1 μm/L	10.3 μm/L
Deficient	35.4 μm/L	10.9 μm/L

Other Pharmacokinetic Genetic Variations

Phenomenon	Drugs	Effects	Geography	Genetics
Dihydropyrimidine dehydrogenase deficiency.	fluorouracil	thymine-uraciluria, stomatitis, ataxia, diarrhea, hair loss	?	AR
Hepatic theophylline biotransformation.	theophylline	gastritis, agitation, seizures, tachycardia	?	AD
Microsomal epoxide hydrolase defect.	diphenylhydantoin	ataxia, nausea, lethargy	?	AD
Thiopurine S-methyltransferase deficiency.	6-mercaptopurine	bone marrow depression	1%	AR

PHARMACODYNAMICS

2. Pharmacodynamic genetic variation is due to
    *   polymorphisms, and
    *   disease-associated drug response abnormalities (idiomorphisms).

*   Glucose 6-phosphate dehydrogenase (G6PD) is required in the glycolytic pathway in the step, glucose 6-phosphate → 6-phosphogluconate, in which it reduces NADP to NADPH, which is required by glutathione reductase in the step, GSSH → GSH.
    *   G6PD deficiency decreases GSH that is required to detoxify free radical metabolites of ingested oxidants, allowing the free radicals to produce brittleness of the erythrocyte membrane, which leads to hemolysis in-vivo.

*   The gene at Xp28 has over 400 allelomorphic forms; most cause G6PD deficiency.
    *   Most are polymorphisms within limited geographic areas.
    *   Over 60 have have been characterized at the DNA level.
    *   Classification is based on clinical severity and enzyme activity.

Geographic Polymorphisms of Common G6PD Allelomorphs

Africa	A-$^{202A/376G}$	India	Kalyan^{949A1}	Mexico	A-$^{202A/376G}$
	A-$^{376G/968C}$		Viangchan^{871A}	Phillippines	Chatham^{1003A}
Algeria	Aures^{143C}	Iran	Mediterranean^{563T}		Chinese3^{493G}
Canary	A-$^{202A/376G}$		Mediterranean^{563T}		Union1^{360T}
Islands	A-$^{376G/968C}$	Israel	Mediterranean^{563T}		Viangchan^{871A}
	Santamaria$^{376G/542T}$	Italy	A-$^{202A/376G}$	Sardinia	Mediterranean^{563T}
	Seattle^{844C}		Mediterranean^{563T}		Seattle^{844C}
China	Canton^{1376T}		Santamaria$^{376G/542T}$	Saudi Arabia	Aures^{143C}
	Chinese4^{392T}		Seattle^{844C}		Mediterranean^{563T}
	Gaohe^{95G}		Union1^{360T}	Southeast Asia	Mahidol^{487A}
	Kaiping^{1388G}	Japan	Ube^{241T}	Spain	A-$^{202A/376G}$
	Mahidol^{487A}		Union1^{360T}		A-$^{376G/968C}$
	Union1^{360T}	Jews*	Mediterranean^{563T}		Aures^{143C}
	Viangchan^{871A}	Jews**	Mediterranean^{563T}		Seattle^{844C}
Costa Rica	Santamaria$^{376G/542T}$	Laos	Kaiping^{1388G}		Union1^{360T}
Egypt	Mediterranean^{563T}		Union1^{360T}	Taiwan	Mahidol^{487A}
Greece	Mediterranean^{563T}		Viangchan^{871A}		

*Askenazi   **Kurdish

Clinical Classes of G6PD Allelomorphs

Class	Proportion	Common examples	% Activity	Clinical
1	34	all rare	9 (0-35)	hereditary non-spherocytic hemolytic anemia
2	26	Mediterranean	4 (0-10)	severe hemolytic crises
3	26	A-, Canton	27 (7-75)	moderate hemolytic crises
4	14	B+, A+	103 (6-105)	mild hemolytic crises
5	1	all rare	400	none

Drugs and Chemicals Known to Cause Hemolytic Crises in G6PD Deficiency

ANALGESICS	ANTIMALARIALS	OTHER AGENTS
Acetaminophen[1]	Primaquine	Fava beans[2,3]
Acetanilid	Pamaquine	Naphthalene
Acetylsalicylic acid[1]	Pentaquine	Methylene blue
Acetophenetidin (Phenacetin)[1]	Quinocide	Phenylhydrazine
Phenazopyridine (Pyridium)	SULFONAMIDES, SULFONES	Ascorbic acid (megadoses)
ANTIBIOTICS	Diphenylsulfone	Quinine[1,2]
Chloramphenicol[1,2]	N-acetylsulfonilamide	Quinidine[1,2]
Furazolidone (Furoxone)	Salicylazosulfapyridine	Niridazole (Ambilhar)
Furmenthol	Sulfacetamide	Nitrites
Nalidixic acid (NegGram)	Sulfamethopyridazine (Kynex)[1]	Toluidine blue
Nitrofurantoin (Furadantin)	Sulfamethoxazole (Gantanol)	Urate oxidase
Nitrofurazone	Sulfanilimide	
	Sulfapyridine	
	Thiazolesulfone	

[1] relatively safe in forms of G6PD deficiency without hereditary non-spherocytic hemolytic anemia
[2] Mediterranean only   [3] DOPA-quinone is the likely culprit

- While drug and chemical exposures are more avoidable, hemolytic crises in G6PD deficiency are most often due to other factors:
  - Infectious diseases are the most frequent: The mechanism is unknown.
  - Neonatal jaundice may be severe, especially in Asians and Mediterraneans.
    - The mechanism is probably hepatocyte G6PD deficiency.

Other Pharmacodynamic Genetic Variations

Phenomenon	Drugs	Effects	Geography	Genetics
Aminoglycoside induced deafness	gentamycin kanamycin neomycin streptomycin tobramycin	ototoxicity	unknown	MT RNR1
Chloramphenicol toxicity	chloramphenicol	aplastic anemia	1/19,000	MT RNR2
Coumarin resistance	coumarin and derivatives	96% less effect	unknown	AD
Malignant hyperthermia. Type 1: ryanodine receptor defect. Type 2: muscle sodium channel alpha (?) Type 3: muscle calcium channel alpha-2	halothane succinylcholine methoxyflurane	hyperthermia, rigidity	unknown	AD
Mydriatic resistance	mydriatics	pupil dilation inadequate for examination.	6%: more frequent with dark irides.	AD

Disease-Associated Drug Response Abnormalities (idiomorphisms)

Disease	Drugs	Effects	Geography	Genetics
Charcot-Marie-Tooth disease	vincristine	neurotoxicity	unknown	AD
Glaucoma: open angle.	steroids	ocular hypertension	unknown	AR
Gout	chlorothiazide cyclosporine	arthritis	unknown	Polygen
Hemoglobins: unstable. Alpha locus: Hasharon, H, Torino. Beta locus: Bushwick, Leiden, M$_{Saskatoon}$, Peterborough, Shepherd's Bush, Zurich	sulfonamides primaquine	hemolysis	unknown	AD
Huntington disease	Levodopa	tremors	unknown	AD
Methemoglobin reductase deficiency	dapsone primaquine chloroquine	methemoglobin-emia	Caucasians: 0.1% Eskimos: frequent Navajos: frequent	AR
Periodic paralysis 1	insulin epinephrine	paralysis	unknown	AD
Porphyria	alcohol barbiturates chlordiazepoxide dichloralphenazone diphenylhydantoin ergot preparations eucalyptol glutethimide griseofulvin imipramine isopropylmepro- bamate meprobamate methprylon methsuximide pyrazolone compounds Sulfonal sulfonamides tolbutamide Trional	neuropathic crisis	Sweden 0.001 (acute intermit-tent type) Bantu: frequent (cutanea tarda type)	AD

GENETIC THERAPEUTICS

3.   Principles of treatment of genetic diseases are those of therapeutics in general:
- The patient or responsible person must be included in discussion and decision-making.
- Therapeutic intervention may be worse than intrinsic recuperative and adaptive capacities.
- Accurate diagnosis is required to assess pathophysiology.
  - Most genetic disorders have phenocopies and extensive genetic heterogeneity.
- Therapeutic effectiveness must be assessed:
  - Few regimens are completely effective.
  - Effectiveness may be different in different forms of a disorder.
  - Effectiveness varies among individuals due to:
    - Genetic background characteristics.
    - Exogenous background characteristics.
    - Intercurrent conditions.
    - Compliance by patient and care-giver.
- Therapeutic acceptability must be assessed.
  - Discomfort and unpleasantness should be minimized.
  - Practicality must be considered.
- Risks to the patient must be assessed:
  - Interactions among pharmaceuticals and other components of the therapeutic regimen.
  - Pharmacogenetic variation in response to therapeutics.
  - Intercurrent conditions may intensify risks.
  - Side effects of some therapeutics may be significant.
- Financial aspects must be assessed.
  - Costs should be determined realistically:
    - Quantity effects on medication costs.
    - Administration may require skilled personnel.
    - Monitoring laboratory tests.
    - Travel to site of therapy, monitoring and medication dispensary.
  - Accomodation to costs may require assistance of outside agencies.
- Continuity must be planned.
  - Some conditions that respond initially are prone to recurrence.
  - Observation for sequelae of disease or therapeutic regimen may be required.
  - Prolonged or continuous therapy is required for many genetic diseases.
  - Sequential manifestations of some genetic diseases require sequential therapy.

- Treatment of the phenotype. Examples:
  - Chondrodystrophies.
    - Orthopedic procedures: osteotomies, straightening, stabilization.
  - Marfan syndrome.
    - Beta-blocker drugs slow the dilatation of the aorta.
  - Pharmacogenetic variations.
    - Avoidance of specific pharmaceuticals.
  - Photosensitive disorders: albinism, xeroderma pigmentosum.
    - Sun screens, protective clothing, indoor occupations.
  - Polyposis coli.
    - Colectomy (prevents cancer).

- Seizures symptomatic of genetic disorders.
  - Anticonvulsants.
- Spherocytosis.
  - Splenectomy minimized the hemolytic anemia.

- Metabolic intervention. Examples:
  - Alternate pathway removal of metabolite.
    - Isovaleric acidemia.
      - Accumulation of isovaleryl-CoA exhausts glycine which would ordinarily detoxify it by forming harmless, readily excreted isovalerylglycine. Treatment with glycine restores this detoxification pathway.
      - Carnitine participates in removal of isovaleryl-CoA through isovalerylcarnitine and is also depleted when isovaleryl-CoA accumulates. Treatment with carnitine restores that pathway and also corrects symptoms of carnitine deficiency.
    - Cystinosis.
      - Therapeutic cysteamine, through disulfide interchange, reacts with insoluble cystine stored in lysosomes to form soluble cysteine and cysteamine-cysteine, which are eventually oxidized and excreted in the urine.
    - Organic acidemias other than isovaleric.
      - Carnitine participates in removal of Co-A esters of the organic acids and their products and is rapidly depleted. Treatment with carnitine restores the excretion pathway and also corrects symptoms of carnitine deficiency.
    - Hemochromatosis.
      - Phlebotomy acts as an alternative pathway to remove iron.
    - Urea cycle disorders.
      - Sodium benzoate diverts nitrogen from urea synthesis by irreversible conjugation with glycine to form hippurate which is excreted in the urine, removing one nitrogen residue per benzoate.
      - Sodium phenylacetate conjugates with glutamine (which was formed from glutamate and an ammonion radical) to form phanylacetylglutamine, also excreted in the urine, removing two nitrogen residues per phenylacetate.
    - Wilson disease.
      - D-penicillamine mobilizes stored copper through an obscure pathway, which results in excretion in the urine.
  - Metabolic inhibition.
    - Familial hypercholesterolemia (LDL receptor defect).
      - Mevinolin (lovastatin) inhibits 3-hydroxy-3-methylglutaryl-CoA reductase in the formation of mevalonate, a rate-limiting reaction in cholesterol synthesis.
    - Gout.
      - Allopurinol, a structural analogue of xanthine, competitively inhibits xanthine oxidase. This lowers the concentration of the reaction product, uric acid, and elevates the less toxic xanthine, producing a salubrious effect.

- Replacement of product. Examples:
    - Adenosine deaminase deficiency.
        - Polyethylene glycol cross-linked bovine adenosine deaminase.
    - Alpha-1 antitrypsin for its deficiency.
    - Biotinidase deficiency
        - Biotin therapy replaces the biotin that would ordinarily have been recovered by the enzyme from biotinylated protein.
    - Endocrinopathies examples:
        - Corticosteroids for adrenogenital syndrome
        - Insulin for diabetes.
        - Growth hormone for hyopituitarism.
        - Thyroxine for hypothyroidism.
    - Gaucher disease 1: macrophage targeted cerebrosidase.
    - Glycogen storage disease type I and II, hypoglycemia.
        - Cornstarch is slowly digested and absorbed as glucose.
    - Hemophilia A: Factor VIII.
    - Hemophilia B: Factor IX.
    - Orotic aciduria, macrocytic anemia due to pyrimidine deficiency.
        - Uridine is a replacement and also supresses acid production, decreasing nephrolithiasis.

- Defective protein activation. Examples:
    - Homocystinuria (some types).
        - Defective cystathione beta-synthetase is partially reactivated by pyridoxine.
    - Lactic acidemia (some types),
        - Thiamine, biotin, or riboflavin partially reacivate enzymes in some cases.
    - Maple syrup urine (some types).
        - Thiamin partially reactivates decarboxylation of branched chain amino scids.

- Transplantation. Examples:
    - Replacement of product:
        - Bone marrow.
            - Lysosomal storage diseases.
            - Beta-thalassemia.
            - Sickle cell disease.
        - Liver.
            - Glycogen storage disease 1.
            - Familial hypercholesterolemia (LDL receptor defect).
            - Ornithine transcarbamylase deficiency.
    - Replacement of organ:
        - Heart:
            - Isolated congenital heart malformations (not part of a lethal syndrome).
        - Kidney.
            - Cystinosis.

- Liver.
  - Alpha-1 antitrypsin deficiency.
  - Hepatorenal tyrosinemia.
- Lung.
  - Cystic fibrosis.

- Gene therapy (replacement). Mostly in the realm of experimentation at present.
  - Abstractions about potential hazards and benefits obscure facts.
    - Utopian: salvation from genetic disease and imperfection.
    - Apocalyptic: dissolution of human values and possibly of humanity.
  - Observations that laboratory technicians working with the Shope papilloma virus had lower arginine levels led to its use in argininemia, the first attempt at gene therapy (1970).
    - Apocalyptic furor prevented publication about success or failure of the attempt.
  - Another attempt at gene therapy involved calcium transfer of DNA into bone marrow cells of two thalassemic patients, followed by partial bone marrow depletion through radiation, then return of the treated marrow cells (1980).
    - The attempt violated ethical guidelines that been established after the first attempt.
      - No benefit was realized by the experimental subjects.
  - A later attempt at gene therapy was sanctioned under all guidelines (1990).
    - A safety-modified vector, tested in previous experiments on patients with advanced melanoma, was successfully used for retroviral insertion of adenosine deaminase (ADA) genes into T lymphocytes of an ADA-deficient patient.
      - Though successful, the treatment must be repeated several times a year because of the limited life-span of T lymphocytes.
  - During the period of development of gene therapy, the Genome Project has revealed extensive complexity of the genome, suggesting many approaches to gene therapy, as well as many challenging hurdles in the way of the realization of any of them. Hundreds of projects are in progress.
    - Transfer of research to the private sector has decreased knowledge dissemination.

BETTER-KNOWN DISEASES FOR WHICH ATTEMPTS ARE BEING MADE TO DEVELOP GENE THERAPY

Disease	Gene	Target	Method
adenosine deaminase deficiency	adenosine deaminase	bone marrow stem cells	retrovirus transfer
cystic fibrosis	CFTR	airway epithelial cells	adenovirus transfer
familial hypercholesterolemia	LDL receptor	hepatocytes	adenovirus transfer
hemophilia B	factor IX	hepatocytes	adenovirus transfer
Duchenne muscular dystrophy	dystrophin	myoblasts	direct injection
ornithine transcarbamalyase deficiency	OCT	hepatocytes	adenovirus transfer
phenylketonuria	PAH	hepatocytes	adenovirus transfer

Additional references

Pharmacogenetics

Beutler E. G6PD Deficiency. Blood 1984;84:3613-3636.

Goth A, Vessell ES. Medical Pharmacology, 11th edition. St Louis: C.V. Mosby, 1984:50-62.

Lentner C (editor). Geigy Scientific Tables. Volume 4. New York: Ciba-Geigy, 1986:289-300.

Mueller RF, Young ID. Emery's Elements of Medical Genetics. 9th edition. New York, Churchill Livingstone, 1995:143-150.

Musa MN, Miescke KJ. Pharmacogenetics of despiramine metabolism. Intl J Clin Pharm Therapeut 1994;32:126-30.

Nebert DW. Polymorphisms in drug-metabolizing enzymes: What is their clinical significance and why do they exist? Am J Hum Genet 1997;60:265-271.

Genetic Therapeutics

Anderson WF. Human gene therapy. Science 1992; 256:808-813.

Beaudet AL, Scriver CR, Sly WS, et al. Introduction to Human Biochemical and Molecular Genetics. New York: McGraw-Hill, 1990.

Cline MJ. Testimony at a hearing before Subcommittee on Investigation and Oversight of the Committee on Science and Technology, U.S. House of Representatives, November 16-18, 1982. Human Genetic Engineering, U.S. Government Printing Office, Committee Print No. 170, 1983, pp442-461.

Graef JW. Manual of Pediatric Therapeutics, 5th edition. Boston: Little, Brown, 1993.

Kolata G, Wade N. Human gene treatment stirs new debate. Science 1980;210:407.

Morgan RA, Anderson WF. Human Gene Therapy. Annu Rev Biochem 1993; 62:191-217.

Morsy MA, Mitani K, Clemens P, et al. Progress toward human gene therapy. JAMA 1993;270:2338-2345.

Naron S (editor). Transplant cures patient's sickle cell disease. St. Jude Rounds, Fall 1995. Memphis, TN: St. Jude Children's Research Hospital, 1995.

Sinsheimer RL. The prospect for designed genetic change. Am Scientist 1969;57:134-142.

Ramsay P. Genetic therapy. A theologian's response. In: Hamilton M (editor). The New Genetics and the Future of Man. Grand Rapids:William B. Eerdmans, 1972: 163-175.

Rogers S, Lowenthal A, Terheggen HG, et al. Induction of arginase activity with the Shope papilloma virus in tissue culture cells from an argininemic patient. J Exp Med 1973;137:1091-1096.

Rosenberg SA, Aebersold P, Cornetta K, et al. Gene transfer into humans. Immunotherapy of patients with advanced melanoma, using tumor-infiltrating lymphocytes modified by retroviral gene transduction. N Engl J Med 1990;323:570-78.

Schmeck H. Virus is injected into 2 children to alter chemical traits. NY Times, September 20, 1970, p 28.

Schuchman EH, Ioannou YA, Rattazzi MC, et al. Neural gene therapy for inherited diseases with mental retardation: Principles and prospects. Ment Ret and Develop Disabil Res Rev 1995; 1:39-48.

Sharma S, Tozer JR. Development of adenovirus vectors for gene therapy. Ment Ret and Develop Disabil Res Rev 1995;:19-26.

Yee J-K. Prospects for using retroviral vectors for human gene therapy. Ment Ret and Develop Disabil Res Rev 1995;1:14-18.

1. Prenatal diagnosis discloses
    *   significant disorders of the fetus in 2% of cases while providing welcome
    *   reassurance in 98% of cases.

Important reference: Weaver DD (1989): <u>Catalogue of Prenatally Diagnosed Conditions</u>.
                   Johns Hopkins, Baltimore.
*   An annotated bibliography of 448 conditions in which at least 1 case has been diagnosed prenatally.

---

*   Each prenatal diagnostic procedure misses some severe congenital disorders
    *   so that between 1/2 and 2/3 are diagnosable.

*   Among indications for prenatal diagnosis are situations in which the
    *   risk of an affected fetus is greater than the
    *   risk that the diagnostic procedure will cause an abortion.

	0 - 7	8 - 15	16 - 40
Expected abortion rates by gestation week*:	15%	3%	1%

*   Expected abortion rates by gestation week*:
    *   Ultrasonography adds no risk.
    *   Other procedures increase risk of abortion.

	Total risks	
Amniocentesis: 0.5%.	3.5%	1.5%
Chorionic villus sampling: 1.5%.	4.5%	2.5%
Percutaneous umbilical blood sampling: 1.9%.	4.9%	2.9%
Fetoscopy: 5%.	8%	6%

*These rates should be multiplied by 1.6 for women with previous spontaneous abortions (Kelly, 1992). Rates of losses of chromosome 21 trisomy fetuses ascertained by amniocentesis at specific gestational ages:

15-17 weeks: 50%	18 weeks: 43.%	19 weeks: 31%	20 weeks: 25%	21-28 weeks: 20%

Maternal age averages 3 years greater in losses of trisomic fetuses ascertained after 17 weeks.

*   Under the above criteria, prenatal diagnosis is indicated when decisions about management of the pregnancy depend on accurate information about the fetus.
    Some conditions currently thought to warrant it include:
    *   maternal age over 35
    *   previous child with chromosomal disorder
    *   structural chromosome aberration in one parent
    *   positive birth defect screening test
    *   family history of neural tube defect
    *   family history of genetic disorder that is diagnosable prenatally
    *   family history of an X-linked disorder
    *   significant possibility of teratogenic disorder that is diagnosable prenatally

*   Maternal epilepsy and diabetes exemplify conditions requiring individual evaluation.
    *   Cumulative factors that may indicate a need for prenatal diagnosis in some cases:
        *   risk of fetal malformation due to the condition itself or its treatment
        *   risk of neonatal problems due to the condition itself or its treatment
        *   risk of inheritance of the condition by the fetus

Problems of the Pregnant Diabetic

Survival: Prior to the availability of insulin, maternal mortality was 50% and infant mortality was 75%. Even after insulin, infant survival was only 54%. Improved medical care of newborns between 1922 and 1974 gradually increased survival to 90%. Newborn intensive care units led to still better survival. Current perinatal mortality rates are obscured by medico-political competition in which manners of counting and calculating are not standardized but is estimated as 0.1% to 0.3% or about twice the rate for non-diabetic pregnancies. Maternal mortality is also obscured but is probably at least 0.001%.

Maternal effects: Pregnancy may precipitate maternal diabetes. It also increases insulin requirements of established diabetics and may accelerate retinopathy, neuropathy or nephropathy of diabetes; some studies show acceleration only when control is poor.

Fetal malformation rates in a recent study:	Total %	CNS	Heart
Insulin-dependent diabetics	18.4	5.3	8.5
Insulin-requiring gestational diabetics	15.1	1.0	9.7
Gestational diabetics	1.8	0.1	0.9
Non-diabetics	2.3	0.34	0.47

Diabetes genes inherited by the fetus, insulin, or the diabetic state: which is the teratogen?
- Getations of women who later develop diabetes produce no excess of fetal malformations.
- The rate of fetal malformations is not correlated with the dose level of insulin.
- First trimester elevation of glycosylated hemoglobin correlates with fetal malformation rate,
  - so hyperglycemia around the time of conception may be at fault.

Fetal malformations highly characteristic of maternal diabetes (all are neural crest-related):
- CNS: holoprosencephaly, hydrocephalus, spina bifida
- Heart: conotruncal heart malformations (double-outlet right ventricle, truncus arteriosus)
- Skeletal: caudal regression (sacrum reduction, vertebral & pelvis anomalies)

Neonatal problems of the infant of the diabetic mother
- Macrosomia (may lead to birth trauma, cesarian section)   >90%
  - Hypoglycemia   33%
  - Hypocalcemia   15%
  - Hyperbilirubinemia   25%
  - Hyperviscosity   15%
  - Respiratory distress, cardiomyopathy, persistent pulmonary hypertension   frequent
- Intrauterine growth retardation   Rare
  - characteristic when mother has diabetic retinopathy or nephropathy
- Transient neonatal diabetes   Rare

Risk of inheritance of diabetes from mother (also see chapter on diabetes):
- IDDM: 2% - 5%
- NIDDM: 5% - 10%
  - Gestational diabetes is usually NIDDM disclosed by pregnancy.
    At least 60% of gestational diabetics later develop NIDDM.

Problems of the Pregnant Epileptic

Fertility: State laws preventing marriage by epileptics existed as late as 1982. At present, marriage rate for female epileptics is 83% that of non-epileptics while for males it is 69%. Fertility rate for male epileptics is normal while for females, it is 69% of normal unless onset of seizures was in the first decade in which case it is 43%.

Maternal effects: Epilepsy is a group of different disorders characterized by seizures. Seizures decrease in frequency in pregnancy in some patients In others, pregnancy may precipitate epilepsy (gestational epilepsy). It may also increase anticonvulsant requirements of established epileptics which can increase seizure frequency; more rarely, status epilepticus may occur. Complications of pregnancy combined with a propensity toward epilepsy may occasionally result in catastrophic status epilepticus during delivery, threatening the lives of both mother and baby.

Fetal malformation rates in a recent study:	Controls	Untreated	Treated
Rates of all congenital malformations (%):	2.14	5	18

Fetal malformations possibly characteristic of maternal epilepsy:
• microcephaly, cleft lip, intrauterine growth retardation

Fetal hazards of a prolonged, uncontrolled maternal seizure (status epilepticus):
• Maternal hypoxia or hypotension may ensue, causing cessation of fetal cerebral blood flow.
• Direct uterine trauma from falling may cause placental hemorrhage, resulting in
  • Inadequate fetal perfusion
  • Focal embolism of fetal structiures.

Neonatal problems of the infant of the epileptic mother:
• most anticonvulsants in newborn serum match maternal levels; valproic acid is higher
  • neonatal depression, 5 - 10%
  • withdrawal, 50%: hyperactivity, myoclonic jerks, sleeplessness, vomiting, yawning, sneezing
• most anticonvulsant drugs depress levels of clotting factors
  • hemorrhagic disease of the newborn occurs in 10%
  • preventable by vitamin K administration to mother before delivery

Teratogenic syndromes due to anticonvulsants. Development may be poor in any of them. Frequency is variable and determined by factors that are discussed in the lesson on teratology.
• hydantoin: hypertelorism, ptosis, low set ears, short nose, fingernail & fingertip hypoplasia
• trimethadione: V-shaped eyebrows, epicanthus, low set ears, dental and palatal anomalies, mental retardation
• valproic acid: brachycephaly, hypertelorism, shallow orbits, flat nose, long philtrum, microstomia, spina bifida
• carbamepazine: Small head, narrow bifrontal diameter, upslanting eyes, short nose, fingernail hypoplasia

Risk of inheritance of epilepsy from mother (see also lesson on epilepsy):
• Risk range is from 5% to 50%, depending on number of relatives with seizures, seizure type, EEG pattern and syndrome association.

2. The risk of chromosome aberrations occurring in the newborn,
   - especially chromosome 21 trisomy, is associated with maternal age.

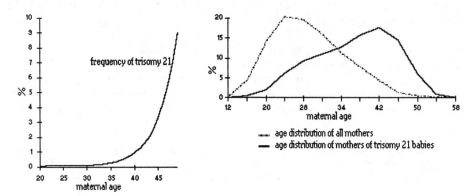

frequency of trisomy 21

...... age distribution of all mothers
—— age distribution of mothers of trisomy 21 babies

Age at delivery	FREQUENCIES Down syndrome		All aberrations		Age at delivery	FREQUENCIES Down syndrome		Alll aberrations	
20	1:1667	0.06%	1:526	0.19%	35	1:385	0.26%	1:204	0.49%
21	1:1667	0.06%	1:526	0.19%	36	1:294	0.34%	1:164	0.61%
22	1:1429	0.07%	1:500	0.20%	37	1:227	0.44%	1:130	0.71%
23	1:1429	0.07%	1:500	0.20%	38	1:175	0.57%	1:103	0.97%
24	1:1250	0.08%	1:476	0.21%	39	1:137	0.73%	1:82	1.22%
25	1:1250	0.08%	1:476	0.21%	40	1:106	0.94%	1:65	1.54%
26	1:1176	0.09%	1:476	0.21%	41	1:82	1.22%	1:51	1.96%
27	1:1111	0.09%	1:455	0.22%	42	1:64	1.56%	1:40	2.50%
28	1:1053	0.09%	1:435	0.23%	43	1:50	2.00%	1:32	3.13%
29	1:1000	0.10%	1:417	0.24%	44	1:38	2.63%	1:25	4.00%
30	1:952	0.11%	1:384	0.26%	45	1:30	3.33%	1:20	5.00%
31	1:909	0.11%	1:384	0.26%	46	1:23	4.35%	1:15	6.67%
32	1:769	0.13%	1:322	0.31%	47	1:18	5.56%	1:12	8.33%
33	1:625	1.16%	1:317	0.32%	48	1:14	7.14%	1:10	10.00%
34	1:500	0.20%	1:260	0.38%	49	1:11	9.09%	1:7	14.29%

- Risks of other chromosome disorders occurring in newborns are
  - less than those of chromosome 21 trisomy but are thought to have similar
  - distributions according to maternal age and specific unusual circumstances.
  - except pericentric inversion in a parent for which
    - the risk of abnormal newborns is 6%, unrelated to parental age.

Unusual circumstances	Risk of Trisomy 21
Mother< 35 years age, previous child with any trisomy	1%
Same, risk to 2nd or 3rd degree relatives	> age specific risk, < 1%
More than 2 trisomies, risk to 2nd or 3rd degree relatives	> age specific risk, > 1%
Mother has translocation 21/13, 21/14, 21/15	15%
Father has translocation 21/13, 21/14, 21/15	5%
Mother has translocation 21/22	10%
Father has translocation 21/22	2%
Either parent has translocation 21/21	100%

3. The most common birth defect screening test is maternal serum alpha-fetoprotein,
    - a fetal albumin that is decreased in concentration when
        - the fetus has a chromosome aberration, or
    - increased in concentration if the fetus has an open neural tube defect
        - or certain other disorders.
    - Concentration is expressed as a multiple of the normal median (MOM).

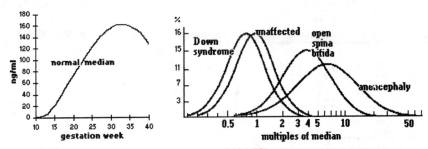

MATERNAL SERUM α-FETOPROTEIN (MSAFP) IN HEALTH AND DISEASE

Weight (lbs)	Factor	Weight (lbs)	Factor	Weight (lbs)	Factor
85-89	0.759	125-129	0.953	165-169	1.199
90-94	0.779	130-134	0.98	170-174	1.234
95-99	0.802	135-139	1.009	175-179	1.27
100-104	0.825	140-144	1.038	180-184	1.307
105-109	0.849	145-149	1.069	185-189	1.345
110-114	0.874	150-154	1.1	190-194	1.384
115-119	0.899	155-159	1.132	195-199	1.424
120-124	0.926	160-164	1.065	>199	1.449

Multiply initial MOM by factor to get true MOM

WEIGHT OF PATIENT AND MSAFP INTERPRETATION

- **Race correction of Maternal Serum α-fetoprotein**
    - Divide initial MOM by 1.12 for final MOM if patient is *African-American*

	0.3	0.4	0.05	0.6	0.7	0.8	0.9	1
0		3.81	2.37	1.66	1.26	1.01	0.84	0.72
0.01		3.61	2.27	1.61	1.23	0.99	0.83	0.64
0.02		3.42	2.19	1.56	1.2	0.97	0.82	0.57
0.03		3.25	2.1	1.52	1.17	0.95	0.8	0.52
0.04		3.09	2.03	1.47	1.15	0.93	0.79	0.48
0.05	5.19	2.95	1.96	1.43	1.12	0.92	0.78	0.45
0.06	4.86	2.81	1.89	1.39	1.1	0.9	0.77	0.42
0.07	4.56	2.69	1.83	1.36	1.07	0.89	0.76	0.4
0.08	4.29	2.57	1.77	1.32	1.05	0.87	0.75	0.38
0.09	4.04	2.47	1.71	1.29	1.03	0.86	0.73	0.36

Find first digit in row 1, second digit in column 1, read factor at intersect: Example: The factor for MOM of 0.41 is 3.61. Multiply the factor by the frequency for the patient's age: For age 40, 3.61 X 1:106 = 3:61:106 = 1:29 = 4%.

EFFECT OF LOW MSAFP ON LIKELIHOOD OF DOWN SYNDROME

Gesta-tion Week	Median values			Condition	Average MOM		
	AFP ng/ml	hCG mIU/ml	uE3 ng/ml		AFP	hCG	uE3
15.0	31.1	34.3	0.61	Down syndrome	0.62	2.0	0.70
15.5	34.5	32.0	0.69	Turner syndrome also (?)			
16.0	36.1	27.0	0.78	Chromosome 18 trisomy	0.44	0.30	0.34
16.5	38.3	24.8	0.88				
17.0	41.0	22.4	0.99				
17.5	43.4	20.9	1.12				
18.0	45.9	19.7	1.26				
18.5	48.4	19.1	1.42				
19.0	51.6	17.7	1.60				
19.5	56.8	17.5	1.80				
20.0	59.4	16.7	2.02				
20.5	62.9	15.7	2.27				

THE TRIPLE SCREEN

Maternal serum unconjugated estriol (uE3) and maternal serum human chorionic gonadotrophin (hCG) can be used in combination with maternal serum α-fetoprotein (AFP) to add accuracy to screening for some conditions. A computer program is used to calculate the combined likelihoods of levels of these analytes and develop odds (affected:unaffected). Corrections for IDDM, weight, race, and multiple gestations are included in the computer calculation.

Barely detectable uE3 levels are indicative of X-linked placental sulfatase deficiency, which manifests after birth in males as ichthyosis with corneal opacities, and, in some cases, anosmia, hypogonadism, mental retardation and skeletal anomalies.

Gestation week	Median AFP
15	33.9
16	37.1
17	40.5
18	45.5
19	55.4
20	68.0
21	88.6
	(ng/ml)

Data from Abbott
Labora tories (1989)
Normal MSAFP

MOM	Adverse Outcome	Abnormalities
2.5-2.9	27%	Open neural tube defect
3.0-3.9	39%	Abdominal wall defect
>4.0	48%	Congenital nephrosis
>6	86%	Renal agenesis
		Retroperitoneal hemorrhage
		Pre-term birth
		-Fetal death
		Triploidy
		Placental hemangioma
		Abruptio placenta

**Outcomes of Pregnancies with
elevated MSAFP** (twins excluded)

MOM	Adverse Outcome	Abnormalities
2.5-2.9	19%	Low birth weight
3.0-3.9	23%	Fetal death
>4.0	25%	Spontaneous abortion
>6	67%	Hydrocephalus
		Heart malformation
		Club feet
		Multiple anomalies

Outcome of Pregnancies with elevated MSAFP in which all amniotic fluid studies were *normal*
(twins excluded)

	2	2.2	2.4	2.6	2.8	3
1.6	925	860	870	920	1000	1150
1.8	530	450	410	395	404	430
2	360	275	230	205	195	195
2.2	275	190	150	125	110	100
2.4	230	150	105	80	70	60
2.6	205	120	82	60	45	40
2.8	195	110	70	45	35	30
3	190	100	60	40	30	20

Find initial MOM value in first row, then find repeat value in column 1. Intersect is denominator of risk. Example: Initial MOM of 2.2, repeat of 2.4 = 150. Likelihood of open neural defect = 1:150.
EFFECT OF REEPEATED MEASUREMENTS OF MSAFP ON RISK OF OPEN NEURAL TUBE DEFECT

MSAFP MOM	Risk if singleton, no IDDM	Risk if singleton, maternal IDDM	Twins*	MSAFP MOM	Risk if singleton, no IDDM	Risk if singleton, maternal IDDM	Twins*
1.0	1:12000	1:3500		2.8	1:160	1:47	1:470
1.1	1:8900	1:2500		2.9	1:130	1:39	
1.2	1:6400	1:1800		3.0	1:120		1:370
1.3	1:4700	1:1300		3.2			1:300
1.4	1:3500	1:1000		3.4			1:240
1.5	1:2700	1:770		3.6	1:53		1:200
1.6	1:2000	1:590		3.8			1:170
1.7	1:1600	1:460		4.0	1:26		1:140
1.8	1:1200	1:360		4.2			1:120
1.9	1:1000	1:280		4.4			1:110
2.0	1:800	1:220	1:1700	4.6	1:14		1:93
2.1	1:640	1:180		4.8			1:82
2.2	1:520	1:140	1:1200	5.0	1:7		1:73
2.3	1:420	1:120		5.2			1:65
2.4	1:340	1:99	1:830	5.4			1:58
2.5	1:280	1:81		5.6			1:53
2.6	1:230	1:67	1:620	5.8			1:48
2.7	1:190	1:56		6.0			1:44

*Average figures. MZ twins are a bit higher and DZ twins are a bit lower.

EFFECT OF INSULIN DEPENDENT DIABETES MELLITUS OR TWINNING ON RISK OF OPEN NEURAL TUBE DEFECT

- Couples of Ashkenazi descent may have had
  - serum hexoseaminidase screening for heterozygosity for Tay-Sachs disease
  - and can be offered prenatal diagnosis if both are heterozygotes.

- Prenatal diagnosis of sickle cell anemia or beta-thalassemia
  - can be offered for heterozygote couples who have been identified by screening,
  - however, ethical questions about this application have arisen
    - because of the homozygote's potential for productive existence.

4. Ultrasonography at 6 weeks allows visualization of
   - cardiac activity, and at
   16 weeks, allows direct visualization of
   - large internal or external anatomic defects and some
   - skeletal dysplasias.

Results	Findings
Oligohydramnios	Renal agenesis
Polyhydramnios	>20% anomalies
Hydrops fetalis	>50% anomalies, >25% arrhythmias or hematologic disorders, >90% mortality
Absence of a normally present structure	Anencephaly, holoprosencephaly, renal agenesis
Presence of additional structures distorting normal contours	Sacrococcygeal teratoma, cystic hygroma
Dilation of a structure behind an obstruction	Hydrocephalus, duodenal obstruction (double bubble), urinary tract obstruction
Herniation through a structural defect	Encephalocoele, omphalocoele, diaphragmatic hernia
Abnormal size of fetus or specific fetal structures	Achondroplasia and other skeletal dysplasias, microcephaly
Absent or abnormal fetal motion	Heart valve defects, dysrhythmias

Prenatal Diagnosis by Ultrasonography

- • Fetuses with abnormal ultrasound findings require
  - • karyotyping by amniocentesis or chorionic villus sampling because
  - • about 20% have chromosome aberrations.

5. Transabdominal amniocentesis is possible around 16 weeks of gestation because
   - • there is a sufficient quantity of amniotic fluid at that time.

- • Amniotic fluid is used most often for alpha-fetoprotein determination and
  - • amniocytes are used for chromosome analysis.

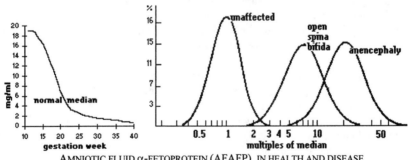

AMNIOTIC FLUID α-FETOPROTEIN (AFAFP) IN HEALTH AND DISEASE

Gestation week	Median AFP
15	16.1
16	14.2
17	13.0
18	11.3
19	9.5
20	6.9
21	5.3

(ng/ml)

Data from Abbott
Labora tories (1989)
Normal AFAFP

MOM*	Neural tube defects	Other abnormalities
2	22%	Abdominal wall defect
3	29%	AChE/PChE < 0.13
4	36%	Congenital nephrosis
5	43%	AChE absent
6	50%	

*Extrapolated from data for >3 and >5 MOM.
AchE = acetylcholinesterase, found in amniotic fluid
in virtually all cases of fetal neural tube defect.
PchE = pseudocholinesterase. AChE/PchE ratio
helps to differentiate other disorders.

**Outcomes of Pregnancies with elevated
amniotic fluid alpha-fetoprotein**

- Amniocytes may also be used to diagnose some rare disorders when it is known
  - that there is a risk that the baby will have a specific disorder, by analyzing for
    - abnormal metabolites,
    - RFLP's, or other
    - genetic markers*.

- Chromosome analysis of amniocytes requires culture of the amniocytes and
  - takes 2 to 3 weeks to complete.

6. Chorionic villus sampling is possible transabdominally at 8 weeks gestation or
    - transcervically at 10 weeks gestation.

- Chorionic villus sampling produces cells
  - that can be analyzed for the same reasons as amniocytes
    - either by direct analysis of chromosomes or
    - by analysis after cell culture for abormal metabolites, DNA & other genetic markers.
  - Also see chapters on Laboratory Diagnosis.

7. Fetoscopy is possible after 17 weeks gestation and allows
    - direct visualization of large external anatomic defects,
    - tissue biopsy (skin, liver) and
    - sampling of fetal blood for diagnosis of
      - fetal infections,
      - chromosome aberrations,
      - certain hematologic disorders and
      - certain metabolic disorders

Complications	Frequencies with:		
	Transabdominal CVS	Transcervical CVS	Amniocentesis
Vaginal bleeding	0.7% (1/143)	10.1% (1/10)	2.5% (1/40)
Vaginal amniotic fluid leakage	?	?	2.5% (1/40)
Oligohydramnios	0.4% (1/250)	?	?
Hematoma	0.3% (1/333)	4% (1/25)	?
Uterine cramping	2.5% (1/40)	?	occasional
Uterine infection	?	0.13% (1/769)	0.1% (1/1000)
Peritonitis	0.3% (1/333)	?	?
Fetal death, miscarriage	1.5% (1/66)	1.5% (1/66)	0.5% (1/200)
Local anesthetic anaphylactic shock	rare	rare	rare
Rh isoimmunization of Rh⁻ patient	rare	rare	rare
Penetrating injury to fetus	rare	rare	rare
Fetal limb defect	1%	1%	rare

Patient Risks of Amniocentesis and Chorionic Villus Sampling (CVS)

Problems	Frequencies with:	
	CVS	Amniocentesis
True fetal mosaicism (confusing results)	.14% (1/714)	0.2% (1/500)
Insignificant fetal mosaicism (false positive results)	?	rare
Mosaicism arising in culture (either false positive or false negative results)	?	0.3% (1/333)
Maternal cell overgrowth in culture (false negative results if fetus is abnormal)	?	0.2% (1/500)
Cells will not grow in culture (no results)	?	1% (1/100)
Overgrowth of non-amniocyte cells that cannot be karyotyped (no results)	?	1% (1/100)

Diagnostic Difficulties of Amniocentesis and Chorionic Villus Sampling (CVS)

8. Percutaneous umbilical blood sampling (PUBS) of the fetus is possible after 17 weeks gestation and is
    * safer and easier than fetoscopy and
    * allows blood sampling for the same purposes.

Additional references:

Abbott Laboratories. Abbott AFP-EIA Monoclonal Package Insert 83-4779/R4, 1979.

Bernstam VA. *Pocket Guide to Gene Level Diagnostics in Clinical Practice*. Boca Raton, FL: CRC Press, 1993.

Bradley LA, Horwitz JA, Dowman AC, et al. Triple marker screening for fetal Down syndrome. Internatl Pediatr 1994;9:168-174.

Crandall BF, Robinson L, Grau P. Risks associated with an elevated maternal serum alpha-fetoprotein level. Am J Obstet Gynecol 1991;165:581-6.

Evans MI. *Reproductive Risks and Prenatal Diagnosis*. Norwalk, CT: Appleton & Lange, 1992.

Filkins K, Russo JF. *Human Prenatal Diagnosis*, 2nd edition. New York, NY: Marcel Dekker, 1990.

Habib ZA. Maternal serum alpha-fetoprotein: Its value in antenatal diagnosis of genetic disease and in obstetric-gynaecological care. Acta Obstet Gynecol Scand (Suppl) 1977;61:1-92.

Hollingsworth DR, Resnik R (editors). *Medical Counseling Before Pregnancy*. New York, NY: Churchill Livingstone, 1988.

Holmes LB. Limb deficiency defects among 125,000 newborns. Abstract 63. Am J Hum Genet 1992;51 (Supplement):A18.

Hook EB, Mutton DE, Ide R, et al. The natural history of down syndrome conceptuses diagnosed prenatally that are not electively terminated. Am J Hum Genet 1995;57:875-81.

Kirkpatrick A, Nakamura RM, Jones OW, et al. Alpha-fetoprotein levels in amniotic fluid and maternal serum as determined by radioimmunoassay: Implications for prenatal diagnosis of fetal neural tube defects. Birth Defects Original Article Series 1977;XIII(3D):259-266.

Knight GJ. Maternal serum a-fetoprotein screening. In: Hommes FA (editor). *Techniques in Diagnostic Human Biochemical Genetics*. New York, NY: Wiley-Liss, 1991.

Kelly J. High maternal serum alpha fetoprotein: Indicator of much more than neural tube defects. The Genetic Letter 1992;2:1-4.

Lilford RJ (editor). *Prenatal Diagnosis and Prognosis*. Boston, MA: Butterworths, 1990.

Liu DTY (editor). *A Practical Guide to Chorion Villus Sampling*. New York, NY: Oxford, 1991.

Macri JN, Weiss RR. The utilization of alpha-fetoprotein in prenatal diagnosis. Birth Defects Original Article Series 1977;XIII(3D):191-199.

Milunsky A. *The Prevention of Genetic Disease and Mental Retardation*. Philadelphia, PA: WB Saunders, 1975.

Milunsky A (editor). *Genetic Disorders and the Fetus. Diagnosis, Prevention and Treatment*. Baltimore, MD: Johns Hopkins, 1992.

Schulman JD, Simpson JL (editors). *Genetic Diseases in Pregnancy. Maternal Effects and Fetal Outcome*. New York, NY: Academic Press, 1981.

Simpson JL. Incidence and timing of pregnancy losses: Relevance to evaluating safety of early prenatal diagnosis. Am J Med Genet 1990;5:165-173.

Wald NJ, Cuckle HS, Densem W, et al. Maternal serum screening for Down's syndrome in early pregnancy. Br Med J 1988;297:883-7.

Wald NJ, Cuckle HS, Densem W, et al. Maternal serum screening for Down's syndrome: The effect of routine ultrasound scan determination of gestational age and adjustment for maternal weight. Br J Obstet Gynaecol 1992;99:141-9.

Wald N, Cuckle HS, Wu t, et al. Maternal serum unconjugated oestriol and human chorionic gonadotrophin levels in twin pregnancies: Implications for screening for Down's syndrome. Br J Obstet Gynaecol 1991;98:9055-8.

Genetic Counseling

1. Genetic counseling is an interaction between counselor and consultand
    *   about genetic transmission or heritability of a disease.

*   A consultand is a person who has
    *   a risk of a genetic disorder in future children,
    *   is capable of reproduction,
    *   has the ability to make reproductive decisions, and has the
    *   freedom to choose among alternative methods of managing a genetic risk.

*   The accuracy of genetic counseling depends on
    *   the accuracy of the phenotype characterization and
    *   the thoroughness of the genealogical inquiry,

Mechanism affecting patient	Risks of having affected children	
	Parent	Patient
Polygenic	2%-16%	2%-16%
Autosomal recessive	25%	Remote
Segregation of heterologous chromosome translocation	5%-15%	50%
Segregation of homologous chromosome translocation	100%	50%
X-linked recessive (male patient)	50% of sons	Remote
Gonadal mosaicism in a parent	Remote to 100%	50%
Compound heterozygosity	25%	Remote
New dominant mutation	Remote	50%
Non-genetic	Remote	Remote

Risks and the Isolated Case (Family History Negative) in approximate order of occurrence

*   Interaction between counselor and non-consultands about genetic matters is
    *   not genetic counseling,
    *   nor are medical encounters with either consultands or non-consultands such as:
        *   diagnostic evaluation (history, physical, genealogy, laboratory);
        *   discussing the nature of the patient's disorder and
        *   its medical consequences to the patient with either patient or relatives.

*. Normals advised to avoid marrying carriers by 10% of carrier parents & 20% of normal parents
* When both found to be carriers, 20% broke engagement
* Both concealed carrier status, resulting in births of affected children
* Marriage and reproduction in spite of carrier status, resulting in affected children.
    REACTIONS TO GENETIC SCREENING (Adapted from Stamatoyannopoulas G [1974])

*   Genetic counseling by a physician is a form of medical evaluation and management,
    *   requiring history-taking, examination or evaluation of examination results, and
        *   medical decision making.

Reactions to birth of an affected child

A. Immediate: disorganization
1. Shock, disbelief, denial, rejection, repression
2. Increasing awareness of loss: sorrow, depression, guilt, anxiety, anger
   a. Peculiar long period of mourning for the lost image of a normal child
   b. Defenses: denial, repression, isolation of affect, avoidance: accompanied by exhaustion, nightmares, psychosomatic illness, rejection of sexual relations, social isolation, reliving of past mourning experiences.
   c. Mature adaptation: acceptance. Achieved by few without genetic counseling. Lasting maladaptive reactions are more common.

B. Long term
1. Sorrow, often lifelong, due to changelessness and unaesthetic quality of the disorder and The symbolism of a defective birth. A natural, not neurotic response.
2. Anger toward doctor, spouse, family, God, self. Latter leads to depression. 79% of mothers of cystic fibrosis children are depressed.
   a. Assuaged by aggressive social activities, fund-raising, sports.
3. Guilt
   a. Worse for carrier of X-linked disorder.
   b. If both parents are carriers, this may lead to psychosexual conflicts.
   c. Worst when child reproaches parents for the misery of his illness.
4. Anxiety: helplessness, outcome can't be altered, anticipation of child's and own death.

C. Effects on parenthood norms

Normal child	**Abnormal child**
Achieve or prove adult status, social identity	Fails proof[+]
Expansion of self, immortality, lineage	Exposes worst, tarnishes lineage[-]
Moral, avoid selfish identity	Self sacrifice[+]
Group ties, affiliation, avoiding loneliness	Need to be needed[+]
Stimulation, novelty, fun	Painful[-]
Creativity, accomplishment, competence	Meet challenges of rearing[+]
Power, influence, effectiveness, values	Test of religious faith[+]
Social comparison and competition	Dashed dreams[-]
Economic utility	Burden[-]
Redefining self along defensible lines	[+]positive influence [-]negative influence

D. Redefining self along defensible lines
1. Compensatory identity: accepting affected child as replacement for expected normal one
2. Trying again for a normal child
3. Maladaptive responses
   a. Cease reproduction
   b. Artificial insemination
   c. Adoption
   d. Sublimation: fostering, scouting
   e. Place blame elsewhere permanently:
      1. Doctor → alienation, malpractice suits
      2. God → agnosticism
      3. Spouse → divorce, new marriage, redefined self.

Adapted from Hollerbach PF (1979): Reproductive attitudes and the genetic counselee. In Hsia YE, Hirschorn K, Silverberg RL, Godmilow l, Eds. Counseling in Genetics. Alan R Liss, New York.

- The aim of genetic counseling is the realization of the
  - fullest potential of the consultand's genetic characteristics.

2. The process of genetic counseling includes at least four steps:
   - explanation of diagnosis
   - discussion of childbearing urges
   - risk analysis
   - formulation of management plan

- The diagnosis is explained in terms of the
  - burden or loss which might arise if an affected child were born.

- During explanation of the diagnosis, it is often necessary to also
  - dispel popular environmental paranoias and to
  - discuss the genetic mechanism of the disorder though these subjects are logically part of standard medical care, not genetic counseling.

- The counselor should determine degree of positive childbearing urge,
  - either personal or vicarious, of the consultand and
  - encourage self-awareness about childbearing.

- To elicit the consultand's childbearing urge, discuss the concept that
  - rights of the individual regarding reproduction take precedence over
  - theoretical "genetic health" of the population.

- The counselor must carefully avoid transference of personal childbearing opinions,
  - either general or specific to the consultand's circumstances.

3. Risk analysis must be tailored to the consultand because same numerical risk
   - may be interpreted as high by some persons or low by others.

- The prior probability is an inference based on prior data while the
  - conditional probability is the probability of a data set given the prior probability.

- In genetic counseling, the prior probability is often that of being either heterozygous or homozygous under an assumed mode of transmission while
  - conditional probabilities are the likelihoods of observed family information or results of laboratory studies.

- The joint probability of an observation is the product of the prior probability and the conditional probability while the
  - marginal probability is the sum of the joint probabilities of all possible observations.

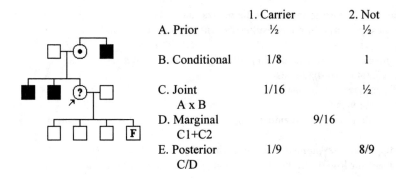

	1. Carrier	2. Not
A. Prior	½	½
B. Conditional	1/8	1
C. Joint A x B	1/16	½
D. Marginal C1+C2		9/16
E. Posterior C/D	1/9	8/9

The patient has an uncle and 2 brothers with muscular dystrophy. She has had 3 normal sons. What is the chance that her male fetus will have muscular dystrophy? The prior probability is the ½ chance that a daughter of a carrier will also be a carrier. The conditional probability is the chance that she would produce 3 normal sons given the prior (½ X ½ x ½ = 1/8 is she is a carrier, 1 x 1 x 1 if not).

AN EXAMPLE OF BAYESIAN ANALYSIS

- Bayes theorem is that the conditional probability can be inverted to allow an evaluation of the prior probability which is called the
  - posterior probability and is calculated for each event by dividing joint probability of that event by the marginal probability.

- When there are sufficient conditional probabilities in a case, Bayesian analysis allows calculation of accurate genetic risks because the posterior probability is
  - the likelihood of the initially inferred prior probability.

- Baseline risks should be used for comparison to the consultand's specific risk:
  - Of pregnancies that last long enough to produce a positive pregnancy test,
    - at least 15% abort spontaneously.
  - Of babies born alive,
    - at least 2% have a major anomaly.
  - From birth to age 60 years, diseases encoded in their genome at conception
    - develop in at least 20% of persons.

Events	Risks	
Death in auto accident per year	1:3700	0.0003
Death from lung cancer - nonsmoker	1:763	0.0013
Death from lung cancer - smoker	1:254	0.0039

Comparative Risks (Murphy EA, Chase GA [1975])

- Pitfalls in risk assessment include:
  - genetic heterogeneity in which
    - diagnosis is correct but amount of risk erroneous
  - phenocopies which have
    - remote genetic risk
  - non-paternity which may have
    - remote genetic risk to one biologic parent if the other is the carrier, or
    - remote biologic risk to either if they are autosomal recessive heterozygotes

- A majority of consultands with a positive childbearing urge will
  - tolerate a risk less than 10% and
  - eschew a risk greater than 20%.

4. Four valid approaches to management of a genetic risk include:
   - reproduce in spite of the risk
   - cease reproduction
   - temporarily suspend reproduction
   - conditional conception based on prenatal diagnosis.

- If a consultand decides to take a risk greater than 10% (often, the disorder is treatable), the counselor should carefully
  - review the counseling with the consultand to ensure understanding, then
  - support the consultand's decision appropriately.

- For consultands who wish to cease reproduction, you must
  - provide contraception or refer them for this purpose;
  - reversible methods are preferable because another reproductive partner
    - might yield a different risk or a different risk interpretation.

- Consultands who have a child with a chronic disorder (often their only child) may
  - eschew reproduction until they are managing well then risk a pregnancy later.

- Conception conditional on satisfactory prenatal diagnosis is applicable when
  - a prenatal test is available
  - therapeutic abortion for this reason is available
  - the consultand condones abortion
  - the health of the consultand is adequate.

- Artificial insemination and other forms of surrogate parenting are poor alternatives for managing a genetic risk because they have
  - the baseline risks plus an
  - unknown amount of risk due to the procedure, plus unique risks, e.g.,
  - claims of surrogate or donor, psychological threat to infertile parent,
  - the total risk approximating the natural risk faced by most consultands.

- Adoptive children are poor alternatives for managing a genetic risk
  because they have
  - the baseline risks plus an
  - unknown amount of risk of gestational pathology as undesired pregnancies and
  - a strong risk of disabling psychological disorder after adolescence,
  - the total risk often exceeding the natural risk faced by most consultands.

- Genetic counseling has been completed satisfactorily when the consultand can
  - confidently arrive at a firm and valid decision about management of the risk,
    - based on his or her own convictions.
  - The counselor must remain non-directive and non-judgmental.

The ***International Classification of Diseases, Clinical Modification***, currently in its ninth edition (**ICD-9-CM**) is the guide to diagnosis coding. Its stated purposes are: (1) retrieval of medical records for education and administration; (2) facilitation of payment for health services; and (3) research into evaluation of utilization patterns, appropriateness of health care costs, epidemiological studies, quality of health care. Those purposes require that the coding be based on the name of the disease that led to the need for medical services. Modifying codes to indicate the manifestation of the disease are included in brackets after the code of the disease. There are either specific or general codes for all diseases that lead to a need for genetic counseling. The modifying code for female consultands is 629.8 and for males, 608.81. Those are the codes for specified disorders of the genital organs of which production of genetically abnormal gametes is definitely one. In systems that do not have room for modifying codes, only the code of the basic disease is used. In two conditions, coding is explicit and modifying codes are not required:

Hemoglobinopathy S: proband: 282.6 relative (sickle trait): 282.5
Cleft palate proband: 749.01 relative (submucous cleft): 749.02

The need for genetic counseling about a disease is definitely a current problem for which patients seek medical care. The **ICD-9-CM** also includes "V" codes that are meant to be used "when a person who has no current problem encounters health care services." Some "V" codes could be construed to be applicable to genetic counseling, including one specifically entitled "Genetic counseling" (V26.3). Careful reading of **ICD-9-CM** indicates that the V26.3 code is intended specifically for genetic counseling as an adjunctive procedure in cases in which a patient has sought medical help in procreating. It is worthwhile to gain general ideas of the person's genetic background and counsel as to the likelihood of an unfortunate outcome of medically-induced procreation. That is quite different from actual physician-patient encounters for genetic counseling about diseases for which the V26.3 code is inappropriate.

DIAGNOSIS CODING

Genetic counseling by a physician or an agent of a physician is an encounter that is covered by Evaluation and Management definitions in ***Physician's Current Procedural Terminology*** (**CPT**). It may be either an inpatient or an outpatient encounter and the level of service depends on the complexity of the problem. Principles are the same as for any other type of encounter between physician and patient. For well-defined problems, the counseling encounter will involve a detailed history, and medical decision making of moderate complexity. An example would be a case of phenylketonuria. Complicated problems with multiple possible causes or outcomes will require a comprehensive history and medical decision making of high complexity. Examples are an isolated case in a family or a case of multiple congenital anomalies.

Genetic counseling by the physician may be accomplished during the same encounter as phenotype characterization and may simply be included among the considerations determining the level of service of that **new patient** encounter. However, phenotype characterization may be complicated and prolonged and may be completed by the physician, with separate codes and fees, prior to genetic counseling. Appropriate codes for subsequent genetic counseling would be those for an **established patient**. It would require from 25 to 60 minutes.

A physician may receive a case for genetic counseling after the phenotype characterization has been completed by another physician or medical agency. That adds a considerable degree of complexity to the encounter because the physician must evaluate not only the case but the accuracy of the phenotype characterization. Physical examination is required for verification. Questions about the diagnosis may occur to the physician during the encounter and further laboratory evaluation may also be required. Appropriate codes would depend on the nature of the relationship with the patient. Usually, the relationship would be a single encounter and would be coded as a **consultation**. Rarely, the referrer may wish to transfer care to the physician and the encounter would be coded as a **new patient**.

CODING OF LEVEL OF SERVICE

Background of counselor	Parents given counseling in sub-specialty clinics, e.g., congenital heart, cystic fibrosis, sickle cell, spina bifida, had virtually no understanding of genetic risks while nearly all counseled for the same disorders in Medical Genetics clinics understood the risks.
Background of consultand	Among impoverished, illiterate Greeks counseled by Greeks about sickle cell anemia, over 90% understood the risks. Among inner city US blacks counseled by blacks, less than 40% understood the risks.
Motivation of consultand	Virtually all self-referred consultands understand and appropriately utilize information gained from genetic counseling. Less than 10% of those who are referred without consent find any interest at all in it.
Research techniques	Investigators in the largest study did not realize that the diagnostic process precedes counseling in Medical Genetics clinics; hence, little or no counseling occurs at the first clinic visit. Nontheless, they found a 50% understanding of the risks after the first visit. They interpreted this as poor performance but it should be interpreted as either invalid or as unexpectedly good performance.

Results of Studies of Factors in Effectiveness of Genetic Counseling

Ethics

5. Ethics is the science of human duty and rules of conduct.
   * It is based upon a synthesis of philosophical and religious views
     * by well-informed, respected, thinking members of a society.
   * It forms the basis of a code of practice which is
     * accepted as reasonable by a majority of members of the society.

   * The specialty of Medical Genetics is now only one generation in duration, and its
     * ethical development has occurred in practice, based on principles of
       * informed consent,
       * informed choice,
       * patient autonomy,
       * confidentiality.

   * Arguments against codification of ethics:
     * Codes are rarely used.
     * Existing international codes are adequate.
     * A code would exclude the views of those whose opinions are in the minority.
     * Ethics is too subjective to codify.
     * Reproductive decisions are too personal
     * Technology changes too fast.
     * A code would lead to an increase in restrictive laws.
     * A code would restrict beneficial research.
     * A code would produce an increase of lawsuits.

   * Arguments in favor of codification of ethics:
     * A code would allay public fear of genetics concerning
       * eugenics, genetic manipulation, genetic engineering and modifying human nature.
     * A code would make genetics accountable to society.
     * A code would protect patients from harm.
     * A code would prevent development of restrictive laws.
     * A code would prevent lawsuits by setting standards that would otherwise be set in court.
     * A code would transmit the moral experience of geneticists to the next generation.
     * A code would improve the image of the profession
     * A code would improve the moral climate of research.
     * A code would have a beneficial influence on public policy.
     * A code would promote international cooperation.

   * A working code of ethics of Medical Genetics.
     * Equitable distribution of genetics services,
       * not dependent on social class or ability to pay, and with
       * priority given to those whose need is greatest.
     * Respect for, and safeguarding of, personal and parental choices in reproduction.

- Confidentiality regarding genetic information of individuals.
    - May be overridden only when four conditions are all met:
        - The individual cannot be convinced to disclose data to relatives.
        - Harm to relatives could be prevented if data were disclosed.
        - Harm to relatives would be serious.
        - Only data relevant to the relative would be disclosed.
- Protection of privacy from institutional third parties.
- Full disclosure of clinically relevant information to patients.
- Prenatal diagnosis only when relevant to health of fetus or mother.
- Acceptance of genetics services must be voluntary.
    - Present services are defined as
        - Prenatal diagnosis.
        - Testing for genetic diseases.
        - Presymptomatic testing.
        - Workplace screening for susceptibility to occupation-related diseases.
        - Genetic counseling.
    - Persons who refuse genetics services must not be stigmatized.
    - Newborn screening need not be voluntary, providing
        - Treatment would prevent harm.
        - Mandating agency provides prompt, affordable treatment.
- Genetic counseling must be non-directive.

- Parts of the working code may not reflect society at large.
    - 62% of medical geneticists favor prenatal diagnosis for sex selection.
    - 44% of the public favors genetic enhancement of intelligence and physique.

6. The eugenics movement of the latter 19th century and early 20th century
    - was an example of aberrant ethics.
    - Among factors that encouraged the eugenics movement were:
        - ignorance, unemployment and economic depression.

- The basis of the eugenics movement was biological determinism, an erroneous concept that
    - human characteristics are constitutional and mainly of genetic origin.
    - Undesirable "biological" characteristics included degeneracy, pauperism, criminality, prostitution, alcoholism, mental illness, mental retardation, epilepsy.
    - The concept was also extended into undesirable ethnicity:
        - Jews, Poles, Russians, southern Europeans, Africans.
    - Undesirable socioeconomic characteristics were also included:
        - unemployment, orphans, homeless persons.

- Negative eugenics was used to minimize transmission of genes for undesirable characteristics, through abortion, sterilization, euthanasia, and genetic discrimination.

- Genetic discrimination is benefit exclusion based on genotype,
    - currently of concern in health insurance, life insurance, and employment.

- Positive eugenics was used to maximize transmission of genes for desirable characteristics (especially a mythical "Aryan" phenotype), through artificial insemination, selective reproduction and genetic favoritism.

- Genetic favoritism is altruism based on genotype.

- Mathematical aspects of the eugenics movement were poorly conceived. Example:
  - Data about intelligence indicate that, using both positive and negative eugenics,
    - an IQ increase of 5 points would have required excluding nearly half of unions,
    - requiring a doubling of family size to sustain the population!

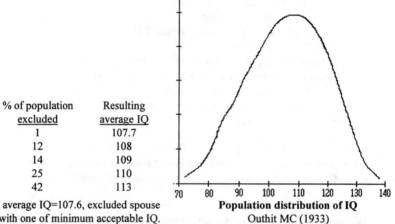

Minimum IQ for reproduction	% of population excluded	Resulting average IQ
70	1	107.7
80	12	108
85	14	109
90	25	110
100	42	113

Assumption: initial average IQ=107.6, excluded spouse would be replaced with one of minimum acceptable IQ.

Population distribution of IQ
Outhit MC (1933)

- Factors that could enable resurgence of eugenics (some mutually related):
  - Ignorance. Education about genetics is scanty and fraught with misconceptions.
  - Unemployment. An increasing problem due to numerous factors.
  - Economic depression. Government sequestration has replaced private.
  - Race. Racial and ethnic enmity is universal, and subcultures are ubiquitous.
  - Psychological responses to birth defects. Disgust leads to discrimination.
  - Stigmatization of carriers of genetic diseases.
  - Public health encroachments on autonomy.
  - Coerced prenatal diagnosis.

- Eugenics in a more enlightened, and more definitive, sense is
  - the science of producing healthy offspring, a basically innocent undertaking,
  - to which Medical Geneticists can contribute through
    - accurate identification of pathogenetic factors,
    - considerately and thoroughly informing patients,
    - advocacy of public enlightenment and education.
  - Medical Geneticists must also actively cultivate ethics
    - to prevent eugenic misuses like those of the past.

Additional references:

Genetic counseling

Emery AEH, Pullen IM (editors). *Psychological Aspects of Genetic Counselling*. New York: Academic Press, 1984.

Epstein CJ, Curry CJR, Packman S, et al. *Risk, Communication and Decision Making in Genetic Counseling*. Birth Defects Original Article Series 1979;15 (5c).

Evers-Kiebooms G, Cassiman J-J, Van Den Berghe H, et al (editors). *Genetic Risk, Risk Perception and Decision Making*. Birth Defects Original Article Series 1987;23 (2).

Fuhrmann W, Vogel F. *Genetic Counseling*, 2nd Edition. Heidelberg Science Library. New York: Springer-Verlag, 1976.

Harper P. *Practical Genetic Counseling*, 3rd Edition. Boston: Wright, 1988.

Capron AM, Lappe M, Murray RF, et al. *Genetic Counseling: Facts, Values, Norms*. Birth Defects Original Article Series 1979;15 (2).

Hsia YE, Hirschorn K, Silverberg RL, et al. *Counseling in Genetics*. New York: Alan R Liss, 1979.

Kelly PT. *Dealing With Dilemma. A Manual for Genetic Counselors*. Heidelberg Science Library. New York: Springer-Verlag, 1977.

Kessler S (editor). *Genetic Counseling. Psychological Dimensions*. New York: Academic Press, 1979.

Lubs HA, de la Cruz F (editors). *Genetic Counseling*. A Monograph of the National Institute of Child Health and Human Development. New York: Raven Press, 1977.

Murphy EA, Chase GA. *Principles of Genetic Counseling*. Chicago: Year Book Medical Publishers, 1975.

Murray RF, Bolden R, Headings VE. Information transfer in counseling for sickle cell trait. Am J Hum Genet 1974;26:63a.

Nora JJ, Fraser FC. *Medical Genetics. Principles and Practice*, 3rd Edition. Philadelphia: Lea & Febiger, 1989.

Reed SC. *Counseling in Medical Genetics*. Philadephia: Saunders, 1955.

Reisman LE, Matheny AP. *Genetics and Counseling in Medical Practice*. St. Louis: CV Mosby, 1969.

Sorenson JR, Swazey JP, Scotch NA (editors). *Reproductive Pasts, Reproductive Futures: Genetic Counseling and Its Effectiveness*. Birth Defects Original Article Series 1981:17 (4).

Stamatoyannapoulas G. Problems of screening and counseling in the hemoglobinopathies. In: Motulsky AG, Lenz W (editors). *Birth Defects: Proceedings of the Fourth International Conference*. Amsterdam: Excerpta Medica, 1974.

Weiss JO, Bernhardt BA, Paul NW (editors). *Genetic Disorders & Birth Defects in Families and Society: Toward Interdisciplinary Understanding*. Birth Defects Original Article Series 1984;20 (4).

Ethics

Durfy SJ. Ethics and the Human Genome Project. Arch Pathol; Lab Med 1993;117:466-469.

Evans MI, Drugan A, Bottoms SF, et al. Attitudes on the ethics of abortion, sex selection, and selective pregnancy termination among health professionals, ethicists, and clergy likely to encounter such situations. Am Jo Obstet Gynecol 1991;164:1092-9.

Fletcher JC. Gene therapy in mental retardation: Ethical considerations. Ment Ret and Dev Disabil Res Rev 1995; 1:7-13.

Garver KL, Garver B. The Human Genome Project and eugenic concerns. Am J Hum Genet 1994; 54:148-58.

Ledley FD. Distinguishing genetics and eugenics on the basis of fairness. Jour Med Ethics 1994; 20:157-64.

Mueller RF, Young ID. *Emery's Elements of Medical Genetics*, 9th edition. New York: Churchill Livingstone, 1995:287:291.

Parker LS. Bioethics for human geneticists: Models for reasoning and methods for teaching. Am J Hum Genet 1994; 54:137-147.

U.S. Congress, Office of Technology Assessment. New developments in biotechnology. Background paper. Public perceptions of biotechnology. OTA-BP-BA-32, Washington DC: U.S. Government Printing Office, 1987:73-74.

Wertz DC, Fletcher JC. Geneticists approach ethics: An international survey. Clin Genet 1993;43:104-110.

Wertz DC, Fletcher JC. Proposed: An international code of ethics for medical genetics. Clin Genet 1993;44:37-43.

Wertz DC, Fletcher JC. Prenatal diagnosis and sex selection in 19 nations. Soc Sci Medicin 1993; 37:1359-66.

BACKGROUND

1. Universal screening of newborns for a disease was the initial public health approach to medical genetics. Though begun around 1950, the guiding principles were not articulated until 1986 [6].
    *   Characteristics of the disorder:
        *   Occurs frequently.
        *   Causes severe functional impairment.
        *   Intervention effective only before clinical diagnosis.
        *   Quantitative or qualitative alteration of a substance that permits differentiation of affected subjects from unaffected.
    *   Characteristics of the test:
        *   Reliable.
        *   Valid.
        *   Adaptable to mass screening.
    *   Characteristics of the screening system:
        *   Mechanism for determining effectiveness of screening test under field conditions.
        *   Prompt collection and analysis of specimens and reporting of positive results.
        *   Physician and patient understanding.
        *   Net economic benefit or effectiveness.

Disease	Incidence	Therapy	Mandated*	Practiced
Sickle cell anemia	1:2,500	+	30	43
Congenital hypothyroidism	1:4,000	+	48	53
Phenylketonuria	1:14,000	+	48	53
Atypical phenylketonuria	1:17,000	+		
Maternal phenylketonuria	1:30,000	+		
Cystinuria	1:15,000	0		
Histidinemia	1:17,000	?	9	
Galactosemia	1:60,000	+	38	43
Argininosuccinic acidemia	1:70,000	+		
Homocystinuria	1:100,000	+	16	21
Hyperglycinemia	1:140,000	+		
Maple syrup urine	1:175,000	+	18	24
Tyrosinemia	1:300,000	?	6	6

* In some states or territories, screening is authorized by regulation or standard of practice.

NEWBORN DISEASES FOR WHICH SCREENING IS AVAILABLE [1]

*   Lousiana law mandates newborn screening for phenylketonuria, congenital hypothyroidism and sickle cell anemia. In 1993 galactosemia screening was removed from the law and substituted with a program to inform about standards of practice for clinical symptoms of galactosemia.
    *   The State Health Department shoulders most of the burden of screening and treatment but the physician remains legally responsible for the outcome.
    *   Duties mandated of the physician:
        *   Obtain, or supervise the obtaining of the blood specimen.
        *   Assist in locating babies with positive results, and in maintaining treatment.
        *   Refer affected babies to specialists and support management regimen.

- Newborn screening programs for metabolic diseases have arisen due to political expediency and pressure from zealots and have only partially met the guiding principles. Though of unquestioned benefit to the affected child, some of their unfortunate characteristics include:
  - Lingering questions about aims and effectiveness.
    - Original aim was "to combat mental retardation" [9].
      - Current stated aim is "to provide testing, counseling and referral [8]," which is the same as the aim of the specialty of Medical Genetics in general.
  - No consideration has been given to the implications of changing incidence.
  - Legislation is proposed yearly on a zealous basis to screen for other diseases.

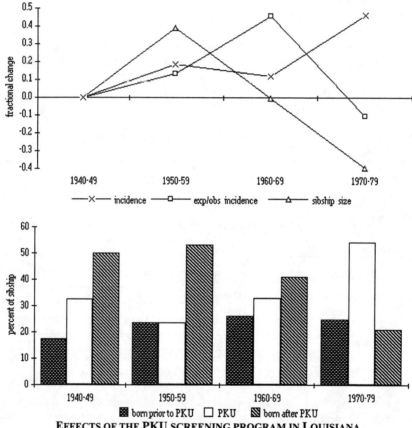

EFFECTS OF THE PKU SCREENING PROGRAM IN LOUISIANA.

80 completed sibships of phenylketonuria probands had sufficient data for tracking 40 years. The probands had 18 affected sibs and 138 unaffected sibs. A precipitous decrease in sibship size led to a gradual increase to only about twice the initial incidence, much less than it would have been if the sibship size had remained the same. Mandated PKU screening began in 1965. To avoid increased incidence, it would be necessary to ascertain all phenylketonuria heterozygotes and limit them to a total of 2 children [14].

- Over-representation of therapeutic benefit:
  In reality, a wide range of responses to therapy is seen due to
  - differing disease alleles which have differing outcomes,
  - differing individual metabolic pathways,
  - differing levels of compliance with therapy.

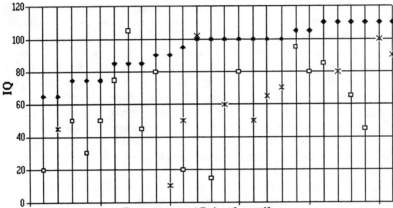

Treatment status: ◆Early □Late ✗None.

Each vertical line represents a sibship. The data points are the IQ scores of individual cases [6].

	Treatment		
	None	Late	Early
% below IQ 85	80	78	31
% average IQ	62	58	94

Treatment regimen, compliance, genetic heterogeneity and other factors result in different results of treatment. Patients treated early do better *on average*. However, IQ of non-treated or late-treated patients correlates with IQ of treated sib. Hence, family resemblance is a strong determinant of IQ even when PKU is present. In about 30% of cases, treatment of PKU does not result in "normal" IQ and in about 20% of cases, non-treatment does not result in mental retardation [7].

EFFECTS OF TREATMENT OF PHENYLKETONURIA

- Exaggerated estimates of cost/benefit ratio:
  - most estimates assume that treatment will avoid institutionalization while in reality modern management rarely includes institutionalization anyway.
  - full cost accounting is not made and major costs are not mentioned, e.g., many hospitals have to hire additional staff to handle the specimens from newborns being discharged on weekends and holidays.

CURRENT STATUS

2. Newborn screening has had best results with phenylketonuria and hypothyroidism which are
   - relatively more common than other metabolic diseases,
   - often amenable to treatment, and
   - have well-defined genetics.

   Little cost is added to screen for galactosemia because it can be done on the same specimen and there are so few positives that little additional work is required for followup, however,
   - individual treatment results are less predictable and
   - genetic aspects are complex.

- Clinical picture of phenylketonuria.
    - Classic: Phenylalanine hydroxyolase deficiency (PAH). Most are asymptomatic in first year, few ever diagnosed without laboratory screening; 25% have eczema and some have a musty odor and depigmentation. Thereafter, delayed development is noticed. Some never walk or talk. Many have seizures. Most have hyperactive, agitated and aggressive behavior. Other common findings are tremor, microcephaly, prominent maxilla with widened interdental spaces and enamel hypoplasia, decalcification of long bones, poor growth. Severe older cases may develop *Schneidersitz*, a sitting posture with incessant rhythmic movements of arms.
        - There is considerable genetic heterogeneity of the phenylalanine hydroxylase locus at chromosome 12q24.1. Phenylketonuria is an autosomal recessive trait so a mutant gene at that locus on one homologue causes no disease. Disease results when both homologues house a mutant gene. Different ethnic groups have characteristic arrays of mutant genes and associated haplotypes which vary in clinical severity.
    - Type IV: dihydrobiopterin reductase (DHPR) deficiency. Inadequate recycling of biopterin (cofactor for PAH, tyrosine hydroxylase & liver enzymes which hydrolize alkyl esters of glycerol). DOPA, folate, serotonin deficiency and ester accumulation → poor feeding, choking, seizures.
    - Type V: deficiency of enzymes of biopterin synthesis (GTP cyclohydrolase, 6-pyruvoyl-tetrahydropterin synthetase). More profound deficit of biopterin. Added symptoms: spasticity, drooling, athetosis, myoclonus.

- Newborn screening for phenylketonuria.
    - Normal serum phenylalanine
        - Premature: 2.0-7.5 mg/dl
        - Newborn: 1.2-3.4 mg/dl
        - Older: 0.8-1.8 mg/dl

Guthrie screening cutoff: 4 mg/dl
- Cases missed by Guthrie
    - 24 hrs   16.1%
    - 48 hrs   2.2%
    - 72 hrs   0.3%
- Improvement over Guthrie:
    - Rescreen around age 7 days with Guthrie.
    - Spectrophotometric phenylalanine method.
    - Serum phenylalanine/tyrosine ratio chromatography

Diagnosis:
- Positive Guthrie: found with all types if baby is on milk.
- State Lab obtains urine neopterin/biopterin in all cases.
    - Neopterin and biopterin are present in type IV, only neopterin is present in type V.
- Documentation and classification. Done under State Program.
    - Plasma and urine chromatography for amino acids

Classification	Phenylalanine hydroxylase	Phenylalanine tolerance	Blood phenylalanine
I Classic	<0.27%	<0.13 mM/kg/day	>25 mg/dl
Mild		0.14-0.3 mM/kg/day	
II	1.5%-34.5%	0.7 mM/kg/day	4-15 mg/dl
III	Like type II but normalize before 18 months age		
IV	Like classic type I but clinically worse & no improvement with diet		
V	Like classic type I but clinically worse & no improvement with diet		

- Clinical picture of congenital hypothyroidism: Most have prolonged jaundice and feeding problems in the nursery. Other frequent problems are enlarged fontanelle and large tongue. Less frequent are decreased activity, hypotonia, hoarse cry, cool dry skin, constipation, umbilical hernia and goiter. Except for those with a large number of these findings or a goiter, they are usually not suspected of having hypothyroidism. Only 10 to 15% are diagnosed clinically. Untreated cases develop short stature and mental retardation.

- Newborn screening for congenital hypothyroidism.
  - Normal newborn   T4:   6.2-22 ug/dl
                             TSH: 3.0-18 uU/ml

  - State lab screening cutoff: T4   < 6 ug/dl
                                         TSH   > 20 uU/ml

  - False positive rates.
    - T4: 0.16%
    - TSH done at age   24 hrs: 6.0%
    -                            96 hrs: 0.05%

  - Types
    - Aplastic thyroid   20%
      Hypoplastic thyroid   13%
      Goitorous cretinism   20%
      Lingual thyroid   25%
      Transient hypothyroidism   17%
      Hypothalamic hypopituitarism   5%

Note: Most types are autosomal recessive traits so family history may be negative for affected relatives. Parents may be consanguineous. A few cases have a severe form of the common polygenic thyroidopathy in which immediate family members may have either hyperthyroidism, hypothyroidism or various forms of thyroiditis. Some cases may have teratogenic or chromosomal syndromes in which there is an array of abnormalities of the CNS and other systems. Excessive dietary iodine taken by the mother has caused some cases.

- Diagnosis flow chart:
  - If T4 is low, do TSH on same filter paper spot.
    - High TSH = hypothyroidism. Treat.
    - Normal or low TSH: do thyroxine-binding globulin (TBG) on same specimen
      - Low TBG = hereditary normal variant - most are X-linked; a few are autosomal dominant. Incidence: 1:10,000.
      - Normal TBG: obtain a repeat filter paper spot and start over. Some babies will have a normal T4 on repeat and need no further observation. Others will have low T4 and a high TSH and will need treatment for hypothyroidism. Some will still have low T4 and TSH and will need evaluation by a pediatric endocrinologist.

- Clinical picture of galactosemia: Abnormalities are usually not noticed at birth in babies with galactosemia though most of them are born with involvement of the lens, liver, kidney and brain. Excessive levels of galactose and galactose metabolites have been found in liver and red cells of galactosemic fetuses as early as 21 weeks gestation. Because glucose can serve as an endogenous source of galactose, red cell concentration of galactose metabolites is elevated in cord blood of the galactosemic fetus even if the mother was on a galactose-free diet throughout pregnancy. In classical cases, feedings of milk after birth lead to food refusal, vomiting and diarrhea. Jaundice ensues rapidly, followed by lethargy, weight loss and hypotonia. E. coli sepsis develops in the second week of life in 50% of classic cases, apparently due to leukocyte toxicity of galactose metabolites. Untreated survivors grow and develop poorly ("failure to thrive"), and evolve nuclear cataracts, hepatic cirrhosis and mental retardation. Older patients express visual-perceptual defect, tremor, ataxia and ovarian failure despite treatment. Cataracts regress with treatment. Wide variation in clinical picture and response to treatment stems from differing genetic types as well as individual variations within genetic types. Individual variant genetic types are so rare that adequate comparison of their clinical pictures has not been done. Without newborn screening, at least 40% of galactosemics who survive the newborn period are not diagnosed clinically by age 1 month and about 25% are still undiagnosed by 4 months age. There is poor correlation between outcome and the age at which treatment was started.

- Newborn screening for galactosemia: The enzyme-linked fluorescent assay of galactose-1-phosphate uridyl transferase that is used for newborn screening shows complete absence of enzyme activity in affected homozygotes. More sensitive tests may reveal a tiny amount of residual activity in some cases. These are all classified as gt genotypes, analysis of the cDNA of the gene reveals a large number of different mutations.

  - A large number of "normal" and "quasi-normal" variants of the enzyme gene exist. Those with 100% activity have been classified as Gt genotypes. The most common varient is the "Duarte" allele, Gt^D.

Genotype	Frequency (%)	Enzyme activity (%)	Phenotype
GtGt	91.2	100	Normal
$GtGt^D$	7.6	75	Normal
Gt^DGt^D	0.16	50	Normal
Gtgt	0.96	50	Normal
Gt^Dgt	0.04	25	Borderline
gtgt	0.0025	0	Galactosemia

- Rarer variants:

		Clinical symptoms	
Variant allele	Enzyme activity in homozygotes	homozygotes	compound (variant/gt) heterozygotes
Berne	40	?	?
Chicago	25	?	yes
Indiana	0 to 40	?	yes
Munster	30	yes	yes
Negro	0	yes	yes
Rennes	7 to 10	yes	yes

Indications for Proband Services

A. Infants with failure to thrive or children with short stature (below 3rd percentile).

B. Patients with a major malformation, e.g., cleft lip/palate, heart defect, absence of a part.

C. Patients with multiple congenital anomalies.

D. Patients who have a syndrome or are suspected of having a syndrome.

E. Small for gestational age babies with anomalies or abnormal measurements.

F. Children with motor or mental delay or regression not due to infection or trauma.

G. Patients with ambiguous genitalia.

H. Patients with suspected inherited diseases of metabolism:
- Fulminant disease in the newborn (asphyxia, sepsis or respiratory distress)
- Involutional neonatal symptoms (vomiting, feeding failure, seizure, lethargy, abnormal tone)
- Patients who develop fluid & electrolyte problems when ill
- Susceptibility to infectious diseases and poor growth and development
- Short stature, epilepsy, mental retardation

I. Patients with suspected chromosome aberrations:
- multiple congenital anomalies
- sex identity problems
- reproductive problems
- behavioral disorders
- mental retardation
- certain malignancies (also used to evaluate therapeutic response).

J. Patients in whose families other relatives have the same disorder as the patient, e.g.:
- bleeding disorder
- blindness
- cerebral palsy
- deafness
- dwarfism
- heart defect
- malformations
- mental retardation
- neuromuscular disorder
- non-nutritional anemia
- seizures

K. Women with primary amenorrhea or unexplained infertility.

L. Couples with a history of a child who died with anomalies.

M. Couples with multiple miscarriages or stillbirths.

N. Consanguineous couples.

O. Certain pregnant women:
- maternal age to be 35 years or older at time of baby's birth.
- previous child with chromosome aberration.
- carriers of balanced chromosome translocations.
- carriers of X-linked disorders, e.g., hemophilia.
- carriers of biochemical or metabolic disorders.
- patient herself has a malformation or a syndrome.
- family history of neural tube defect.
- MSAFP less than 0.6 or greater than 2.0 MOM.

Modified from: Cherry FF, Trachtman L, Braud SM, et al. *Procedure Manual. Genetic Diseases Program.* New Orlenas, LA: Louisiana Department of Health and Human Resources, 1983:8.

3.   Other Public Health genetics services:
  * Extended screening for phenylketonuria for persons not previously tested.
    * Women in prenatal clinics.
    * Mentally retarded persons.
    * Family members of known cases.
    * Recipients of Handicapped Children's Services.
  * Management of metabolic diseases.
    * Confirmatory tests.
    * Monitoring plasma levels of patients on dietary treatment of metabolic diseases.
    * Issuance of special formulas for infants with metabolic diseases.
      * Requires attendance to Tulane Hayward Genetics Center in New Orleans, as well as strict adherence to treatment guidelines.
  * Sickle cell anemia services.
    * Pilot screening programs for women in prenatal clinics and family planning clinics.
    * Family studies when indicated.
    * Centralized tracking of cases and suspected cases.
    * Medical services.
      * Sickle cell anemia clinics in hospitals in the state system.
      * Nursing supervision through local Health Units.
  * "Proband services" through Regional Genetics Clinics throughout the state.
    * Medical evaluation, laboratory testing and genetic counseling for a wide range of conditions.
      * Professional staff are under contract from academic institutions but support staff and clinic facilities derive from regional health units.
      * Patients requiring more extensive services may be referred to the institution.
      * Services are coordinated with other specialties and ancillary professionals.
    * Services do not extend to relatives but are available through the institution.

THE FUTURE: RETRENCHMENT OR IMPROVEMENT?

4.   Provision of medical care for genetic diseases to promote public health is at a crossroads.
  * Historically, services gradually transfer to the general health care system as it acquires the capabilities. This is occurring in regard to Medical Genetics at present.
    * Medical genetics services under public health are less satisfactory to the consumer.
      * Less than 25% recalled receiving medical genetics services [10,14].
        * Of those, 60% found the services of some benefit (15% of original group).
      * Approximately 50% of patients receiving the same services in other public settings recalled the service,
        * and 50% found the services beneficial (25% of original group).
        In a private care environment, 100% of patients recalled receiving services,
        * and 90% found the services beneficial (90% of original group).
    * Most of these differences appear to relate to motivation, i.e., when the need is perceived by the system rather than the patient, the service may not be valued by the patient [14].
  * Commercialization of medical care in the late 20th century has produced competitive compartmentalizations of patient populations. This may reverse historical tendencies.

- Medical genetics problems have a unique epidemiology which must be considered in planning either for provision of services or for prevention.

- Spontaneous mutation initiates the process of genetic disease causation.
  - This type of mutation differs from induced mutation in that it reflects physiochemical limitations of processes that maintain DNA integrity.
  - Within each species, the spontaneous mutation rate is constant and is a recognizable characteristic of a species [11].
  - Since induced mutation plays no part in genetic disease etiology,
    - services provided in correlation with mutagen locations are not more likely to reach significant proportions of patients,
    - nor can genetic disease incidence be lowered by decreasing exposure to mutagens.

- Primordial order (mostly random mating) would keep genetic diseases at basal rates.
  - Submicroscopic mutations usually occur in heterozygous form and most are recessive.
    - Due to the haploid state of the gamete, there is a slight differential survival of gametes bearing the normal gene which results in loss of the mutant gene in a few generations.
  - Visible mutations as well as submicroscopic dominant mutations are lost from the population, and polygenic diseases are kept at basal rates, because of:
    - Limited survival of newborns.
    - Limited ability to reproduce.

- Departures from primordial order promulgate mutations within a population and increases frequencies of all genetic diseases. The departures are inter-related. The vehicle in most cases is departure from random mating, especially assortative mating.
  - Reproductive dominance.
    - Group living.
    - Conquest.
  - Consanguineous mating.
    - Geographic or cultural reproductive isolation.
  - Altruism.
    - Medical care, especially that of the newborn and infant.
    - Fraternalization.

Some genetic diseases are accorded more public significance.
  - Numerical significance may be inversely related to accorded significance.
    - Non-genetic disorders, though formerly more significant, have waned.
    - Polygenic disorders are the least understood but the most significant.
    - Disorders due to submicroscopic mutations are of intermediate significance.
    - Disorders due to visible mutations are of less significance but are well known because their graphical nature promotes ease of comprehension.

	Affected	Etiologic factors			
		Submicroscopic mutations	Visible mutations	Polygenic	Non-genetic
Neonatal screening	0.2	100			
Handicapped Children	3	24	1	74	1
Spina bifida	*0.1*		*1*	*97*	*1*
Muscular dystrophy	*0.001*	*100*			
Hemophilia	*0.001*	*100*			
Blindness	*0.01*	*44*	*2*	*44*	*10*
Deafness	*0.01*	*44*	*2*	*44*	*10*
Neonatal intensive care	0.1	25	10	60	5
Mental retardation	0.5	25	10	60	5
Total	3.8				
Cumulative significance [Σ(affected X etiology)]		107	9	258	6

MEDICAL GENETICS PUBLIC HEALTH PROBLEMS, THEIR ETIOLOGIES AND SIGNIFICANCES.
The Affected column contains approximate population incidences of the disorders. Numbers are
percentages: overall percentage to the left, component percentages to the right. The non-genetic
category comprises dysmorphological conditions. Interpretation examples: The Handicapped
Children category comprises 3% of all births. 24% are due to submicroscopic mutations, 1% due to
visible mutations, 74% polygenic, and 1% non-genetic. In the Non-genetic column, cumulative
significance is estimated by multiplying the number in the Affected column by the number in the
Etiologic factor column, then summing. Handicapped children 3 x 1 = 3, Neonatal intensive care 0.1
x 5 = 0.5, Mental retardation 0.5 x 5 = 2.5, sum = 6. The chart indicates that the two most significant
causes of Medical Genetics Public Health problems are submicroscopic mutations and polygenic
diseases.

	Physiological submicroscopic mutations	Morphological submicroscopic mutations	Chromosome aberrations	Polygenic
Current program	D	D	D	D
Biochemical tests	P(2)D			
Chromosome tests			P(1)D(2)	
Screening physical exam		D(2)	D(2)	D(2)
Genetic registry	P(2)	P(2)	P(1)	P(2)
Extended genealogy	P(2)	P(2)	P(1)	P(2)
Genetic counseling	P	P(2)	P(2)	P(2)

Public health approaches to genetic diseases. D=diagnostic (medical care), P=preventive,
(1)=applicable only to rare familial cases, (2)=underutilized.

Underutilized Public Health approaches that promote the public health (medical care):
* expanded screening physical examination of newborns and pre-schoolers which
  * would supplement the standard examination with
    * measurements of all body parts for which standards exist [2],
    * retinal visualization,
    * dermatoglyphics recording,
    * photographs of any physical abnormalities found.
  * Definitive diagnosis of any abnormalities that are found.
    * Imaging of brain and other internal organs are the most important, followed by
    * neurological electrodiagnostic tests,
    * echocardiography, and
    * access to a complete panel of medical specialists.
  * Louisiana's unique coordinated medical care system of public hospitals, academic medical institutions and private health care facilitates these approaches.

* Laboratory testing - often unavailable through local health care providers or too costly.
  * Biochemical testing for genetic disorders
  * DNA testing for genetic disorders
  * Karyotyping for chromosome disorders

Underutilized Public Health approaches to prevention of genetic diseases.
* Anything like primordial order is impossible.
* Some approaches may not be palatable. High utilization of elective abortion of chromosomally abnormal fetuses has produced chromosome aberration frequency below basal level in at least one metropolitan area but has poor utilization in most areas [4].
* A centralized registry of genetic diseases, which facilitates tracing of genetic diseases to
  * segments of the population with the greatest departure from random breeding.
* Extended studies of the genealogies of probands, which
  * identify persons who have excessive potential of abnormal progeny [3].
* Genetic counseling for relatives of reproductive age, which permits
  * informed reproductive decisions by persons who have excessive potential of abnormal progeny.

The combined use of the last three is both acceptable and highly effective. Research models show only occasional instances of uncooperativeness, of failure to recall services, of unappreciativeness, or of failure to act appropriately upon indications of genetic risk [5,12].

* Laboratory testing can also be preventive by
  * identifying relatives of probands who have excessive potential of abnormal progeny.

Additional references:

1. Council of Regional Networks for Genetic Services. National Newborn Screening Report, 1991.

2. Hall JG, Froster-Iskenius UG, Allanson JE. *Handbook of Normal Physical Measurements.* New York: Oxford, 1989.

3. Harper AE. Potential contributions of genetic epidemiology. Genet Epidemiol 1988;5:203.

4. Heuther C, Karam S, Priest J, et al. Utilization of prenatal chromosome diagnosis and its impact on reducing births with Down syndrome in metropolitan Atlanta and southwest Ohio. Am J Hum Genet 1991;49(Supplement):471.

5. Hill TW. Louisiana: a genetic gold mine. Medical World News, 1972; February 11.

6. Holtzman NA. Genetic screening: criteria and evaluation - A message for the future. In: Carter TP, Willey AM (editors). *Genetic Disease Screening and Management.* New York: Alan R. Liss, 1986.

7. Hsia DYY, Holtzman NA. A critical evaluation of PKU screening. In McKusick VA, Claiborne R (editors). *Medical Genetics.* New York: Hospital Practice Publishers, 1973.

8. Louisiana Department of Health and Human Resources (1983): Procedure Manual. Genetic Diseases Program.

9. Louisiana Revised Statutes 40:1299. Acts 1964, No. 1269,1.

10. Sorenson JR, Swazey JP, Scotch NA (editors). *Reproductive Pasts, Reproductive Futures: Genetic Counseling and Its Effectiveness.* Birth Defects Original Article Series 1981;17 (4).

11. Suzuki DT, Griffiths AJF, Miller JH, Lewontin RC. Chapter 7. An Introduction to Genetic Analysis. *Gene Mutation,* 2nd Edition. New York: WH Freeman, 1981.

12. Thurmon TF. The Primary Prevention Program. A part of the yearly progress report on Grant number CE-39 to the National Foundation-March of Dimes, 1976.

13. Thurmon TF, Robertson KP, Paddison P. Genetic counseling and the non-motivated Consumer. Am J Hum Genet 1978;30:70A.

14. Thurmon TF, Ursin SA. Phenylketonuria Trends. Am Hum Genet 1984;36:182S.

15. Further references about phenylketonuria:

• Eisensmith RC, Woo SLC. Molecular basis of phenylketonuria and related hyperphenylalaninemias: mutations and polymorphisms in the human phenylalanine hydroxylase gene. Hum. Mutat. 1992;1:13-23.

• Guthrie R. Blood screening for phenylketonuria. JAMA 1961;178:863.

• Knox WE. Phenylketonuria. In: Stanbury JB, Wyngaarden JB, Fredrickson DS (editors). *The Metabolic Basis of Inherited Disease,* 3rd edition. New York, NY: McGraw-Hill,1972:266-295.

• Tyfield LA, Stephenson A, Cockburn F, et al. Sequence variation at the phenylalanine hydroxylase gene in the British Isles. Am J Hum Genet 1997;60:388-96.

16. Further references about screening:

• Bickel H, Guthrie R, Hammersen G, editors. *Neonatal Screening for Inborn Errors of Metabolism*. New York: Springer-Verlag, 1980.

• Carter TP, Wiley AM , editors. *Genetic Disease. Screening and Management*. New York: Alan R. Liss, 1986.

• Committee for the Study of Inborn Errors of Metabolism. *Genetic Screening. Programs, Principles, and Research*. Washington, D.C.: National Academy of Sciences, 1975.

• President's Commission for the Study of Ethical Problems in Medicine and Biomedical and Behavioral Research. *Screening and Counseling for Genetic Conditions. A Report on the Social and Legal Implications of Genetic Screening, Counseling and Education Programs*. Library of Congress card number 83-600502. Washington, D.C.: U.S.Government Printing Office, 1983.

• Reichardt JK, Levy HL, Woo SL. Molecular characterization of two galactosemia mutations and one polymorphism: Implications for structure-function analysis of human galactose-1-phosphate uridyltransferase. Biochemistry 1992;31:5430-5433.

• Rodenstock IW, Childs B, Simopoulos AP. *Genetic Screening. A Study of the Knowledge and Attitudes of Physicians*. Washington, D.C.: National Academy of Sciences, 1975.

• Schild S. Psychological issues in genetic counseling of phenylketonuria. In Kessler S. *Genetic Counseling. Psychological Dimensions*. New York: Academic Press, 1979.

• Scriver, C.R., Beaudet, A.L., Sly, W.S., Valle, D., Editors. *The Metabolic Basis of Inherited Disease*, 6th edition. New York: McGraw-Hill, 1989.

16. Appreciation is expressed to Mr. Charles Myers, Administrator of the Louisiana Genetic Diseases Program, for review of the manuscript of this chapter and for helpful comments and additions.

Data for these charts were compiled from the publications listed in Additional References. The graphic charts were re-plotted and smoothed in order to standardize the terminology as percentiles. In each case, the resulting curves were analyzed in order to identify theoretical extremes near the ends of the distributions. The lowest point identified was 0.001 percentile, and the highest, 99.999 percentile. Measurements within that range have normalcy potential, especially when the measurements of close relatives are similar, while measurements outside of that range are seldom normal. Blood pressure is described in standard deviations, above +2 standard deviations regarded as hypertension. A theoretical third standard deviation was also plotted.

Within the theoretical normal range, percentiles are relative. Their value is to allow tracking and to identify incongruencies. One critical exception is the use of mid-arm muscle circumference to recognize malnutrition. Persons with normal nutrition seldom have values below fifth percentile. Young children below the third percentile usually require parenteral nutrition for recovery.

Cultural and genetic differences are known to affect these anthropological data. Only striking, practical and well-documented differences are included here. Some that could be of clinical value are not well documented. An example is palpebral fissure width. African heritage is known to produce a considerable increase. That could lead to failure of diagnosis of the alcohol syndrome; however, there are not enough data available for a graphic chart.

The graphics charts that are included here pertain to body parts for which measurements may be considered a part of a routine physical examination. Lack of standardized expressions of these measurements makes diagnosis of dysmorphic conditions a matter of dead-reckoning or gestalt. By contrast, variable expression is so common that normal measurements of a part known to be affected by a dysmorphic condition does not totally rule it out. Hence, the charts are meant to be used with discretion in order to provide concrete statements about physical characteristics.

The references include other graphic charts that can help in analyzing growth in syndromes that affect one or another of the parameters upon which graphics charts are based. Also in the references are graphics charts of numerous other body parts that might not be typically measured as a part of a routine physical examination but might need analysis in order to recognize a specific syndrome.

List of charts:

Newborn: head circumference, weight, length, leg length	Testis length
Head circumference	Triceps skin fold
Weight	Mid arm circumference
Height	Mid arm muscle circumference
Leg length (lower segment)	Middle finger length
Inner canthal	Palm length
Interpupillary	Arm length
Outer canthal	Foot length
Palpebral fissure width	Bone age
Cornea diameter	Tooth eruption
Nose length	Blood pressure
Philtrum	Total cholesterol
Intercommisural width	HDL cholesterol
Ear length	LDL cholesterol
Body mass index	Triglycerides
Chest circumference	Dermatoglyphics
Internipple distance	Normal traits
Penis length	

Newborn

Head circumference

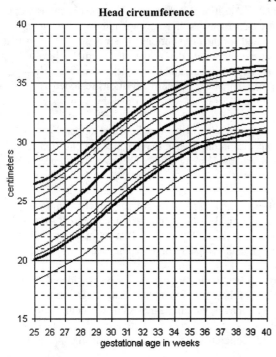

Weight

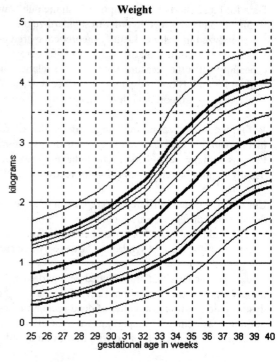

Length

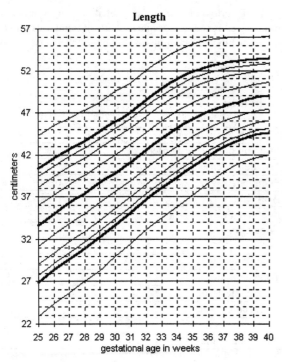

Leg length (lower segment)

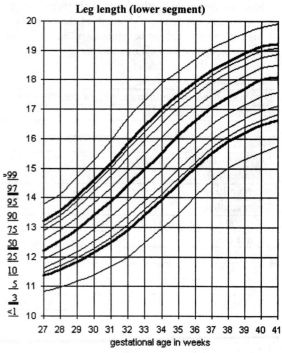

Head Circumference

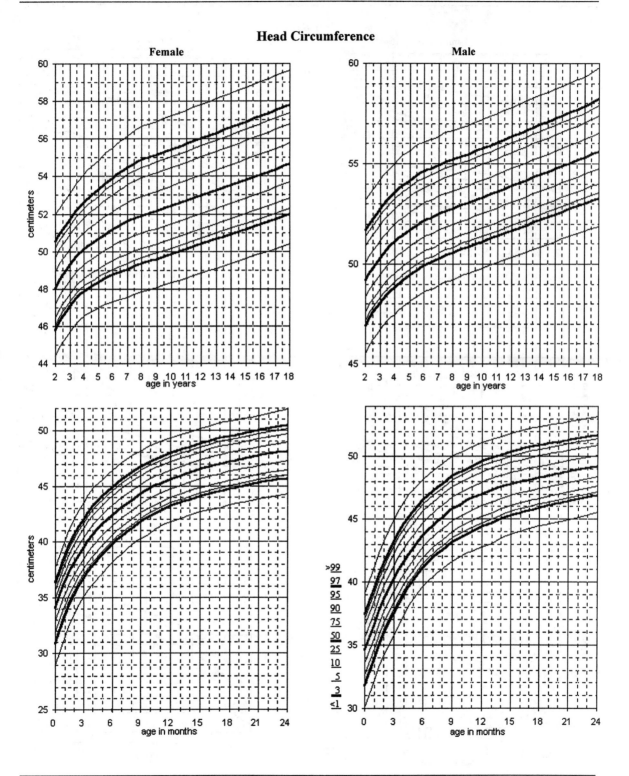

Weight

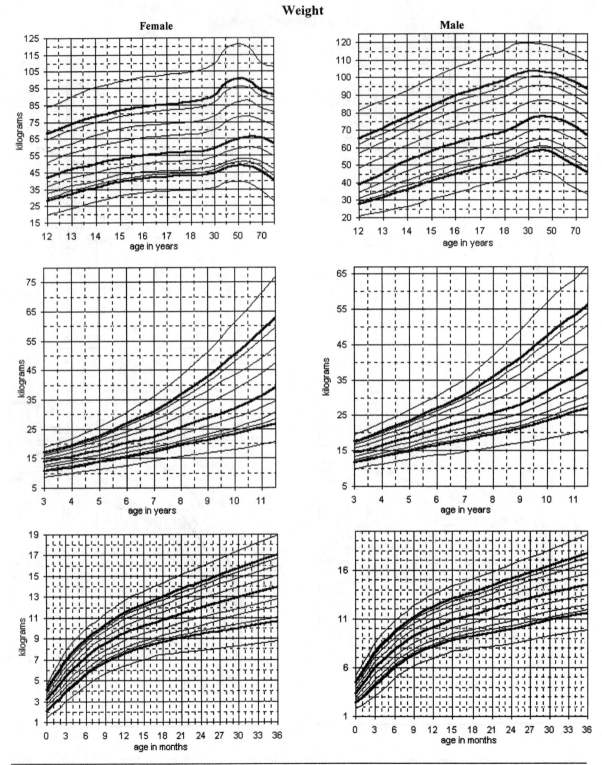

Height

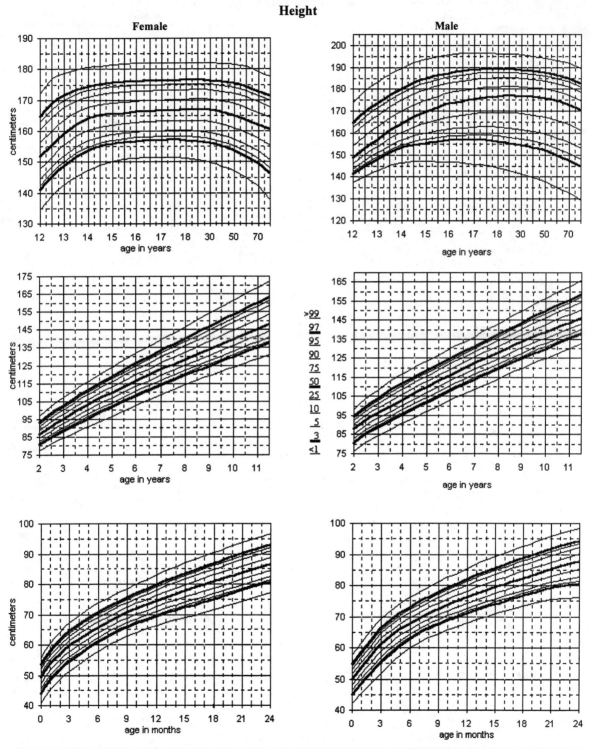

Leg length

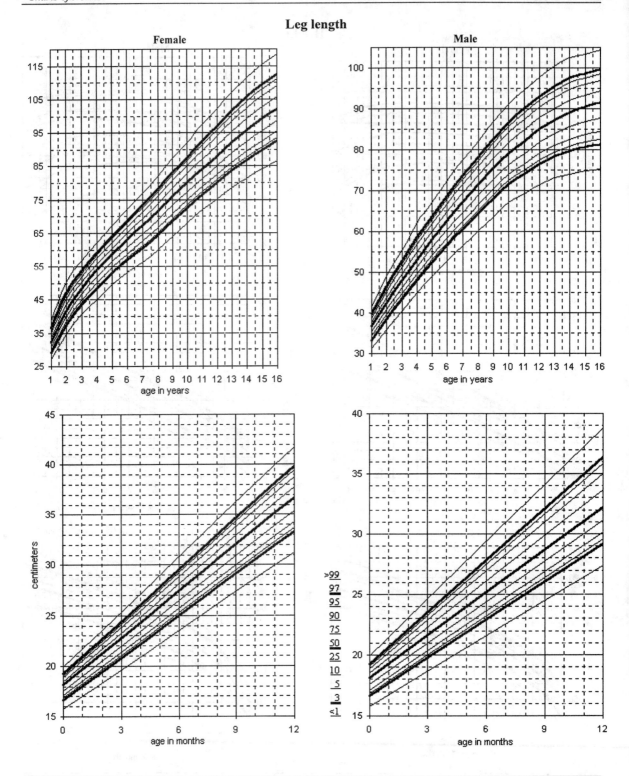

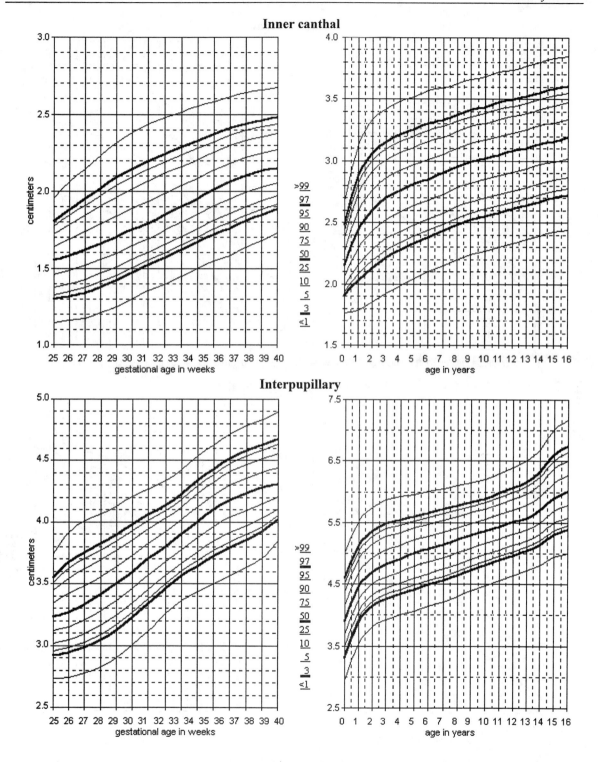

Inner canthal

Interpupillary

Outer canthal

Palpebral fissure width

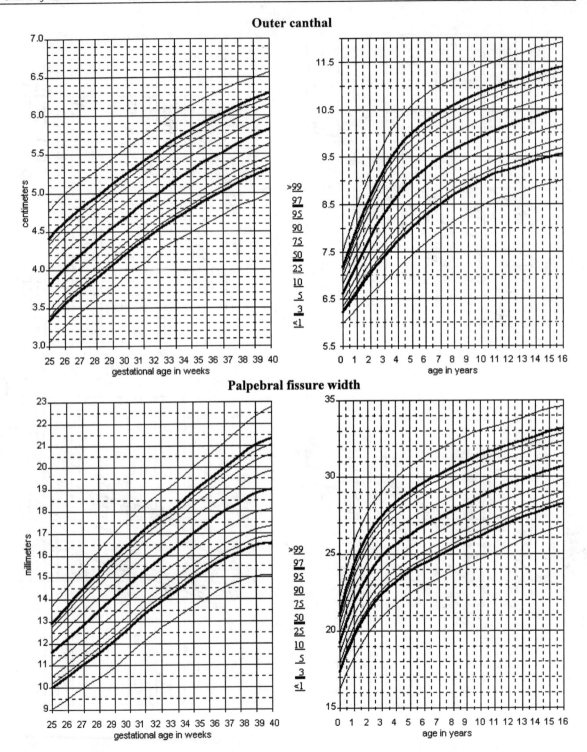

Cornea diameter: Newborn 10 mm, Adult 11.8 mm, Microcornea < 10 mm, Megalocornea 13 - 18 mm.

Nose length

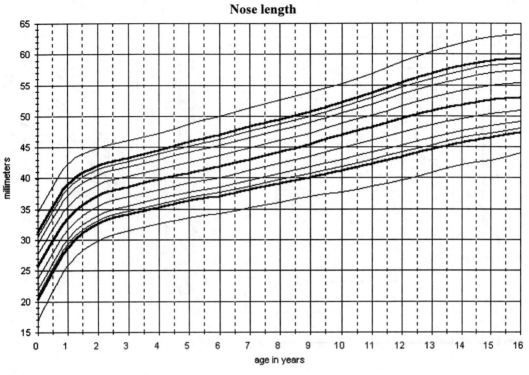

Philtrum

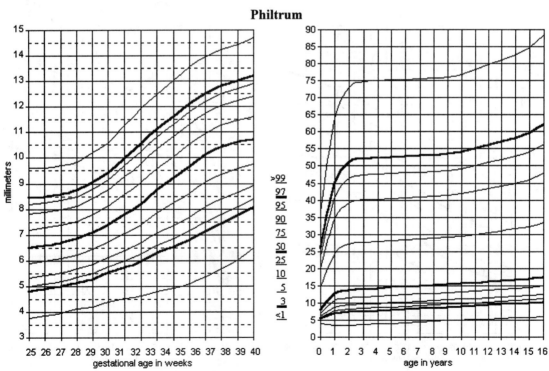

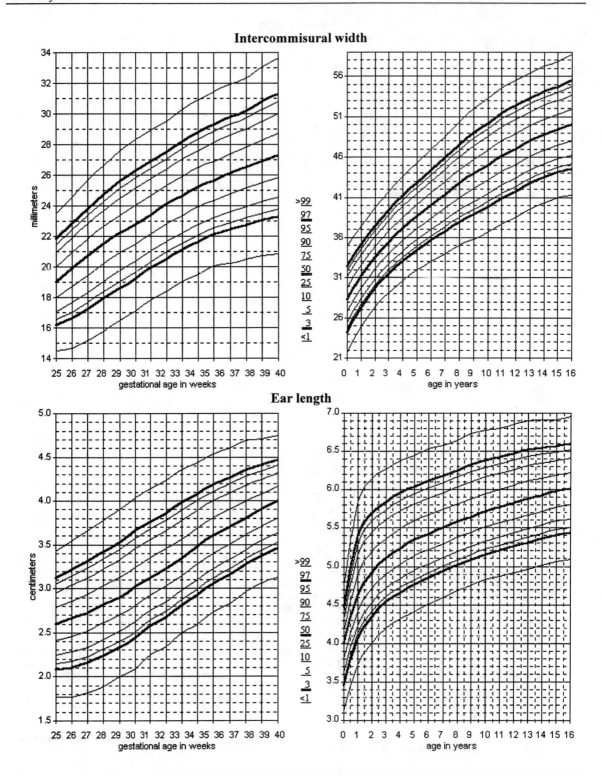

Intercommisural width

Ear length

- **Body Mass Index** (weight/height^2 X 100)

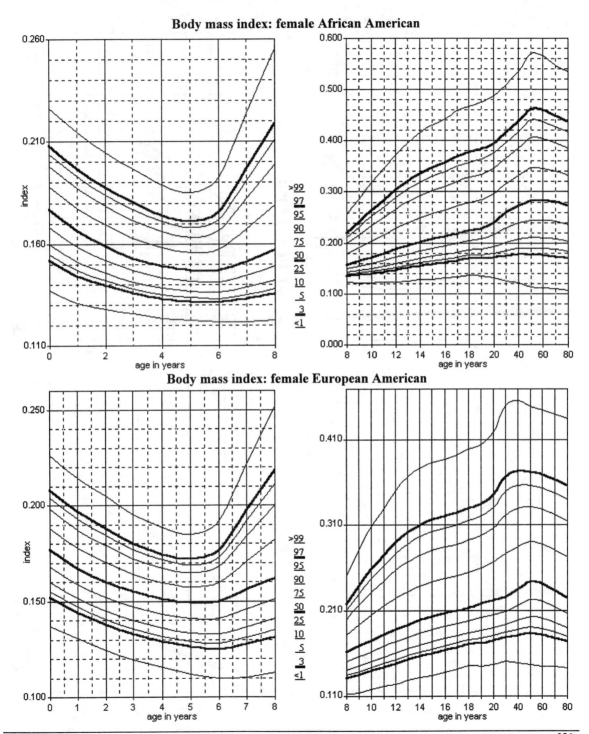

- **Body Mass Index** (weight/height^2 X 100)

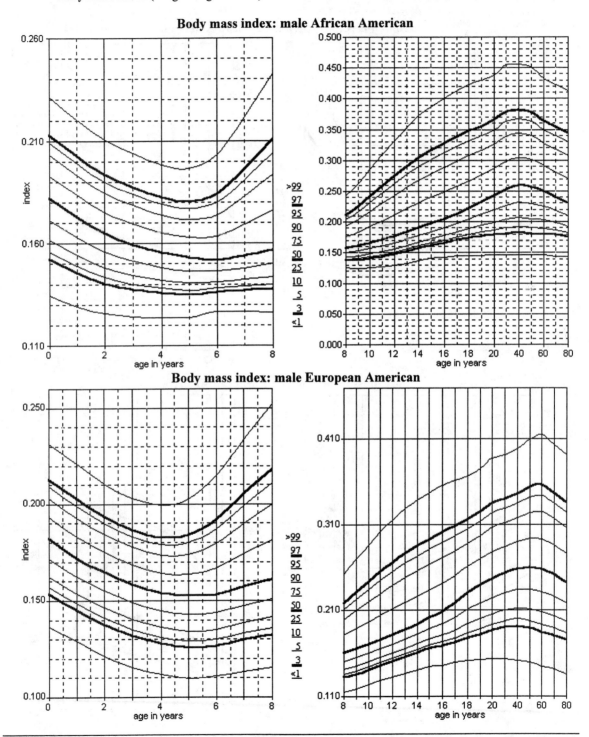

Body mass index: male African American

Body mass index: male European American

Chest circumference

Internipple distance

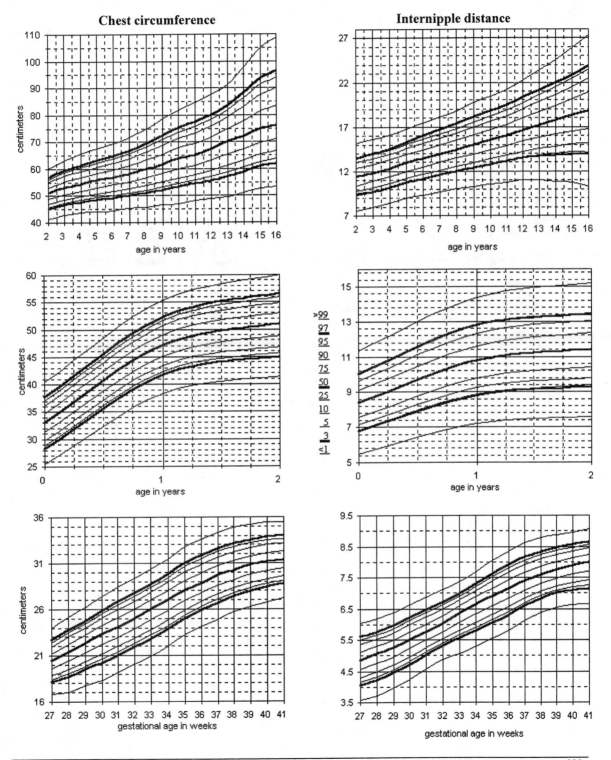

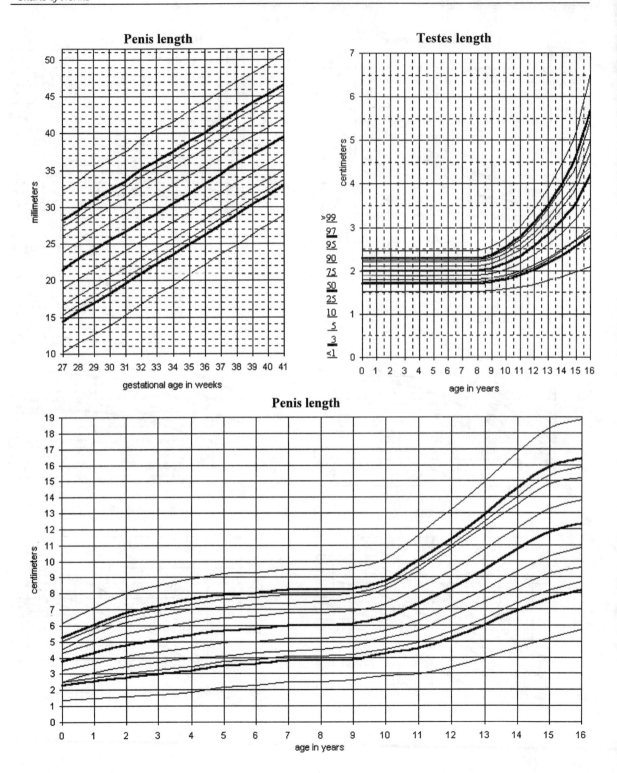

Penis length

Testes length

Penis length

Triceps skin fold: female

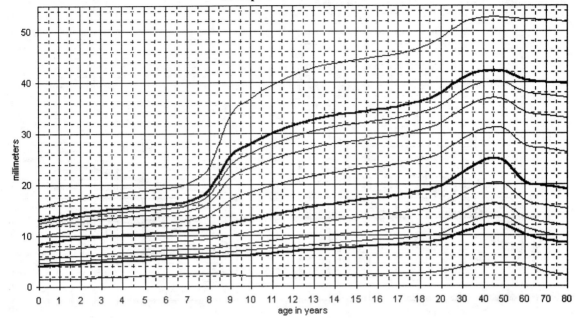

Triceps skin fold: male

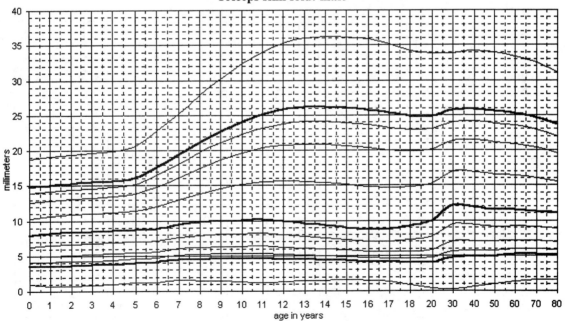

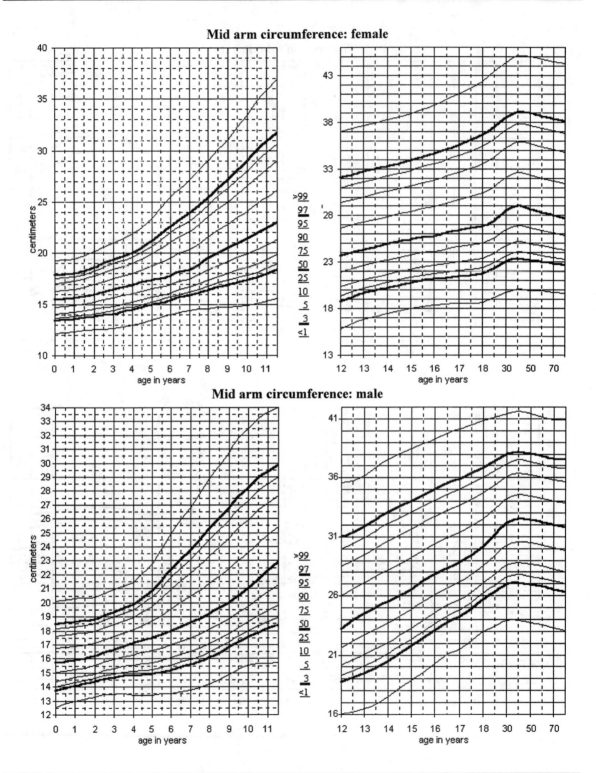

- **Mid-Arm Muscle Circumference** $(((10 \times mac)-(3.14 \times tsf))/10)$

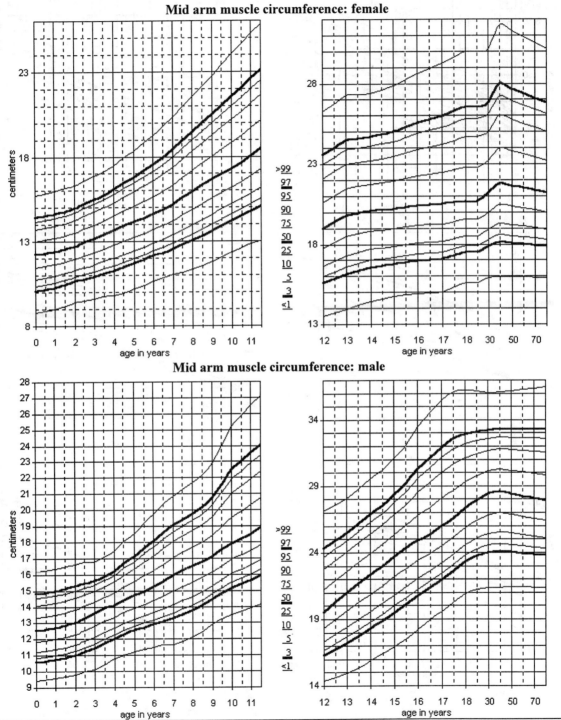

Mid arm muscle circumference: female

Mid arm muscle circumference: male

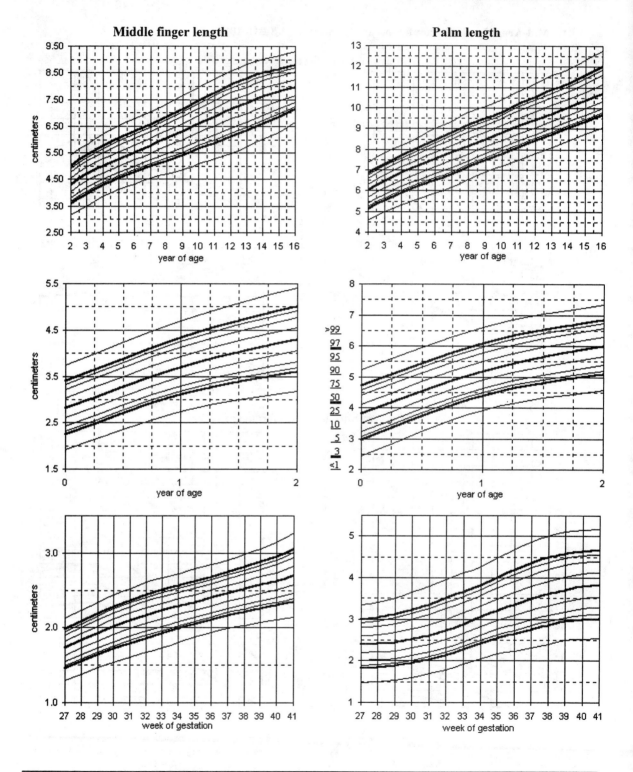

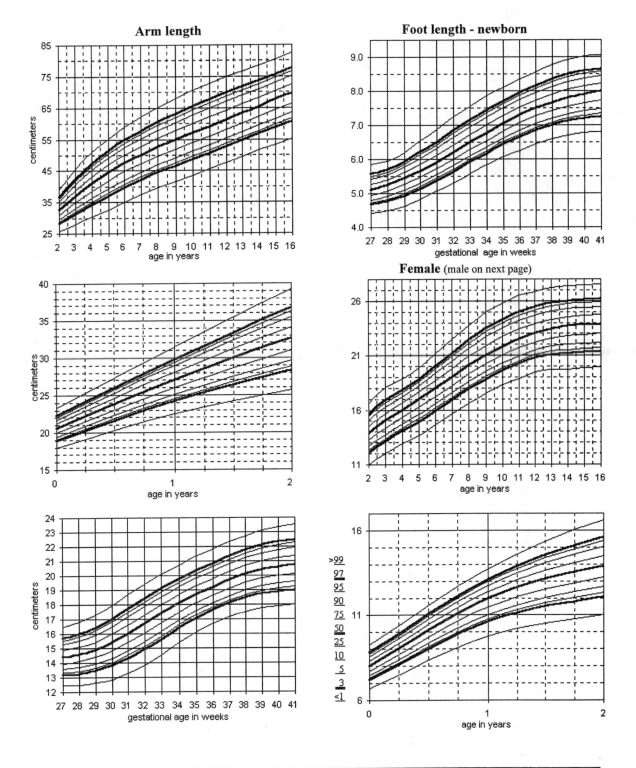

Arm length

Foot length - newborn

Female (male on next page)

Foot length - male

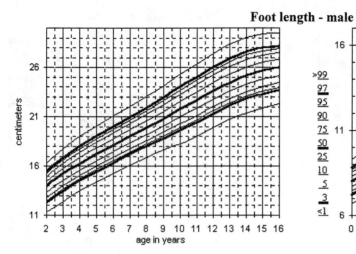
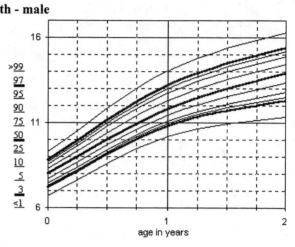

Bone age

Age	Site	Ossification center
Birth	knee	epiphyses: proximal tibial, distal femoral
	ankle	talus, calcaneus, cuboid
1 year	wrist	capitate, hamate, distal radius epiphysis
	shoulder	humerus head epiphysis
	hip	femur head epiphysis
	ankle	external cuneiform, tibia distal epiphysis
2 years	shoulder	humerus greater tuberosity
	elbow	humerus capitellum
	ankle	fibula distal epiphysis
3 years	wrist	triquetrum, epiphyses: phalanges, metacarpals
	ankle	internal cuneiform, metatarsal epiphysis
4 years	wrist	lunate
	hip	greater trochanter epiphysis
	knee	fibula proximal epiphysis
	ankle	navicular, middle cuneiform
5 years	wrist	trapezium, navicular
	elbow	radius proximal epiphysis
	knee	patella

Tooth eruption

	deciduous			permanent
	lower	*average*	*upper*	*average*
central incisor-lower	4.5 m	8m	10m	6-7 y
central incisor-upper	6 m	9.5 m	12 m	7-8 y
lateral incisor-upper	8.5 m	11.5 m	14 m	5-6 y
lateral incisor-lower	9 m	12 m	16 m	7-8 y
first molar-upper	12 m	15 m	18 m	10-11 y
first molar-lower	12 m	15.5 m	18.5 m	10-12 y
canine-lower	14.5 m	18 m	22 m	9-11 y
canine-upper	14.5 m	18 m	22 m	11-12 y
second molar-lower	22 m	26 m	30 m	11-13 y
second molar-upper	22 m	26 m	30 m	10-12 y

Blood pressure

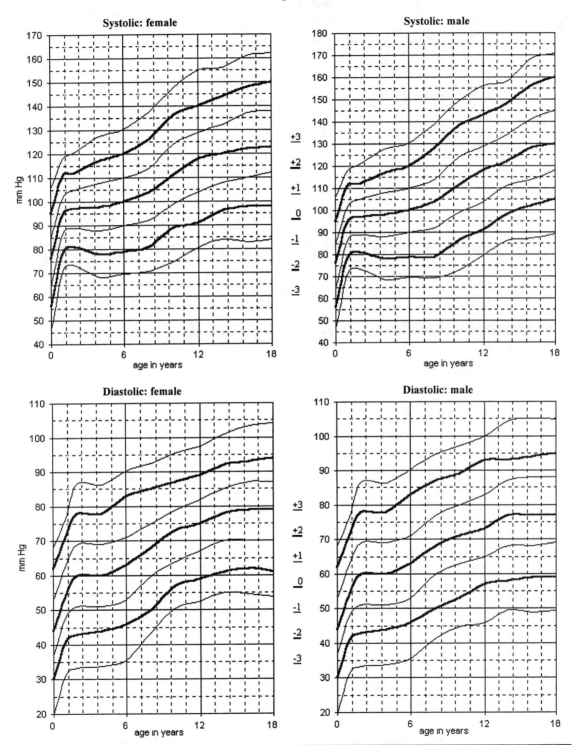

NORMAL VALUES

Total Cholesterol: Male

Age group

	0-1	5-9	10-14	15-19	20-24	25-29	30-34	35-39	40-44	45-49	50-54	55-59	60-64	65-69	>70
5%	114	125	124	118	118	130	142	147	150	163	156	161	163	166	144
10%	125	131	131	123	126	137	152	157	160	171	168	172	170	174	160
25%	137	141	144	136	142	154	171	176	179	188	189	188	191	192	185
50%	151	153	160	152	159	176	190	195	204	210	211	214	215	213	214
75%	171	168	173	168	179	199	213	222	229	235	237	236	237	250	236
90%	186	183	188	183	197	223	237	248	251	258	263	260	262	275	253
95%	203	189	202	191	212	234	258	267	260	275	274	280	287	288	265

Total Cholesterol: Female

Age group

	0-1	5-9	10-14	15-19	20-24	25-29	30-34	35-39	40-44	45-49	50-54	55-59	60-64	65-69	>70
5%	112	131	125	118	121	130	133	139	146	148	163	167	172	167	173
10%	120	136	131	126	132	142	141	149	156	162	171	182	186	179	181
25%	139	151	142	140	147	158	158	165	172	182	188	201	207	212	196
50%	156	164	159	157	165	178	178	186	193	204	214	229	226	233	226
75%	172	176	171	176	186	198	199	209	220	231	240	251	251	259	249
90%	189	190	191	198	220	217	215	233	241	256	267	278	282	282	268
95%	200	197	205	207	237	231	228	249	259	268	281	294	300	291	280

HDL Cholesterol: Male

Age group

	0-1	5-9	10-14	15-19	20-24	25-29	30-34	35-39	40-44	45-49	50-54	55-59	60-64	65-69	>70
5%		38	37	30	30	31	28	29	27	30	28	28	30	30	31
10%		42	40	34	32	32	32	31	31	33	31	31	34	33	33
25%		49	46	39	38	37	38	36	36	38	36	38	41	39	40
50%		54	55	46	45	44	45	43	43	45	44	46	49	49	48
75%		63	61	52	51	50	52	49	51	52	51	55	61	62	56
90%		70	71	59	57	58	59	58	60	60	58	64	69	74	70
95%		74	74	63	63	63	63	62	67	64	63	71	74	78	75

HDL Cholesterol: Female

Age group

	0-1	5-9	10-14	15-19	20-24	25-29	30-34	35-39	40-44	45-49	50-54	55-59	60-64	65-69	>70
5%		36	37	35	33	37	36	34	34	34	37	37	38	35	33
10%		38	40	38	37	39	40	38	39	41	41	41	44	38	38
25%		47	45	43	44	47	46	44	48	47	50	50	51	49	48
50%		52	52	51	51	55	55	53	56	58	62	60	61	62	60
75%		31	58	61	62	63	64	64	65	68	71	73	75	73	71
90%		67	64	68	72	74	73	74	79	82	84	85	87	85	82
95%		73	70	74	79	83	77	82	88	87	92	91	92	98	92

NORMAL VALUES

LDL Cholesterol: Male

	0-1	5-9	10-14	15-19	20-24	25-29	30-34	35-39	40-44	45-49	50-54	55-59	60-64	65-69	>70
								Age group							
5%		63	64	62	66	70	78	81	87	98	89	88	83	98	88
10%		69	72	68	73	75	88	92	98	106	102	103	106	104	100
25%		80	81	80	85	96	107	110	115	120	118	123	121	125	119
50%		90	94	93	101	116	124	131	135	141	143	145	143	146	142
75%		103	109	109	118	138	144	154	157	163	162	168	165	170	164
90%		117	122	123	138	157	166	176	173	186	185	191	188	188	182
95%		129	132	130	147	165	185	189	186	202	197	203	210	210	186

LDL Cholesterol: Female

	0-1	5-9	10-14	15-19	20-24	25-29	30-34	35-39	40-44	45-49	50-54	55-59	60-64	65-69	>70
								Age group							
5%		68	68	59	57	71	70	75	74	79	88	89	100	92	96
10%		73	73	65	65	75	77	81	84	89	94	97	105	99	108
25%		88	81	78	82	90	91	96	104	105	111	120	126	125	127
50%		98	94	93	102	108	109	116	122	127	134	145	149	151	147
75%		115	110	111	118	126	128	139	146	150	160	168	168	184	170
90%		125	126	129	141	148	147	161	165	173	186	199	191	205	189
95%		140	136	137	159	164	156	172	174	186	201	210	224	221	206

Triglycerides: Male

	0-1	5-9	10-14	15-19	20-24	25-29	30-34	35-39	40-44	45-49	50-54	55-59	60-64	65-69	>70
								Age group							
5%		28	33	38	44	45	46	52	56	56	63	60	56	54	63
10%		34	37	43	50	51	57	58	69	65	75	70	65	61	71
25%		39	46	53	61	67	76	80	89	88	94	85	84	78	87
50%		48	58	68	78	88	102	109	123	119	128	117	111	108	115
75%		58	74	88	107	120	142	167	174	165	178	167	150	164	152
90%		70	94	125	146	171	214	250	252	218	244	210	193	227	202
95%		85	111	143	165	204	253	316	318	279	313	261	240	256	239

Triglycerides: Female

	0-1	5-9	10-14	15-19	20-24	25-29	30-34	35-39	40-44	45-49	50-54	55-59	60-64	65-69	>70
								Age group							
5%		32	39	36	37	42	40	40	45	44	53	59	57	56	60
10%		37	44	40	42	45	45	47	51	55	58	65	66	64	68
25%		45	53	52	60	57	55	61	66	71	75	80	78	86	83
50%		57	68	64	80	76	73	83	88	94	103	111	105	118	110
75%		74	85	85	104	104	104	115	116	139	144	163	143	158	141
90%		103	104	112	135	137	140	170	161	180	190	229	210	221	189
95%		126	120	126	168	159	163	205	191	223	223	279	256	260	289

DERMATOGLYPHICS TERMINOLOGY

A	arch		t	axial triradius just distal to wrist crease
A^t	tented arch		t_b	axial triradius in lower Hy
a	triradius at base of index finger		t'	axial triradius 1/3 down palm
atd	angle formed by joining a, t, and d triradii		t"	axial triradius 2/3 down palm
D	distal		tfrc	total finger ridge count
d	triradius at base of little finger		W	whorl
F	fibular		Wd	double loop whorl
Hl	sole proximal to hallux, "ball of foot"		Wl	loop whorl
Hy	hypothenar area		1	thumb
Hx	hallux		2	index finger
L	loop		3	middle finger
P	proximal		4	ring finger
R	radial		5	little finger
SC	simian crease		I	area between 1 and 2
SL	sidney line		II	area between 2 and 3
T	tibial		III	area between 3 and 4
Th	thenar area		IV	area between 4 and 5

DERMATOGLYPHICS NORMS

FINGERS

Normal frequency (%)

Area:	1	2	3	4	5	
Pattern: UL	60	37	72	52	80	
RL	1	20	2	2	1	
W	35	30	17	44	17	increased in male
A	4	13	9	2	2	increased in female

tfrc: Males 145 (s 51), females 127 (s 52)

symmetry: Right and left ridge counts correlate for 3 or 4 fingers

Right and left patterns correlate for 2 or 3 fingers

PALM

Only parallel lines are found in the majority of normal persons. For most areas, figures are available only for presence or absence of any pattern. For the hypothenar area, frequencies of individual patterns are known.

Normal frequency (%)

Area:	I	II	III	IV	Th	Hy
Pattern: Any	3	4	46	50	6	38
UL						5
RL						20
PL						1
W						2
Wd						10

simian crease: Unilateral: 5%, bilateral: 2%

symmetry: Bilateral presence of a pattern: 30% (not necessarily the same).

Bilateral t': 35%, bilateral t": 3%.

triradii: Distal and hypothenar axial triradii are unusual.

atd angle: Normally less than 90°. Becomes greater when t is distal.

SOLE

Normal frequency (%)

	Pattern:	A	FA	PA	TA	DL	FL	TL	W
Area:	Hx	7					80	5	8
	Hl		5	2	2	52	1	10	28

Normal Morphologic Traits

McKusick number*
↓

102350 Acromial dimples	139600 Hairy elbows
102350 Acromial dimples	139630 Hairy nose tip
106240 Anisocoria	139650 Hairy palms and soles
106600 Anodontia partial (hypodontia)	142500 Heterochromia irides
107800 Arcus cornae (senilis)	145400 Hypertelorism (Greig)
110000 Blepharochalasis	147250 Incisors fused
210750 Blond hair	147300 Incisors long
114600 Canine teeth absence	147400 Incisors shovel shaped
114700 Carabelli anomaly	149100 Knuckle pads
116850 Catatrichy	155200 Line mediosternal
117900 Cervical rib	151630 Lip upper median nodule
118000 Cervical vertebral bridge	152600 Lunulae fingernail
119000 Cleft chin	153470 Macrocephaly
124300 Darminian point of pinna	309630 Metacarpal 4-5 fusion
124400 Darwinian tubercle	157200 Midphalangeal hair
125550 Dermal ridges off end	161500 Nasal groove transverse
125540 Dermal ridges patternless	161600 Navicular bone accessory
125570 Dermatoglyphic arches	163600 Nipples inverted
125580 Dermatoglyphic finger ridge count	163700 Nipples supernumerary
125590 Dermatoglyphic fingerprint pattern	164000 Nose potato shape
125900 Diastema	165670 Ossified ear cartilage
126100 Dimples facial	168500 Parietal foramina
126500 Double nail fifth toe	261400 Peronius tertius muscle absence
126550 Doughnut lesion of skull	161100 Pigmentation fingernail bed
128400 Ear flare	163100 Port wine stain of neck
128500 Ear folding	176700 Prognathism mandibular
129100 Ear movement	177800 Pseudopapilledema
128700 Ear pits	266300 Red hair
128800 Ear without helix	228980 Retina fleck benign
128900 Earlobe attachment	181300 Scapula vertebral border contour
128950 Earlobe crease	137400 Scrotal tongue
131500 Epicanthus	185200 Striae distensae
133500 Exchondrosis of pinna	187050 Teeth natal
227240 Eye color	187000 Teeth odd shapes
133800 Eyebrow whorl	274200 Thumb hyperextensible
110000 Eyelid fold Nordic	189000 Toe fifth phalanges number
145100 Eyelid hyperpigmentation	189150 Toe fifth rotated
133900 Facial asymmetry in crying	189200 Toes relative length
134000 Facial hypertrichosis	189300 Tongue curling, rolling, folding
136100 Finger length	275250 Tongue pigmented papillae
137000 Futcher line	192400 Vein pattern anterior thorax
139450 Hair curly	194000 Widow's peak
191480 Hair uncombable	
139400 Hair whorl	
194300 Hair wooly	

*McKusick VA. *Mendelian Inheritance in Man. Catalogues of Autosomal Dominant, Autosomal Recessive, and X-linked Phenotypes*, 10th edition. Baltimore: The Johns Hopkins Press, 1992.

Normal Physiologic Traits

McKusick number*
↓

103800	Alder anomaly
103600	Analbuminemia
108320	Artichoke taste modification
108400	Asparagus component excretion
108980	Atrioventricular conduction time
109160	Azotemia familial
109600	Beeturia
210100	beta-aminosiobutyric excretion urine
103600	Bisalbuminuria
211100	Bombay phenotype
115300	Carotenemia
117800	Cerumen variation
136540	Chromosome fragile site 10q23
136620	Chromosome fragile site 10q25
136560	Chromosome fragile site 11q13
136630	Chromosome fragile site 12q13
136570	Chromosome fragile site 16p12
136580	Chromosome fragile site 16q22
136660	Chromosome fragile site 17p12
136590	Chromosome fragile site 20p11
136610	Chromosome fragile site 2q11
136650	Chromosome fragile site 3p14.2
136640	Chromosome fragile site 9q32
136670	Chromosome fragile sites other
304300	Cyanide anosmia
220150	Dalmatian hypouricemia
126180	Discrimination sensory
130200	EEG 14 & 6/sec spike
130300	EEG frontoprecentral beta groups
130400	EEG occipital slow beta waves
229250	Freesia anosmia
229800	Fructosuria
138070	Glucoglycinuria
233100	Glycosuria renal
234000	Hageman factor deficiency
139900	Handedness
141800	Hemoglobin alpha locus 1 variants
141850	Hemoglobin alpha locus 2 variants
141860	Hemoglobin alpha locus 3 variants
141940	Hemoglobin beta locus 1 pseudogene
141900	Hemoglobin beta locus variants
142000	Hemoglobin delta locus variants

142100	Hemoglobin epsilon locus variants
142200	Hemoglobin epsilon locus variants
142250	Hemoglobin gamma locus 2 variants
142270	Hemoglobin gamma locus regulator
142240	Hemoglobin theta locus 1 variants
142309	Hemoglobin variants other
142310	Hemoglobin zeta locus variants
142300	Hemoglobin zeta pseudogene
306600	Hemolysis of trypsinized erythrocytes
144100	Hyperhidrosis gustatory
240400	Hypoascorbemia
241500	Hypophosphatasia III
242600	Iminoglycinuria
207000	Isobutyric anosmia
243400	Isoniazide inactivation
243450	Isovaleric anosmia
250700	Methemoglobinemia
157600	Mirror movements
254150	Musk anosmia
159420	Mydriasis
169400	Pelger-Huet anomaly
260800	Pentosuria
261500	Peroxidase/phospholipid deficiency eosinophils
171200	Phenylthiocarbamide tasting
182100	Secretor factor
270350	Skunk anosmia
301700	Smell blindness
314200	TBG variants
190100	Trembling chen
191200	Tune deafness
191500	Undritz anomaly
314380	Unique green
194320	Woronets trait

*McKusick VA. *Mendelian Inheritance in Man. Catalogues of Autosomal Dominant, Autosomal Recessive, and X-linked Phenotypes,* 10th edition. Baltimore: The Johns Hopkins Press, 1992.

Additional references

Cronk CE, Roche AF. Race and sex specific reference data for triceps and subscapular skin folds and weight/stature^2. Am J Clin Nutr 1982;35:347-354.

Feingold M, Bossert WH. Normal values for selected physical parameters. Birth Defects Original Article Series 1974; 10:13.

Gurney JM, Jeliff DB. Arm anthropometry in nutritional assessment: nomogram for rapid calculation of muscle circumference and cross-sectional muscle and fat areas. Am J Clin Nutr 1973;26:912-915.

Hall JG, Froster-Iskenius UG, Allanson JE. *Handbook of Normal Physical Measurements*. New York: Oxford, 1989.

Hamill PVV. NCHS growth charts, 1976. Monthly Vital Statistics Report 1976;25 (3).

Hammer LD, Kraemer HC, Wilson DM, et al. Standardized percentile curves of body-mass index for children and adolescents. Am J Dis Childr 1991;145:259-263.

Lauer RM, Burns TL, Clarke WR. Assessing children's blood pressure - considerations of age and body size. The Muscatine Study. Pediatrics 1985;75:1081-1090.

Lee J, Burns TL. Genetic dyslipoproteinemias associated with coronary atherosclerosis. In Pierpont ME, Moller JH, (editors). *Genetics of Cardiovascular Disease*. Boston: Martinus Nijhoff Publishing, 1986.

Lieberman E. Hypertension in Childhood and Adolescence. CIBA Symposia 1978;30(3). CIBA Pharmaceutical Co, Summit, NJ.

Merlob P, Sivan Y, Reisner SH. Anthropometric measurements of the newborn infant (27 to 41 gestational weeks). Birth Defects Original Article Series 1984; 20:7.

Saul RA, Skinner SA, Stevenson RE, et al. Growth references from conception to adulthood. Proceedings of the Greenwood Genetic Center 1988: Supplement 1.

Schaumann B, Alter M. *Dermatoglyphics in Medical Disorders*. New York: Springer-Verlag, 1976.

Suskind RM, Varma RN. Assessment of nutritional status of children. Pediatrics In Review 1984;5:195-202.

Wilkins RW, Hollander W, Chobanian AV. *Evaluation of Hypertensive Patients*. CIBA Symposia 1972;24(2). CIBA Pharmaceutical Co, Summit, NJ.

Two events in the late 1990's crystallized various techniques of record keeping in the field of Medical Genetics. One was the publication of *Documentation Guidelines for Evaluation and Management Services* in the USA in 1997 by the Health Care Financing Administration (HFCA). Though it originated as a mechanism to allow fair auditing, the document was formulated with participation of the American Medical Association whose interest was the quality of medical care. The other event was a gradual standardization of the format of genealogical data that was facilitated by widespread interest at all levels.

Form 1 resulted from adaptation of several medical genetics forms to those changes. Consistent with the HFCA *Guidelines*, change and evolution of the form is anticipated. The current version is indicated by the notation just below the triple line at the far right. This form is most useful in the practice of Medical Genetics. It serves to collate data and to ensure that the multiple needs of clinical practice are met, including investigation and documentation.

It should to be used by the Medical Geneticist or his/her representative for the recording of data that are obtained about an individual during a clinical encounter or a clinical investigation. Rarely, a patient, or a patient's representative may be able to use the first two parts of the form directly. This is most likely when that person is familiar with genealogical investigation. However, the form is not meant to be routinely distributed to patients or relatives prior to appointments in a Medical Genetics Clinic.

The redundant nature of genealogical data requires careful thought so that there are neither unnecessary duplications nor omissions of data. Identifying data are required on each form but other data should not be repeated if present on a preceding form. Clinical data should be repeated on forms from subsequent encounters only as required to summarize and characterize the current state of the case. Optimal use of the forms requires inventory of data during an initial encounter and accuracy checking during subsequent encounters. Updating is often required.

The items on the form are fairly inclusive. Most of them ultimately prove to be of value in the evaluation and management of most cases; however, it should not be assumed that all items are *required*. During a particular clinical encounter, relatively few data may be available for recording. Copies of the form may be used under the general copyright permission of this publication (not sold). The form in the pocket version must be enlarged with an enlarging copier before use. A full-size double-sided version is available from the author.

The first part of the form (down to single solid line) is for identifying data. The second part of the form (between single line and double line) is equivalent to a standard genealogical data form. In a medical setting, the third section (between double line and triple line) serves for recording referral source, sources of payment for services, and legal responsibility. The section of the form below the triple line is for medical use. It conforms to the HFCA *Guidelines*. Consistent with the guidelines, there are expanded parts that apply to the field of Medical Genetics.

An individual form should be devoted to each person who is present at an encounter. Most data will be entered into the proband's form. Very little may be needed on the forms of other persons. For example, consider the case of a dysmorphic baby (proband) who is the product of the only pregnancy of both parents who themselves have no medical problems. The parents' forms may require only their names, work telephone numbers, information about their parents, information about their occupations, and a statement under DIAGNOSIS, MANAGEMENT such as "No visible anomalies. Reproductive risk due to dysmorphic baby." This documents that they were present and that examination of them was limited to inspection. The proband's form documents counseling content.

When the form is used to extend a genealogical evaluation, the first two parts are used for each person. If the baby in the above example had Down syndrome, it might be of interest to obtain a list of all pregnancies produced by each of the grandparents with each of their spouses to develop a count of specific spontaneous abortions that could be indicative of a balanced translocation. Variable expression, incomplete penetrance, X-linkage and translocation may result in informative data among collateral relatives. In those cases, it might be worthwhile to complete a form for each offspring of grandparents who lived to reproduce. Extending still further, a form could be completed for each sib and half sib of grandparents. In purely genealogical uses, a form may be completed without a face-to-face encounter with a person by using public or private records.

In order to prevent illicit use of data, care must be taken to protect information about living persons. Even posthumous data can be problematic in cases of contested parentage. Without legal consent, copies of completed forms should not be released to anybody except the persons who themselves provided the data. In a medical setting, there are standard practices in this regard. In other settings, it is advisable to consult an attorney.

Collated data from copies of Form 1 completed on all family members can be the basis of a genealogical chart generated either by hand or electronically. When dealing with an easily ascertained phenotype, this will allow a reliable estimation of mode of inheritance. More often than not, it provides instead an investigative framework, and it is necessary to examine and test relatives for the phenotype before a mode of inheritance can be estimated. Relatives at risk for having affected progeny may also be identified in the course of an investigation.

When there is a strong bias favoring autosomal recessive inheritance, Form 2 can be used to efficiently record data pertaining to consanguinity. It is most often used in double-sided format. The name of mother of the proband is placed in position one on one side, and the name of the father of the proband in position one on the other side. In cases of unknown etiology, speculative use of Form 2 allows an estimation of the likelihood of autosomal recessive inheritance, because most clinically significant consanguinity occurs within these five generations.

These forms integrate with the data structure known as CONTACTS. The forms themselves can serve as a manual file system when filed alphabetically by name. The data can also be computerized on virtually any platform, permitting compact storage with rapid recall and analysis. The CONTACTS system includes other forms that facilitate documentation. Coding (ICD and CPT) and recording of tasks and time devoted to a case may be of particular interest. Copies are available from the author.

Central to the CONTACTS system is the concept of the proband-related genealogy. It answers an age-old question of how to manage the voluminous data that result from genealogical investigations by providing a numerical system that keys all relatives and keeps them in order. Each number is "reserved" for each relative whether or not they exist so assignments can be made upon ascertainment without waiting for a completed set. In a manual file system, index cards can filed by number for a cross reference.

The base number is the proband number. It is simply a number from an accession series in which female probands are numbered with odd numbers and male probands with even numbers. Hence, the first female proband in the record set is 1, the second 3, the third 5, etc. The number below represents the 1172nd female proband:
2345

Other relatives are given the proband number plus a relating number indicating the relationship to the proband based on a standard Germanic genealogy chart. A decimal point is used to separate the Proband number and the Relating number. The first 3 positions after the decimal point represent the direct ancestor through whom lineage is traced. For accuracy, the genealogy is traced through females when possible.

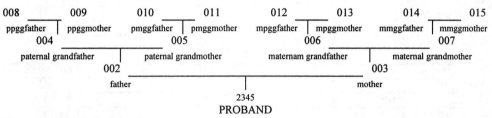

Hence, the proband's father is:
2345　.　002

Note that the first 3 positions of the R number can be all zero's, designating simply the proband but superfluous. However, they are necessary for designating the proband's spouse. In the above example, the proband's first spouse would be
2345　.　000　　　1

For purposes of this numbering system, the term, "spouse," is defined as a person with whom there has been a legal marriage, _**OR**_ with whom a pregnancy has been produced.

The relating numbers can be extended into relatives of the spouse by adding 2 zero's and reverting to the above format for ancestors. The spouse's maternal grandmother would be
2345　.　000　　　100　　　007

To construct relating numbers of progeny, the 2 positions after the spouse are used in a format similar to proband numbers, i.e., sequential odd numbers for males and even numbers for females, in birth order. The numbers are read in groups of 3, the first (s) being the spouse in order of reproduction and the next 2 (oo) being the offspring by that union.
2345　.　000　　soo　　soo　　soo　　soo　　soo　　soo　　soo　　soo

The number below represents the second son of the proband's father by the father's second spouse:
2345　.　002　　204

If the spouse's maternal grandmother had 2 sons by her third spouse, the second son would be
2345　.　000　　100　　007　　304

The proband can also be numbered to aid in thinking about numbers of other relatives:
2345　.　003　　103

This would indicate that the proband is the second daughter born to the union of her mother and her first spouse. Hence, the proband's half brother who is the first son born to the union of her mother with her second spouse would be:

2345 . 003 202

Some practice may be required to become adept at proband numbers but some quick references follow:

Relative	R number
Father	002
Mother	003
Paternal grandfather	004
Paternal grandmother	005
Maternal grandfather	006
Maternal grandmother	007
Spouse	0001
Spouse's Father	000100002
Spouse's Mother	000100003
Spouse's Paternal grandfather	000100004
Spouse's Paternal grandmother	000100005
Spouse's Maternal grandfather	000100006
Spouse's Maternal grandmother	000100007
Brother and second son of mother by her second spouse	003204
Sister and second daughter of mother by her third spouse	003303
Second son by second spouse	000204
Neice and first daughter of half brother through mother (her second son by her first spouse) by his second spouse	003104201

This numbering system allows numerical specification of anybody in a genealogy. Though not unique, the proband related number is specific; i.e., a number always represents only one person and no other, though a person may have several numbers depending on the relatives through whom the genealogy is traced.

Records numbered in this manner can be entered into a computer file in real-time at random, allowing the use of clerks instead of data-processing personnel. Sorting the proband-related numbers in the computer file results in grouping by family and degree of relationship.

In clinical work, limited to living persons, most of the numbers are simple. One is usually interested only in maintaining records on persons actually contacted and these are usually quite few.

A classic example is a situation in which a baby with seizures is examined in an intensive care nursery. The mother may be examined also, but several days later while visiting the baby, and the father in clinic a month later. His sister is in a special school and thought to have the same problem as the baby. She is examined some weeks later during a trip to the school. It is found that she is really a half-sister with tuberous sclerosis inherited from her father who had a mild case. She is the second daughter born to the union of the father's mother with her third spouse.

During this interval 233 other families are evaluated and their records entered into the computer data base in real time. A simple sort rapidly brings up all records of the family of the baby:

Proband:	2345			
Father	2345	.	002	
Mother:	2345	.	003	
Aunt:	2345	.	005	303

Broader uses are also possible, such as entering computer data about all persons identified in a series of genealogies. For example, this might be undertaken if one were studying the lineage of all persons attending a specialty clinic for a specific hereditary condition in a geographic area, the object being to contact those persons and determine the efficiency of dissemination of information about genetic risks. Some persons might be in several genealogies. Sorting of the computer files both by name and PR number followed by cross-tabulation can allow rapid analysis.

Adopted children are usually not biological relatives so they are ordinarily not considered in this system. However, there are at least 2 situations in which it may be worthwhile to record them: (1) There is a suspicion that the adopted child is actually a biological child. (2) In the course of a contact, the adopted child receives some service that we are obliged to record.

An example would be a prenatal patient, the only daughter of her biological parents, being evaluated and counseled about the age-related risk of Down syndrome in her progeny, accompanied by a stepsister who is the adopted child of the woman's parents and who also wants counseling. An adoptive relationship is signified by placing a **plus sign** in the first position of the R number. So, here, it is +03101 to indicate that the stepsister was the first adoptive daughter adopted by the adoptive mother and her first spouse. The P number would be that of the patient.

Adoptive parents of a patient may be coded with an R number of +02 for the father and +03 for the mother. This would be required only if neither is a biological parent. If one is a biological parent, the other is coded as the appropriate spouse of that parent. Hence, the third spouse of the mother when the patient was a product of the first spouse would have an R number of 0033 . Recall that her first spouse, the father of the patient, would have an R number of 002 .

Succedents may be coded in a similar manner: The first daughter adopted by the patient and her third spouse would have the R number +00301 .

The special + codes apply only to legal adoptions by non-biological relatives. Standard codes for biological relatives are used even if they have legally adopted a child who is a relative. In situations where the child is living with a non-relative but not legally adopted, the only record kept in this system is that of guarantor.

This numbering strategy would degenerate for adoptive relationships through relatives more distant than 5th degree. Little significance would seem to pertain to such relationships except on a population basis. For population use, it is possible to devote six digits to the ancestor through whom lineage is traced instead of three, encompassing all of recorded history.

Additional references:

Thurmon TF, Robertson KP, Ursin SA: CONTACTS: a microcomputer program for storage and analysis of clinical data from medical genetics units. Demonstration at Southern Genetics Group Meeting, Shreveport, LA, 7/23/82.

FORM 1. Complete one of these forms to triple line for PATIENT.
Also complete a form to double line for EACH relative present.
"MAIDEN" name (women only) is the surname at birth.

/ /					
First, middle, MAIDEN, last name	Birth date	Soc sec no	City and State of birth	Sex Race	Years of school

How are you	Address			City	ST	ZIP code
related to the patient?		Telephones: HOME: ( )	WORK: ( )		OTHER: ( )	
What medical						
problems do you have?						

	Birth date	Soc sec no	City and State of birth	Years of school	Marriage date
	/ /				/ /
Your FATHER: First, middle, last name	Birth date	Soc sec no	City and State of birth	Years of school	
	/ /				Marriage date
Your MOTHER: First, middle, MAIDEN, last name	Birth date	Soc sec no	City and State of birth ,	Years of school	

"Spouse" means a person to whom you were married OR with whom you produced one or more pregnancies.

	Birth date	Soc sec no	City and State of birth	Years of school	Marriage date
	/ /				/ /
Your first spouse: First, middle, MAIDEN, last name	Birth date	Soc sec no	City and State of birth	Years of school	Marriage date
	/ /				/ /
Your second spouse: First, middle, MAIDEN, last name	Birth date	Soc sec no	City and State of birth	Years of school	Marriage date
	/ /				/ /
Your third spouse: First, middle, MAIDEN, last name	Birth date	Soc sec no	City and State of birth	Years of school	Marriage date
	/ /				/ /
Your fourth spouse: First, middle, MAIDEN, last name	Birth date	Soc sec no	City and State of birth	Years of school	Marriage date
	/ /				/ /
Your fifth spouse: First, middle, MAIDEN, last name	Birth date	Soc sec no	City and State of birth	Years of school	Marriage date

PREGNANCIES YOU HAVE PRODUCED

No.	sex	length of pregnancy ↓	Birth date	Name of child if any	Abnormality at birth or later in life	Other parent name or spouse #
1			/ /			
2			/ /			
3			/ /			
4			/ /			
5			/ /			
6			/ /			
7			/ /			
8			/ /			
			/ /			
			/ /		**Attach a separate page to list more spouses or more pregnancies.**	

(   )

Doctor or Agency who sent you here	Title/Institution	Telephone

Address of referring Doctor or Agency	City	ST	ZIP code

Telephones of guarantor ↓

Guarantor (guardian) if patient is a child who lives apart from parents	Soc sec no	Relationship to patient	HOME ( )
			WORK ( )
Address of guarantor	City	ST ZIP code	OTHER ( )

Employer of patient or of guarantor	Occupation - circle: patient or guarantor

Address of employer	City	ST	ZIP code	Medicaid/Medicare numbers
Medical insurance company:			Ins company Phone: ( )	
Full name of policyholder:			Policy/Group numbers:	

☙ **DO NOT WRITE BELOW THIS LINE** ☙   980715FORM 1

PROBLEM (complaint, location, quality, severity, duration, timing, context, modifying factors, associated signs & symptoms):

REVIEW Constitutional (growth, fever, weight loss):

Eyes, ears, face, head:
Mouth, nose, throat:
Cardiovascular, pulmonary:
Gastrointestinal:
Genitourinary:
Musculoskeletal, limbs:
Neurologic, psychiatric:
Integument (+ breasts):
Hematologic, lymphatic:
Allergic, immunologic, endocrine:

PAST HISTORY GESTATION G....P....A... Bleed (T1,2,3)...... Wgt chg ±lbs....... Thyroid (+,-,0)... Bld prs (+,-,0)... Diab (+,0)...
   Abdominal surgery (+,0)... Alcohol (+,0)... Tobacco (+,0)... Diet...
   Meds, Rec drugs, Other...
NEWBORN..Paternal age....... Maternal age....... Gestation wks....... Head......., ...% Length......., ...% Weight......., ...%
   Apgars (5,10)......, ... Hosp days...... Abns..
Postnatal ILLNESSES, OPERATIONS, INJURIES

FAMILY HISTORY (medical events & diseases which bear on patient's case)
Genealogy chart

SOCIAL HISTORY (age appropriate past and current activities)

EXAMINATION Span....... Waist....... BP supine sys......., ...% sit sys......., ...% stand sys......., ...% Pulse..... reg (+,-)..
Head......., ...% Hgt......., ...% Temp.......   dias......., ...%   dias......., ...%   dias......., ...% Resp.....reg (+,-)..
Wgt......., ...% BMI......., ...% Chest......., ...% Intnip......., ...% Penis......., ...% Testis R......., ...% L......., ...%
Inner canth......., ...% Interpup......., ...% Outer canth......., ...% Nose......., ...% Philtrum......., ...% Mouth......., ...%
Palpebral RIGHT......., ...% LEFT......., ...% Cornea R......., ...% L......., ...% Ear RIGHT......., ...% LEFT......., ...%
RIGHT Arm......., ...% Palm......., ...% Middle finger......., ...% Middle finger/Palm..... Hand/Height.....   Conicity.....
        TSF......., ...% MAC......., ...% MAMC......., ...% Foot......., ...% Foot/Height....... Leg......., ...% Up/Lo seg...
LEFT Arm......., ...% Palm......., ...% Middle finger......., ...% Middle finger/Palm..... Hand/Height.....
        TSF......., ...% MAC......., ...% MAMC......., ...% Foot......., ...% Foot/Height....... Leg......., ...% Up/Lo seg...
general (development, nutrition, habitus, deformities, grooming)

head   face
eyes
ears, nose, mouth, throat
dentition
neck
chest   back
respiratory
cardiovascular
abdomen
perineum
lymphatic
musculoskeletal
arm   hand
leg   foot
neurologic
psychiatric
integument
dermatoglyphics

DIAGNOSIS, MANAGEMENT
differential (#)
course
Rx & changes
referrals & consultations

DATA
current (ordered, reviewed)
old (ordered, reviewed)
discussed
interpreted

RISKS OF COMPLICATIONS, MORBIDITY, MORTALITY
comorbidity
invasive (ordered, performed, referred)

COUNSELING, COORDINATION Time: Content:

FORM 2   Chart No. _____

For each person indicated, list
full name, which, for women, is
the full maiden name followed
the surname of the legal spouse,
if any, at time of succedent's
birth.

Use position 1 for the PATIENT
or proband. If the patient is a
pregnant woman, complete
another chart using position 1 for
FATHER OF THE BABY.

In the spaces below the names,
list date, city and state of
birth, and of death, if dead.

8
father of No. 4

4
father of No. 2

9
mother of No. 4

2

father of No. 1

10
father of No. 5

5
mother of No. 2

11
mother of No. 5

1

12
father of No. 6

6
father of No. 3

13
mother of No. 6

3

mother of No. 1

14
father of No. 7

7
mother of No. 3

15
mother of No. 7

16
father of No. 8   con't on chart No. ____

17
mother of No. 8   con't on chart No. ____

18
father of No. 9   con't on chart No. ____

19
mother of No. 9   con't on chart No. ____

20
father of No. 10   con't on chart No. ____

21
mother of No. 10   con't on chart No. ____

22
father of No. 11   con't on chart No. ____

23
mother of No. 11   con't on chart No. ____

24
father of No. 12   con't on chart No. ____

25
mother of No. 12   con't on chart No. ____

26
father of No. 13   con't on chart No. ____

27
mother of No. 13   con't on chart No. ____

28
father of No. 14   con't on chart No. ____

29
mother of No. 14   con't on chart No. ____

30
father of No. 15   con't on chart No. ____

31
mother of No. 15   con't on chart No. ____

_____
Patient to whom you are related

_____
Relationship

Chart No. _____

For each person indicated, list
full name, which, for women, is
the full maiden name followed
the surname of the legal spouse,
if any, at time of succedent's
birth.

Use position 1 for the PATIENT
or proband. If the patient is a
pregnant woman, complete
another chart using position 1 for
FATHER OF THE BABY.

In the spaces below the names,
list date, city and state of
birth, and of death, if dead.

16
father of No. 8   con't on chart No. _____

8
father of No. 4

17
mother of No. 8   con't on chart No. _____

4
father of No. 2

18
father of No. 9   con't on chart No. _____

9
mother of No. 4

19
mother of No. 9   con't on chart No. _____

2
father of No. 1

20
father of No. 10   con't on chart No. _____

10
father of No. 5

21
mother of No. 10   con't on chart No. _____

5
mother of No. 2

22
father of No. 11   con't on chart No. _____

11
mother of No. 5

23
mother of No. 11   con't on chart No. _____

1

24
father of No. 12   con't on chart No. _____

12
father of No. 6

25
mother of No. 12   con't on chart No. _____

6
father of No. 3

26
father of No. 13   con't on chart No. _____

13
mother of No. 6

27
mother of No. 13   con't on chart No. _____

3
mother of No. 1

28
father of No. 14   con't on chart No. _____

14
father of No. 7

29
mother of No. 14   con't on chart No. _____

7
mother of No. 3

30
father of No. 15   con't on chart No. _____

15
mother of No. 7

31
mother of No. 15   con't on chart No. _____

_____
Patient to whom you are related

_____
Relationship

980715FORM2

KEY:

Name of disorder.	Synonyms.		
BDE number	McKusick number	ICD code	Trait type*

Cardinal findings are listed in this part. This is a brief characterization meant to facilitate rapid recognition and comparison. More complete discussions and literature references may be found in the publications listed in Additional References. Some of these disorders are caused by specific gene loci or other etiologic factors. Others have been found in sufficient numbers that there is a reasonable likelihood that their features represent a syndrome. Many more disorders exist in too few cases to implicate a specific gene locus or other etiologic factor or to prove that their features form a syndrome. Some disorders of that type are described in the BDE [Buyse ML (editor). *Birth Defects Encyclopedia.* Cambridge, MA: Blackwell Scientific, 1990]. Also described in the BDE are some syndromes that may represent chance conjunction of more than one disorder in a patient. That is especially prone to occur in population isolates.

*Trait types:

AD	Autosomal Dominant	AR	Autosomal Recessive	XD	X-linked Dominant	XR	X-linked Recessive
C	Chromosomal	S	Sporadic	I	Infectious agent	E	Environmental agent

Note: An Index of these listings begins on page 379.

Note: An Index of these listings begins on page 379.

Aase-Smith syndrome. Cleft palate-contractures-Dandy-Walker malformation.
| 3029 | 147800 | 759.8 | AD |
Broad forehead, blepharophimosis, ptosis, short nose, retrognathia, cleft palate, absent finger flexion creases, club foot, Dandy-Walker malformation, and in some cases, contractures of elbows, wrists, knees and fingers.

Ablepharon-macrostomia.
| 2777 | 200110 | 759.8 | AR |
Low-set ears, absent eyebrows, eyelids and eyelashes, macrostomia, hypoplastic teeth, hypoplastic nipples, hypoplastic genitalia, thick dry skin which on palms produces mild syndactyly and finger flexion, thin hair.

Achondroplasia and Swiss agammaglobulinemia. Metaphyseal chondrodysplasia-thymolymphopenia.
| 0655 | 200900 | 759.8 | AR |
Lymphopenia, agammaglobulinemia, thymic hypoplasia, rhizomelia, metaphyseal chondrodysplasia, poor fetal growth, short stature, poor postnatal growth, death in infancy. Some cases have adenosine deaminase deficiency, ectodermal dysplasia.

Acrodysostosis syndrome.
| 0016 | 101800 | 759.8 | AD |
Brachycephaly, short nose with anteverted nares, prognathism, distal shortening of limbs, short broad hands with wrinkled dorsal skin, cone- shaped phalangeal epiphyses, mental retardation, poor fetal growth, short stature, poor postnatal growth, arthritis.

Adams-Oliver syndrome. Aplasia cutis congenita-transverse limb defect.
| 0459 | 100300 | 759.8 | AD |
Central areas of the scalp are thinned or there may be an ulcerated scalp defect and an underlying skull defect may be associated; transverse limb defects such as aphalangia of terminal phalanges, adactylia, acheiria, apodia or transverse hemimelia.

Albinism-deafness syndrome.
| 0030 | 30700 | 270.2 | XR |
Nerve deafness and partial or total albinism. When the albinism is partial, the skin has a variegated appearance ("piebald"). Heterozygotes may have partial manifestation.

Albinism with hemorrhagic diathesis. Hermansky-Pudlak syndrome.
| 0033 | 203300 | 270.2 | AR |
Oculocutaneous albinism and bleeding diathesis due to defective platelet aggregation. Pulmonary fibrosis may be found in some cases. Reticuloendothelial cells contain abnormal pigment granules, and platelet-dense bodies are markedly deficient. Platelet ADP release is deficient.

Alcohol syndrome.
| 0379 | | 760.71 | E |
Poor fetal growth, poor postnatal growth, microcephaly, blepharophimosis, short nose,

indistinct philtrum, thin smooth upper lip, atrial or ventricular septal defect, short distal palmar crease, aberrant joint functions, neuronal heterotopia, tremulousness, mental retardation.

Alopecia-anosmia-deafness-hypogonadism, Johnson neuroectodermal syndrome.
2765   147770   759.8   AD
Congenital alopecia, hyposmia, hypoplastic ears, conductive deafness, hypogonadotrophic hypogonadism and in some cases, mental retardation.

Alopecia-mental retardation.
2783   203650   759.8   AR
Congenital alopecia, microcephaly, low birth weight, mental retardation.

Alopecia-seizures-mental retardation. Shokier syndrome.
3031   104130   759.8   AD
Congenital alopecia, psychomotor seizures, periodontal disease, mental retardation.

Alopecia-skeletal anomalies-mental retardation.
2782   203550   759.8   AR
Congenital alopecia, poor fetal growth, poor postnatal growth, short stature, microcephaly, joint contractures, tubular bone fusions.

Aminopterin syndrome.
0380   760.79   E
Poor fetal growth, poor postnatal growth, short stature, cranial dysplasia, bulbous head, hypertelorism, micrognathia, mesomelia, talipes equinovarus.

Amniotic band syndrome. ADAM complex.
0874   217100   762.8   S
Variable associations of anencephaly, placenta attached to head or abdomen, unusual facial clefting, facial distortion, eye malformation, unusual cleft lip/palate, choanal atresia, ear malformation, craniosynostosis, abdominal and thoracic wall defects, short umbilical cord, omphalocoele, polydactyly, syndactyly, phocomelia, amputation, limb hypoplasia, constriction bands around limbs and digits.

Anemia and triphalangeal thumb. Aase syndrome.
2028   205600   759.8   AR
Poor postnatal growth, short stature, triphalangeal thumb, congenital hypoplastic anemia which improves with age, and in some cases, radial hypoplasia, leukopenia.

Angelman syndrome. Happy puppet syndrome.
2086   105830   759.8   AD
Postnatal microbrachycephaly with flat occuput, large mandible, macrostomia, frequent smiling, tongue thrusting, paroxysmal laughter, absent speech, wide-based ataxic gait with jerky limb movements and hand flapping, psychomotor retardation, hypotonia, hyperreflexia, hyperkinesis, seizures, hypopigmentation. EEG shows symmetrical, synchronous, monorhythmic high amplitude bilateral spike and wave pattern with 2/sec slow wave component. Visible or submicroscopic deletions within the q11-q13 band of the maternally derived chromosome 15 causes some cases while others appear to be due to paternal uniparental isodisomy of chromosome 15.

Anus-hand-ear syndrome.
0072   107480   759.8   AD
Microtia, satyr ear or lop ear; sensorineural deafness; triphalangeal thumb, supernumerary thumb or broad thumb; anal stenosis, anterior anus placement or imperforate anus; and, in some cases, bony anomalies of wrist and ankle, metatarsal fusion, hypoplastic toes.

Asplenia-polysplenia syndrome. Asplenia with cardiovascular anomalies. Ivemark syndrome.
0092   208530   759.8   AR
Either asplenia or polysplenia. Asplenia may be partial or total, and is associated with epiarterial bronchi, bilateral tri-lobed lungs, bilateral morphologic right atria, pulmonary and systemic venous anomalies, complex heart malformation, symmetric liver, intestinal malrotation with stomach on either side. Findings with polysplenia are similar, with the following exceptions: hyparterial bronchi, bilateral bilobed lungs, and bilateral morphologic left atria.

Asymmetric crying face syndrome.
2035   125520   759.8   AD
Congenital hypoplasia of depressor anguli oris muscle producing asymmetry when crying, ventricular septal defect, and, in some cases, microcephaly, mental retardation.

Bardet-Biedl syndrome.
2363   209900   759.8   AR
Poor fetal growth, poor postnatal growth, short stature, pigmentary retinopathy, genital hypoplasia,

hypogonadotrophic hypogenitalism, polydactyly, obesity, mental retardation.

Biemond II syndrome.
3034   210350   759.8   AR
Iris coloboma, postaxial polydactyly, hypogenitalism and hypotonia are noted at birth. Obesity and mental retardation begin in the first year of life.

Blepharochalasis and double lip. Ascher syndrome.
0111   109900   743.62   AD
Sagging eyelids, a fold in the upper lip elicited by muscular contraction causing it to appear double, and in some cases, non-toxic goiter.

Blepharophimosis-ptosis-epicanthus inversus.
2103   110100   759.8   AD
Blepharophimosis, ptosis, epicanthus inversus, often with obstructive vision defect.

Bloom syndrome.
0112   210900   757.39   AR
Poor fetal growth, poor postnatal growth, short stature, small head, malar hypoplasia, photosensitivity, telangiectasia, erythema, leukemia, excessive chromosome breaks and sister chromatid exchanges.

Borjeson-Forssman-Lehmann syndrome.
2272   301900   759.8   XR
Small head, large ears, blepharophimosis, fleshy face, nystagmus, retinal malfunction, cryptorchidism, hypogonadotrophic hypogonadism, seizures, decreased EEG alpha waves, mental retardation.

Bowen Hutterite syndrome.
2422   211180   759.8   AR
Microcephaly, prominent nose, micrognathia, finger 5 radial clinodactyly, rocker-bottom foot, cerebellar hypoplasia, lethargy, death in infancy.

Branchiootorenal dysplasia. BOR syndrome.
2224   113650   759.8   AD
Cup-shaped ear with anteverted pinna, hypoplasia of cochlear apex, sensorineural deafness, prehelical pit, brachial cleft fistula, renal dysplasia, urinary malformation.

Brachydactyly and hypertension.
      112410   759.8   AD
Hypertension, short metacarpals and phalanges.

Bullous dystrophy with macules. Epidermolysis bullosa dystrophica - macular type.
302000   757.39   XR
Bullae form without trauma, and leave scars. Depigmented macules form on hands, feet, and face, and pigmented macules form on trunk. Other features include hairlessness, microcephaly, short stature, mental retardation, short hands, tapered fingers, onychodystrophy, acrocyanosis, and death in childhood.

Carbamazepine syndrome.
2991   760.79   E
Low birth weight, small head size, onychodystrophy, neural tube defects.

Cataract-dental syndrome. Nance-Horan syndrome.
2119   302350   759.8   XR
Congenital nuclear cataracts, microcornea, high nasal bridge, Hutchinsonian or cone-shaped incisors, supernumerary teeth, diastema, prominent anteverted pinnae, short metacarpals, developmental disorder. Posterior Y-sutural cataracts, small corneas and slightly reduced vision in heterozygous females.

Cataract-ichthyosis syndrome.
0131   212400   743.3   AR
Cortical cataract and skin changes typical of ichthyosis vulgaris.

Catel-Manzke syndrome. Stevenson syndrome. Hyperphalangy.
2194   302380   759.8   XD
Cleft palate, micrognathia, radial deviation of index finger at the metacarpophalangeal joint due to accessory first phalanx ossification center, ulnar deviation of index finger at the first interphalangeal joint due to hypoplastic second phalanx, and, in some cases, heart malformation, vertebral anomalies and clubfoot.

Caudal regression syndrome.
3211   182940   759.8   S
Defect or absence of lumbar vertebrae, sacrum, coccyx; denervation deficit of legs, bladder and rectum; dysplasia of pelvis and hips; genitourinary dysplasia; imperforate anus.

Cerebrocostomandibular syndrome.
0138   117650   759.8   AD
Microcephaly, micrognathia, neonatal respiratory distress, posterior rib gap defects on X-ray, death in infancy.

Cerebro-hepato-renal syndrome. Zellweger syndrome.
0139   214100   759.8   AR
High forehead, flat face with flat supraorbital ridges, epicanthus, Brushfield spots, redundant neck skin, camptodactyly, flexion contractures of fingers, simian crease, heart malformation, hepatomegaly, decreased fetal motion, neonatal hypotonia, areflexia, and death in infancy. Laboratory findings include albuminuria, hypoprothrombinemia and absence of liver peroxisomes. X-ray shows particulate chondral calcification, especially of patella. Pathologic findings include macrogyria, polymicrogyria, hypoplastic corpus callosum, intrahepatic biliary dysgenesis, and renal glomerular cysts.

Cerebrooculofacioskeletal syndrome. COFS syndrome.
0140   214150   759.8   AR
Microcephaly, hypotonia, eye malformation, large ears, prominent nose, overhanging upper lip, micrognathia, wide-spaced nipples, arthrogryposis, kyphoscoliosis, osteoporosis, neuronal heterotopia, poor postnatal growth, death in childhood.

Charge association.
2124   214800   759.8   S
Coloboma of retina or iris, ear malformation, sensorineural deafness, choanal atresia, retrognathia, heart malformation, hypoplastic genitalia, mental retardation, poor postnatal growth.

Chediak-Higashi syndrome.
0143   214500   288.8   AR
Decreased pigmentation of hair and eyes, photophobia, nystagmus, and in most cases, hepatosplenomegaly and lymphadenopathy. There is a propensity to purulent infections and lymphoma. Hematologic findings include neutropenia and large eosinophilic peroxidase-positive inclusion bodies in myeloblasts and promyelocytes. Ultrastructure studies show large lysosomal granules in leukocytes, and giant melanosomes in melanocytes.

Cholestasis with peripheral pulmonary stenosis. Arteriohepatic dysplasia. Alagille syndrome.
2084   118450   759.8   AD
Broad forehead, bulbous tip of nose, pointed chin, posterior embryotoxon, retinal pigmentary changes, pulmonic valvular and peripheral stenosis, neonatal jaundice, "butterfly" vertebrae, caudad narrowing of

interpeduncular distance, areflexia, mental retardation. Liver biopsy shows a paucity of intrahepatic bile ducts. SGPT is chronically elevated.

Chondrodysplasia punctata-asymmetric. Chondrodysplasia calcificans congenita.
2730   302950   756.59   XD
Asymmetric limb shortening, scoliosis, flat facies, follicular atrophoderma, sparse coarse hair, and in some cases, ichthyosiform skin dysplasia, joint contractures, cataract, frequent infections, poor postnatal growth, short stature and developmental disorder. X-ray shows irregular asymmetric particulate chondral calcification during infancy.

Chondrodysplasia punctata-mild. Chondrodysplasia calcificans congenita. Conradi-Hunermann syndrome.
0153   118650   759.59   AD
Flat facies, short nose, and in some cases, poor postnatal growth, short stature, developmental disorder. X-ray shows irregular symmetric particulate chondral calcification, especially of tarsus, during infancy.

Chondrodysplasia punctata-rhizomelic. Chondrodysplasia calcificans congenita.
0154   215100   756.59   AR
Symmetrical rhizomelia, flat nasal bridge, short nose, long philtrum, joint contractures, neonatal respiratory distress, poor postnatal growth, short stature, mental retardation, and death in infancy. In some cases, ichthyosiform skin dysplasia is present. X-ray shows particulate chondral calcification during infancy and metaphyseal flaring.

Chromosome 01q42 to qter deletion.
2429   758.3   C
Poor fetal growth, poor postnatal growth, short stature, microcephaly, fine sparse hair, epicanthus, low nasal bridge, short nose with anteverted nares, prognathism, positional foot deformity, hypospadias, mental retardation, high-pitched cry, seizures. Usually a spontaneous mutation.

Chromosome 01q25 to qter duplication.
        758.5   C
Poor fetal growth, poor postnatal growth, short stature, deep-set eyes, low-set malformed ears, pointed nose with anteverted nares, small mouth, re-trognathia, conotruncal heart malformation, hypoplastic thymus, absent gallbladder, long tapering fingers, renal malformation,

cryptorchidism, hirsutism, death in infancy. Usually due to segregation from a balanced rearrangement in a parent.

Chromosome 01q32 to qter duplication.
2426   758.5   C
Poor fetal growth, poor postnatal growth, short stature, bulbous head, prominent forehead, large anterior fontanelle, low nasal bridge, downward eye slant, retrognathia, redundant neck skin, long overlapping fingers and toes, wide-spaced nipples, conotruncal heart malformation, mental retardation, death in infancy. Usually due to segregation from a balanced rearrangement in a parent.

Chromosome 01q25 to q32 duplication.
2428   758.5   C
Deep-set eyes, broad nasal bridge, small mouth, retrognathia, low-set ears, camptodactyly, overlapping fingers, heart malformation, developmental disorder. Usually due to segregation from a balanced rearrangement in a parent.

Chromosome 01 ring.
                     758.5   C
Poor fetal growth, poor postnatal growth, short stature, mental retardation. Usually a spontaneous mutation.

Chromosome 02p23 to pter duplication.
2132   758.5   C
Poor fetal growth, short stature, poor postnatal growth, microcephaly, high forehead, strabismus, epicanthus, short nose with anteverted nares, low nasal bridge, large malformed ears, retrognathia, long trunk, dolichostenomelia, excessive number of digital arches, clinodactyly of fifth finger, mental retardation, hypotonia. Usually due to segregation from a balanced rearrangement in a parent.

Chromosome 02q23 to q32 deletion
2349   758.5   C
Microcephaly, low-set ears, downward eye slant, microphthalmia, cataracts, corneal opacity, prominent nose, maxillary hypoplasia, micrognathia, cleft palate, dental anomalies, finger contractures, wide separation of toes 1 & 2, heart malformation, mental retardation, poor fetal growth, short stature, poor postnatal growth, death in infancy. Usually a spontaneous mutation.

Chromosome 02q34 to qter duplication.
2348   758.5   C

Microcephaly, plagiocephaly, frontal bossing, low-set ears, hypertelorism, short nose with anteverted nares, low nasal bridge, long philtrum, cleft palate, retrognathia, clinodactyly, distal palmar axial triradius, low total finger ridge count, heart malformation, clitoral hypertrophy, mental retardation, hypotonia, poor fetal growth, short stature, poor postnatal growth, death in infancy. Usually due to segregation from a balanced rearrangement in a parent.

Chromosome 03p25 to pter deletion.
2431   758.5   C
Microcephaly, dolichocephaly, low-set malformed ears, ptosis, upward eye slant, triangular face, synophrys, hypertelorism, epicanthus, short thick nose, retrognathia, pectus excavatum, hypoplastic genitalia, finger 5 clinodactyly, mental retardation, poor fetal growth, short stature, poor postnatal growth. Usually due to segregation from a balanced rearrangement in a parent.

Chromosome 03p25 to p26 duplication.
2432   758.5   C
Microcephaly, brachycephaly, large ears, hypertelorism, small nose, macrostomia, cleft lip/palate, small chin, excessive number of digital whorls, heart malformation, intestinal malformation, hypoplastic genitalia, cryptorchidism, mental retardation. Usually due to segregation from a balanced rearrangement in a parent.

Chromosome 03q21 to qter duplication.
2430   75.85   C
Plagiocephaly, irregular cranial sutures, low-set malformed ears, low-set thick eyebrows, hypertelorism, upward eye slant, glaucoma, corneal opacity, long eyelashes, low nasal bridge, short nose with anteverted nares, long philtrum, thick upper lip, retrognathia, cleft palate, webbed neck, wide-spaced nipples, short limbs, hand and foot malformations, broad thumbs, genital malformation, renal malformation, heart malformation, hypertrichosis, mental retardation, hypotonia, seizures.Usually due to segregation from a balanced rearrangement in a parent.

Chromosome 04p16 to pter deletion. Wolf-Hirshhorn syndrome.
0164   758.3   C
Microcephaly, dolichocephaly, frontal bossing, simple ears, hypoplastic orbits, ptosis, iris coloboma, strabismus, nasal bridge level with forehead, prominent broad nasal bridge,

hypertelorism, epicanthus, down-turned mouth, short philtrum which appears to arise in nares, retrognathia, cleft lip/palate, heart malformation, hypoplastic genitalia, anomalies of vertebrae and ribs, long thin fingers with hyperconvex nails, excessive number of digital arch patterns, simian crease, hypoplastic dermal ridges, distal axial triradius, dimples on elbows and knees, club foot, scalp defects, hypotonia, seizures, mental retardation, poor fetal growth, short stature, poor postnatal growth, death in infancy. Usually a spontaneous mutation.

Chromosome 04p distal duplication.
2433   758.5   C
Microcephaly, large ears with prominent antihelix, strabismus, blepharophimosis, hypertelorism, prominent glabella, broad nasal root, synophrys, small round nose, long indistinct philtrum, prominent chin, faint vermillion border of upper lip, anomalous teeth, short neck, low posterior hairline, wide-spaced nipples, scoliosis, anomalies of the vertebrae and ribs, hypoplastic genitalia, hypospadias, cryptorchidism, camptodactyly, polydactyly, simian crease, distal axial triradius, excessive number of digital whorl patterns, positional deformities of hands and feet, hypertonia followed by hypotonia, stupor, seizures, mental retardation, delayed osseous maturation, poor fetal growth, short stature, poor postnatal growth, death in childhood. Usually due to segregation from a balanced rearrangement in a parent.

Chromosome 04q partial deletion. Chromosome 04 ring.
2435   758.3   C
Large ears with flattened architecture and pointed upper helix, hypertelorism, low nasal bridge, short nose, retrognathia, cleft palate, heart malformation, renal malformation, cubitus valgus, radial arm and hand malformations, malposition of toes, sacral dimple, mental retardation, poor fetal growth, short stature, poor postnatal growth, death in childhood. Usually a spontaneous mutation.

Chromosome 04q distal duplication.
2434   758.3   C
Microcephaly, receding forehead, prominent metopic suture, large low-set ears with folded upper helix, blepharophimosis, nasal bridge level with forehead, epicanthus, prominent philtrum, pursed mouth with protruding upper lip and dimple below lower lip, short neck, wide-spaced nipples, heart malformation, cryptorchidism, renal malformation,

malformed thumb, simian crease, hypotonia, seizures, mental retardation, poor fetal growth, short stature, poor postnatal growth, death in childhood. Usually due to segregation from a balanced rearrangement in a parent.

Chromosome 05p15 deletion. Cri du chat syndrome.
0163   758.3   C
Strabismus, epicanthus, round flat face in infancy, facial asymmetry, hypertelorism, low nasal bridge, retrognathia, high-pitched "mewing" cry, heart malformation, scoliosis, small hands and feet, excessive number of digital arches and whorls, simian crease, hypotonia followed by hypertonia, mental retardation, poor fetal growth, short stature, poor postnatal growth. Usually a spontaneous mutation.

Chromosome 05p partial duplication.
2436   758.5   C
Broad forehead, prominent occiput, low-set ears, upward eye slant, epicanthus, hypertelorism, prominent nasal bridge, anteverted nares, prognathism, macroglossia, heart malformation, long fingers, excessive number of digital ulnar loops, hypotonia, seizures, mental retardation, short stature, poor postnatal growth. Usually due to segregation from a balanced rearrangement in a parent.

Chromosome 05q12 to q22 deletion.
2544   758.5   C
Brachycephaly, narrow forehead, frontal bossing, low nasal bridge, anteverted nares, prominent philtrum, short neck, hip dysplasia, club foot, mental retardation, short stature, poor postnatal growth. Usually a spontaneous mutation.

Chromosome 05q31 to qter duplication.
2437   758.5   C
Microcephaly, low-set malformed ears, upward eye slant, strabismus, hypertelorism, epicanthus, long indistinct philtrum, thin upper lip, small mouth, heart malformation, clinodactyly, mental retardation, short stature, poor postnatal growth. Usually due to segregation from a balanced rearrangement in a parent.

Chromosome 06p distal duplication.
2438   758.5   C
Microcephaly, high forehead, flat occiput, low-set malformed ears, blepharophimosis, ptosis, epicanthus inversus, hypertelorism, prominent nasal bridge, bulbous nose, retrognathia, pointed chin, small mouth, heart malformation, small

dysfunctional kidneys, mental retardation, poor fetal growth, short stature, poor postnatal growth, death in infancy. Usually due to segregation from a balanced rearrangement in a parent.

Chromosome 06q partial duplication.
2439   758.5   C
Microcephaly, brachycephaly, malformed ears, downward eye slant, low nasal bridge, anteverted nares, long philtrum, retrognathia, bow-shaped mouth, clinodactyly, tapered fingers, excessive number of digital arches, simian crease, dimples about elbows and knees, mental retardation, poor fetal growth, short stature, poor postnatal growth. Usually due to segregation from a balanced rearrangement in a parent.

Chromosome 06 ring.
2440   758.5   C
Microcephaly, low-set malformed ears, wide nasal bridge, epicanthus, wide philtrum, short neck, vertebral anomalies, mental retardation, poor fetal growth, short stature, poor postnatal growth. Usually a spontaneous mutation.

Chromosome 07p22 deletion.
2447   758.3   C   °
Microcephaly, craniosynostosis, low-set ears, prominent nose, limited jaw movement, heart malformation, simian crease, mental retardation. Usually a spontaneous mutation.

Chromosome 07q partial deletion.
2443-5   758.3   C
Microcephaly, frontal bossing, low-set malformed ears, bulbous nose tip, cleft lip/palate, hernia, genital malformation, simian crease, hypotonia, mental retardation, short stature, poor postnatal growth. Usually a spontaneous mutation.

Chromosome 07q32 to qter duplication.
2442   758.5   C
Prominent occiput, frontal bossing, low-set malformed ears, blepharophimosis, eye malformation, hypertelorism, short nose, retrognathia, macroglossia, cleft palate, short neck, dystonia, mental retardation, poor fetal growth, short stature, poor postnatal growth. Usually due to segregation from a balanced rearrangement in a parent.

Chromosome 08p21 to pter deletion.
2450   758.3   C

Microcephaly, narrow cranium, epicanthus, retrognathia, prominent long upper lip, short neck, wide-spaced nipples, heart malformation, genital malformation, cryptorchidism, distal axial palmar triradius, mental retardation, poor fetal growth, short stature, poor postnatal growth. Usually a spontaneous mutation.

Chromosome 08p partial duplication.
2449   758.5   C
Microcephaly, low-set ears, strabismus, wide face, epicanthus, prominent nasal bridge, down-turned mouth, heart malformation, hypoplastic nails, short fingers, clinodactyly, camptodactyly, hyperextensible phalangeal joints, absent flexion creases on fingers, simian crease, absence of corpus callosum, mental retardation, short stature, poor postnatal growth. Usually due to segregation from a balanced rearrangement in a parent.

Chromosome 08q2 to qter duplication.
2449   758.5   C
Prominent forehead, hypertelorism, retrognathia, sternum malformation, heart malformation, cryptorchidism, vertebral malformation, clino-dactyly, camptodactyly, malposition of toes, joint stiffness, narrow shoulders and hips, distal axial palmar triradius, mental retardation. Usually due to segregation from a balanced rearrangement in a parent.

Chromosome 08 trisomy.
0157   758.8   C
Prominent forehead, large malformed ears, deep-set eyes, strabismus, broad nasal bridge, anteverted nares, retrognathia, thick everted lower lip, sternum malformation, accessory ribs, urinary tract malformation, cryptorchidism, vertebral malformation, narrow shoulders and hips, long limbs, limited elbow supination, long or short fingers, camptodactyly, clinodactyly, hypoplastic nails, deep furrows on palms and soles, excessive number of digital arches, hypothenar whorl, thenar whorl, halluceal whorl, absent patella, malposition of toes, hypertonia, poor speech development, poor coordination, mental retardation, short stature, poor postnatal growth. Usually a spontaneous mutation, mosaic with a normal cell line.

Chromosome 09p to 22pter deletion.
2231   758.3   C
Trigonocephaly, prominent forehead, metopic ridge, low-set malformed ears with attached or absent lobule, broad nasal bridge, epicanthus, short nose

with anteverted nares, long philtrum, broad neck, wide-spaced nipples, heart malformation, omphalocoele or umbilical hernia, hypoplastic labia, hypospadias, long fingers with supernumerary flexion creases, excessive number of digital whorls, distal axial palmar triradius, hyperconvex "square" nails, long toes, mental retardation, hypotonia. Usually due to segregation from a balanced rearrangement in a parent.

Chromosome 09p13 to pter duplication.
2451   758.5   C
Microcephaly, brachycephaly, persistent metopic suture in infancy, large ears, eccentric pupils, strabismus, hypertelorism, prominent nasal bridge, fleshy nose, short upper lip, downturned mouth, everted lower lip, asymmetric smile, short neck, narrow upper thorax, wide-spaced nipples, hypogonadism, lordosis or scoliosis, simian crease, excessive number of digital arches, long palms, brachymesophalangy, clinodactyly, malposition of thumb, hypoplastic nails, mental retardation, poor speech development, poor coordination, delayed osseous maturation, poor postnatal growth. Usually due to segregation from a balanced rearrangement in a parent.

Chromosome 09q12 to q21 deletion.
                       758.3   C
Low-set ears, hypertelorism, short nose with anteverted nares, prominent philtrum, retrognathia, narrow vermillion border of upper lip, mental retardation. Usually a spontaneous mutation.

Chromosome 09q partial duplication.
2453   758.5   C
Microcephaly, low-set malformed ears, deep-set eyes, small face, prominent forehead, retrognathia, small mouth, protruding upper lip, narrow hips, long thin malpositioned fingers and toes, limited joint motion, mental retardation, poor fetal growth. The duplication is of the distal half of 9q, with similar proportions due to segregation from a balanced rearrangement in a parent, or to spontaneous mutation.

Chromosome 09 ring.
2454   758.5   C
Microcephaly, trigonocephaly, malformed ears, exophthalmos, hypoplastic midface, epicanthus, anteverted nares, retrognathia, obliteration of Cupid's bow of upper lip, heart malformation, genital malformation, excessive number of digital whorls, mental retardation, hypotonia, poor fetal

growth, short stature, poor postnatal growth. Usually a spontaneous mutation, mosaic with other cell lines.

Chromosome 09 trisomy.
2452   758.5   C
Microcephaly, dolichocephaly, prominent forehead, low-set malformed ears, blepharophimosis, deep-set eyes, prominent nose, prominent cheeks, retrognathia, heart malformation, cryptorchidism, vertebral anomalies, multiple dislocations, limited motion of phalangeal joints, simian crease, mental retardation, hypotonia, poor fetal growth, short stature, poor postnatal growth. Usually a spontaneous mutation, mosaic with a normal cell line.

Chromosome 10p13 to pter deletion.
2457   758.3   C
Low-set malformed ears, ptosis, low nasal bridge, broad nose, epicanthus, retrognathia, cleft lip/palate, wide-spaced nipples, heart malformation, genital malformation, urinary tract malformation, mental retardation, poor fetal growth, short stature, poor postnatal growth, death in infancy. Usually a spontaneous mutation.

Chromosome 10p partial duplication.
2456   758.5   C
Dolichocephaly, high prominent forehead, backswept scalp hair, low-set large malformed ears, long palpebral fissures, small face, broad nasal bridge, short nose, high arched eyebrows, retrognathia, cleft lip/palate, heart malformation, thrombocytopenia, genital malformation, renal malformation, flexion deformity of hands, club foot, mental retardation, hypotonia, poor fetal growth, short stature, poor postnatal growth, death in childhood. Usually due to segregation from a balanced rearrangement in a parent.

Chromosome 10q24 to qter duplication.
2455   758.5   C
Microcephaly, high prominent forehead, low-set ears, blepharophimosis, ptosis, round flat face, hypoplastic midface, thin eyebrows, epicanthus, low nasal bridge, short nose with anteverted nares, long philtrum, retrognathia, short neck, heart malformation, cryptorchidism, renal malformation, scoliosis, joint laxity, hammer toe hallux, simian crease, clinodactyly, mental retardation, poor fetal growth, short stature, poor postnatal growth, death in infancy. Usually due to segregation from a balanced rearrangement in a parent.

Chromosome 11p13 partial deletion.
2245   758.3   C
Prominent forehead, cranial asymmetry, aniridia and other eye malformations, ptosis, hypertelorism, prominent nasal bridge, ambiguous genitalia, mental retardation, and in some cases, Wilm's tumor. Usually a spontaneous mutation.

Chromosome 11p partial duplication.
2459   758.5   C
Frontal bossing, prominent forehead, strabismus, nystagmus, hypoplastic supraorbital ridges, broad nasal root, low nasal bridge, short nose, cleft lip/palate, dysphonic cry, hypogonadism, broad fingers and toes, simian crease, mental retardation, hypotonia, spastic paraplegia, poor postnatal growth. Usually due to segregation from a balanced rearrangement in a parent.

Chromosome 11q23 to qter deletion.
0162   758.3   C
Scaphocephaly or trigonocephaly, metopic ridge, low-set ears with prominent antihelix, strabismus, hypertelorism, broad nasal root, low nasal bridge, epicanthus, short nose with anteverted nares, indistinct philtrum, retrognathia, heart malformation, genitourinary malformations, narrow vermillion of upper lip, clinodactyly, irregular brachydactyly, simian crease, mental retardation, poor speech development, poor fetal growth, short stature, poor postnatal growth. Usually a spontaneous mutation.

Chromosome 11q23 to qter duplication.
0161   758.5   C
Microcephaly, low-set ears, broad nose, short nose with anteverted nares, long prominent philtrum, retrognathia, horizontal crease under lower lip, cleft palate, short neck, malformed clavicles, wide-spaced nipples, heart malformation, gastrointestinal malformation, urinary tract malformation, small penis, malformed hips, lax skin, mental retardation, poor fetal growth. Usually due to segregation from a balanced rearrangement in a parent.

Chromosome 12p11 to p13 partial deletion.
2461   758.3   C
Microcephaly, prominent occiput, large low-set ears, high arched eyebrows, retrognathia, heart malformation, cryptorchidism, clinodactyly, narrow hands, mental retardation, poor fetal growth, short stature, poor postnatal growth. Usually a spontaneous mutation.

Chromosome 12p12 to pter partial duplication.
2130   758.5   C
Turricephaly, low-set ears, nystagmus, hypoplastic midface, broad nasal bridge, short nose with anteverted nares, long philtrum, retrognathia, everted lower lip, short neck, short sternum, broad hands, simian crease, flat feet, mental retardation, hypotonia, infantile corpulence. Usually due to segregation from a balanced rearrangement in a parent.

Chromosome 12p tetrasomy mosaicism. Pallister-Killian mosaic syndrome.
2189   758.9   C
Prominent forehead, upward eye slant, hypertelorism, flat nasal bridge, epicanthus, short nose with anteverted nares, indistinct philtrum, everted lower lip, variegate hypopigmentation, hydrocephalus ex vacuuo, mental retardation, hypotonia followed later by contractures. The tetrasomy is due to a supernumerary isochromosome of 12p, usually found only in skin and due to spontaneous mutation.

Chromosome 13q14 to qter deletion.
0167   758.3   C
Microcephaly, large ears, retinoblastoma, hypotelorism, flat face, strabismus, heart malformation, urinary tract malformation, genital malformation, lumbar focal vertebral agenesis, synostosis of metacarpals 4 and 5, hypoplastic thumbs, holoprosencephaly. Usually a spontaneous mutation.

Chromosome 13q21 deletion.
0167   758.3   C
Retinoblastoma, prominent maxilla, short hypoplastic thumbs, hypoplastic phalanges, polydactyly, psychomotor retardation. Similar proportions are due to dominant transmission from a parent, or to spontaneous mutation.

Chromosome 13q31 to q32 deletion. Chromosome 13 ring.
0167   758.3   C
Microcephaly, trigonocephaly, frontal bossing, low-set ears, eye malformation, hypertelorism, epicanthus, prominent maxilla, urinary tract malformation, genital malformation, absent thumbs, hypoplastic phalanges, metacarpal 1 hypoplasia, metacarpal 4-5 fusion, mental retardation, poor postnatal growth. Usually a spontaneous mutation.

Chromosome 13q32 to q34 deletion. Chromosome 13 ring.

2465   758.3 C

Microcephaly, trigonocephaly, large ears, eye malformation, protruding central incisors, imperforate anus, urinary tract malformation, genital malformation, poor postnatal growth. Usually a spontaneous mutation.

Chromosome 13q14 to pter duplication.

2464   758.5 C

Microcephaly, prominent forehead, retrognathia, microstomia, persistent fetal hemoglobin, clinodactyly, simian crease, mental retardation. Similar proportions are due to segregation from a balanced rearrangement in a parent, or to spontaneous mutation.

Chromosome 13q13 to qter duplication.

2463   758.5 C

Microcephaly, prominent forehead, low-set malformed ears, curly eyelashes, microphthalmia, epicanthus, delayed dentition, persistent fetal hemoglobin, hernias, renal malformations, polydactyly, simian crease, capillary hemangiomata, mental retardation. Similar proportions are due to segregation from a balanced rearrangement in a parent, or to spontaneous mutation.

Chromosome 13 trisomy. Patau syndrome.

0168   758.1 C

Microcephaly, receding forehead, low-set malformed ears, microphthalmia, hypotelorism, cleft lip/palate, heart malformation, excessive number of neutrophil projections, persistent embryonic and fetal hemoglobins, urinary tract malformation, cryptorchidism, "saddlebag" scrotum, bicornuate uterus, postaxial polydactyly of hands and feet, flexion contracture of fingers, narrow hyperconvex fingernails, excessive number of digital radial loops, simian crease, rocker bottom feet, hallucal arch fibular, or S, or loop tibial, glabellar capillary hemangioma, scalp ulceration, deafness, seizures, mental retardation, arrhinencephaly, holoprosencephaly, poor fetal growth, short stature, poor postnatal growth, death in infancy. Usually a spontaneous mutation, due either to nondisjunction or to an unbalanced rearrangement.

Chromosome 14pter to q23 duplication.

0165   758.5 c

Microcephaly, broad nasal bridge, prominent nose, retrognathia, long upper lip with faint philtrum and Cupid's bow, sagging outer edges of lower lip, cleft palate, short neck, heart malformation, cryptorchidism, vertebral malformation, limb malformation, mental retardation, seizures, poor fetal growth, short stature, poor postnatal growth. Usually due to segregation from a balanced rearrangement in a parent.

Chromosome 14 trisomy.

2547   758.5 C

Broad nose, retrognathia, wide mouth, cleft palate, heart malformation, mental retardation, poor postnatal growth. Usually a spontaneous mutation, mosaic with another cell line.

Chromosome 15pter to q21 duplication.

2548   758.5 C

Type I: mental retardation, hypotonia, seizures. Type II: Low-set ears, blepharophimosis, almond-shaped eyes, telecanthus, strabismus, wide-spaced high eyebrows lacking an arch, mental retardation, poor postnatal growth. Similar proportions are due to segregation from a balanced rearrangement in a parent, or to spontaneous mutation.

Chromosome 15 distal duplication.

2131   758.5 C

Prominent forehead, epicanthus, retrognathia, mental retardation, poor postnatal growth. Usually due to segregation from a balanced rearrangement in a parent.

Chromosome 15 ring.

2468   758.5 C

Microcephaly, mental retardation, poor fetal growth, short stature, poor postnatal growth. Usually a spontaneous mutation.

Chromosome 16q partial duplication.

2470   758.5 C

Plagiocephaly, hypoplastic mandible, heart malformation, intestinal malrotation, cryptorchidism, hypoplastic phalanges, sclerotic tufts on distal phalanges, malposition of fingers and toes, mental retardation, poor fetal growth, short stature, poor postnatal growth, death in infancy. Usually due to segregation from a balanced rearrangement in a parent.

Chromosome 18p partial deletion.

0158   758.3 C

Microcephaly, low-set large malformed ears, strabismus, ptosis, hypertelorism, low nasal bridge, epicanthus, short upper lip with faint Cupid's bow, short webbed neck, wide-spaced nipples, hernias, simian crease, tapered fingers, clinodactyly, cubitus valgus, mental retardation, poor fetal growth, short stature, poor postnatal growth, and in some cases, cebocephalus or cyclocephalus, microphthalmia, arrhinencephaly, heart malformation, and hormone deficiencies. Usually a spontaneous mutation.

Chromosome 18q21 to qter deletion.
0159   758.3   C
Microcephaly, prominent antitragus and antihelix, atretic ear canals, deep-set eyes, strabismus, glaucoma, tapetoretinal degeneration, optic atrophy, midfacial hypoplasia, prominent mandible, faint Cupid's bow and philtrum, short upper lip, cleft lip/palate, wide-spaced nipples, heart malformation, hypoplastic genitalia, dimples on elbows and knees, long fingers with prominent tips, excessive number of large composite digital patterns, mental retardation, hypotonia, seizures, poor fetal growth, short stature, poor postnatal growth. Usually a spontaneous mutation.

Chromosome 18 ring.
2473   758.5   C
Microcephaly, eye malformation, midfacial hypoplasia, epicanthus, cleft palate, short webbed neck, narrow upper thorax, excessive number of digital whorls, poor fetal growth, short stature, poor postnatal growth, and in some cases genital malformation, limb malformation, cebocephaly, arrhinencephaly. Usually a spontaneous mutation.

Chromosome 18 trisomy. Edwards syndrome.
0160   758.2   C
Microcephaly, dolichocephaly, prominent occiput, faunesque ears, epicanthus, small face, small chin, short webbed neck, short sternum, heart malformation, renal malformation, cryptorchidism, gastrointestinal malformation, flexion deformity of fingers, overlapping fingers, simian crease, excessive number of digital arches, hypoplastic nails, narrow malformed hips, short dorsiflexed hallux, rocker bottom feet, hypertonia, mental retardation, poor fetal growth, short stature, poor postnatal growth. Usually a spontaneous mutation.

Chromosome 19q13 to qter duplication.
2474   758.5   C
Microcephaly, prominent glabella, ptosis, flat face, hypertelorism, small nose with anteverted nares, downturned oral commissures, cleft palate, short neck with excess skin, wide-spaced nipples, diaphragmatic hernia, heart malformation, hypoplastic gall bladder, intestinal malrotation,

polycystic kidneys, hypospadias, clinodactyly, bifid thumb, mental retardation, seizures, hypotonia, apnea, poor fetal growth, short stature, poor postnatal growth, death in infancy. Usually due to segregation from a balanced rearrangement in a parent.

Chromosome 20p11 to pter duplication.
2475   758.5   C
Prominent cheeks, telecanthus, epicanthus, short nose with anteverted nares, small chin, dental malformation, wide-spaced nipples, heart malformation, vertebral malformation, malposition of thumb, hip malformation, coarse scalp hair, mental retardation, excessive growth. Usually due to segregation from a balanced rearrangement in a parent.

Chromosome 20 ring.
                  758.5   C
Mental retardation, aberrant behavior, seizures. Usually a spontaneous mutation.

Chromosome 21q21 to pter deletion.
                  758.3   C
Prominent forehead, low-set malformed ears, large auditory canals, blepharophimosis, microphthalmia, broad nasal bridge, long upper lip, cleft palate, heart malformation, renal malformation, skeletal malformation, flexion deformity of fingers, overlapping fingers, mental retardation, cerebral malformation, poor fetal growth, short stature, poor postnatal growth. Usually a spontaneous mutation.

Chromosome 21 monosomy. Chromosome 21 ring.
0170   758.5   C
Microcephaly, protuberant occiput, frontal bossing, epiblepharon, microphthalmia, broad prominent nasal bridge, retrognathia, long upper lip, small mouth, heart malformation, thrombocytopenia, hypogammaglobulinemia, gastrointestinal malformation, renal malformation, hypospadias, cryptorchidism, skeletal malformation, mental retardation, poor fetal growth, short stature, poor postnatal growth. Usually a spontaneous mutation.

Chromosome 21 trisomy. Down syndrome.
0171   758   C
Brachycephaly, flat occiput, flat forehead, small ears, Brushfield spots, lens opacity, midfacial hypoplasia, low nasal bridge, epicanthus, open mouth with protruding tongue, short neck, heart malformation, duodenal atresia, hernias, small penis, short broad hands and feet, mesobrachydactyly of

finger 5, wide space between toes 1 and 2, simian crease, excessive number of digital ulnar loops, distal axial palmar triradius, deafness, nystagmus, mental retardation, poor fetal growth, short stature, poor postnatal growth. Usually a spontaneous mutation.

Chromosome 22q partial deletion.
2537   758.3   C
Ptosis, low nasal bridge, epicanthus, syndactyly, mental retardation, hypotonia. Usually a spontaneous mutation.

Chromosome 22q proximal duplication. Cat eye syndrome.
0544   758.5   C
Preauricular tags, malformed ears, coloboma, hypertelorism, heart malformation, anal atresia, genital malformation, mental retardation. Usually a spontaneous mutation.

Chromosome 22 ring.
2477   758.5   C
Almond-shaped eyes, hypertelorism, epicanthus, mental retardation. Usually a spontaneous mutation.

Chromosome 22 trisomy.
2478   758.5   C
Microcephaly, low-set malformed ears, preauricular tags, anteverted nares, long philtrum, retrognathia, cleft palate, imperforate anus, hernias, small penis, cryptorchidism, finger-like thumb, long fingers, malformed hips, mental retardation, hypotonia, poor fetal growth, short stature, poor postnatal growth. Usually a spontaneous mutation.

Chromosome triploidy.
0169   758.5   C
Large fontanel, low-set ears, eye malformation, hypertelorism, low nasal bridge, retrognathia, heart malformation, renal cystic dysplasia, hypoplastic genitalia, finger 3 to 4 syndactyly, simian crease, talipes equinovarus, adrenal hypoplasia, hydrocephalus, holoprosencephaly, mental retardation, poor fetal growth, short stature, poor postnatal growth, large hydatiform placenta, death in infancy.

Chromosome X monosomy. Turner syndrome.
0977   758.6   C
Low posterior hairline, large ears, webbed neck, broad shieldlike chest with wide-spaced nipples, cubitus valgus, lymphedema, poor fetal growth, short stature, poor postnatal growth, and in some cases, coarctation of aorta, distal palmar axial triradius, mental retardation, Hashimoto thyroiditis, and after puberty, elevated gonadotrophins. A few are mosaic with another cell line. If the mosaic line is XX, fertility may be near normal. If it is XY, there is a propensity toward gonadoblastoma after age 20 years. A few have X isochromosome, Xp deletion, Xq deletion, or X ring. Usually a spontaneous mutation.

Chromosome X polysomy.
3006-7   758.8   C
Epicanthus, hypertelorism, low nasal bridge, coarse face, oval face, heart malformation, menstrual disorders, radioulnar synostosis, narrow shoulders, schizophrenia, mental retardation. The phenotype is loosely correlated with the number of X chromosomes - those with XXX are usually mildest, and may have a normal phenotype, while those with XXXXX are usually severely affected. Usually a spontaneous mutation.

Chromosome XXY syndrome. Klinefelter syndrome.
0556   758.8   C
Eunuchoid proportions, passive aggressive personality, small testes, and after puberty, gynecomastia. Some are mentally retarded. After puberty, azoospermia and elevated gonadotrophins are found. A few are mosaic with another cell line. If the mosiac cell line is XY, fertility may be near normal. Those mosaic with an abnormal cell line have characteristics associated with that line. A few have XXYY karyotype, and those have worse mental retardation and antisocial behavior. Usually a spontaneous mutation.

Chromosome XYY syndrome.
2552   758.8   C
Prominent glabella, long ears, large teeth, abrupt behavior, poor coordination, tallness due to excessive growth in mid-childhood. Some cases have antisocial behavior, mental retardation, and genital malformation.

Cleft lip-palate, ectodermal dysplasia, syndactyly. Rosselli-Gulienetti syndrome.
0179   225000   759.8   AR
Cleft lip-palate, scarring alopecia, congenital adhesions of eyelids and labia, kissing ulcers in areas of skin approximation, syndactyly, hypohydrosis, hypodontia, mental retardation.

Cleft lip-palate and popliteal pterygium.

0818   119500   759.8   AD
Cleft lip/palate, popliteal pterygium, syndactyly, hypoplastic genitalia, cryptorchidism, bifid scrotum, and in some cases mucous cysts of lower lip, ankyloblepharon filiforme adnatum, accessory buccal frenulae.

Cleidocranial dysplasia. Yunis-Varon syndrome.
2405   216340   759.8   AR
Macrocrania, cranial suture diastasis, micrognathia, retracted and poorly defined lips, absent clavicles, absent thumbs and distal phalanges of fingers, hypoplasia of proximal phalanx and absence of distal phalanx of hallux, pelvic dysplasia, hip dislocation.

Cloacal dysgenesis with female virilization.
3161   759.8   S
Female (46,XX) with perineal structures simulating phallus and scrotum but no perineal opening; imperforate anus; vesicovaginal fistula; uterus malformations; renal agenesis, dysplasia or hydronephrosis; oligohydramnios; pulmonary hypoplasia; renal failure; early death.

Cocaine syndrome.
2603   760.72   E
Poor fetal growth with limb, heart and neural tube defects.

Cockayne syndrome II.
2787   216410   759.8   AR
Microcephaly, cryptorchidism. During the first year: cataracts, sunken eyes, deafness, sparse hair, kyphosis, flexion contractures, swallowing dysfunction, poor fetal growth, short stature, poor postnatal growth, death in infancy or early childhood.

Coffin-Lowry syndrome.
0190   303600   759.8   XD
Prominent forehead, hypertelorism, pugilistic nose, anteverted nares, large ears, patulous lips, large mouth, tapered fingers, pectus carinatum, hypotonia, and mental retardation, short stature, poor postnatal growth. X-ray shows drumstick terminal phalanges.

Coffin-Siris syndrome. Fifth digit syndrome.
2025   135900   759.8   S
Small head with sparse hair, coarse face, full lips, hypoplastic or absent fifth digits, lax joints, radial dislocation, hypotonia, mental retardation, poor fetal growth, poor postnatal growth.

Cornelia de Lange syndrome.
0242   122470   759.8   AD
Microbrachycephaly, synophrys, long eyelashes, flat nasal bridge, small nose, anteverted nares, thin lips, micromelia, simian crease, posterior placement of thumb, flexion contracture of elbow, genital hypoplasia, cryptorchidism, low growling cry, hypertonia, mental retardation, poor fetal growth, short stature, poor postnatal growth.

Cranioectodermal dysplasia.
2127   218330   759.8   AR
Dolichocephaly, rhizomelia, brachydactyly, sparse hair, dental anomalies, osteopenia, poor fetal growth, short stature, poor postnatal growth.

Craniosynostosis with radial defects. Baller-Gerold syndrome.
0231   218600   759.8   AR
Oxycephaly, radial aplasia, short and curved ulna, and in some cases conductive hearing loss, malformation of some carpals and metacarpals, hypoplastic thumb, vertebral malformation, anteriorly placed or imperforate anus, short stature, poor postnatal growth.

Crome syndrome.
2162   218900   759.8   AR
Congenital cataracts, seizures, mental retardation, short stature, poor postnatal growth, death in infancy. Pathological findings include encephalopathy and renal tubular necrosis.

Cryptophthalmos syndrome. Fraser syndrome.
2271   219000   759.8   AR
Cryptophthalmos, anterior hairline fused with lateral eyebrow, ear malformation, notched small nares, partial cutaneous syndactyly, hypospadias, cryptorchidism, bicornuate uterus, vagina:atresia.

Curly hair-ankyloblepharon-nail dysplasia syndrome. CHANDS.
3039   214350   759.8   AR
Ankyloblepharon, hypoplastic nails, curly hair.

Cytomegalovirus syndrome.
0381   760.2   E
Usually asymptomatic but about 15% later have deafness. A tiny proportion is born with variable combinations of poor fetal growth, hepatosplenomegaly, thrombocytopenia, hemolytic anemia, microcephaly and cerebral calcifications.

Deafness-congenital-Marshall type.

0261   154780   759.8   AD
Low nasal bridge, anteverted nares, hypertelorism, congenital cataracts, myopia, sensorineural deafness.

Deafness-congenital-vitiligo-achalasia.
0275   221350   759.8   AR
Sensorineural deafness, poor postnatal growth, vitiligo, muscle wasting, and achalasia.

Deafness-congenital with onychodystrophy.
DOORS syndrome.
0262   220500   759.8   AR
Congenital sensorineural deafness, onychodystrophy, and in some cases triphalangeal thumb, hypoplastic terminal phalanges, excessive number of digital arch patterns, mental retardation.

Deafness-congenital with onychodystrophy.
2034   124480   759.8   AD
Congenital sensorineural deafness, coniform teeth, partial anodontia, syndactyly, small dystrophic nails. Sweat electrolytes are elevated.

Diabetes syndrome.
2498   760.7   E
Poor fetal growth, neural tube defect, conotruncal defect, caudal regression.

DiGeorge syndrome. CATCH-22 syndrome.
0943   188400   279.11   S
Hypertelorism, mongoloid eye slant, short philtrum, ear malformation, hypoplastic or aplastic thymus, hypoplastic or absent parathyroid, aortic arch anomalies, tetralogy of Fallot, ventricular septal defect, hypocalcemia, seizures, cellular immunodeficiency, severe infectious disease, death in infancy. Most cases have microscopic or molecular deletions at chromosome 22q11.2. Deletions of other chromosome sites have been found in some cases instead. The Shprintzen syndrome or the velocardiofacial syndrome may result from the similar deletions.

Digito-reno-cerebral syndrome.
2792   222760   759.8   AR
Absent distal phalanges of fingers and toes, microcephaly, renal dysplasia, hydrocephalus ex vacuuo.

Dilantin syndrome.
0382   760.79   E
Large fontanel, hypertelorism, low nasal bridge, short nose, bowed upper lip, cleft lip/palate, hypoplasia of distal phalanges, small nails, excessive

digital low arches, finger-like thumb, hip dislocation, hirsutism, poor fetal growth, poor early development.

Dubowitz syndrome.
0299   223370   759.8   AR
Microcephaly, nasal bridge level with forehead, blepharophimosis with lateral telecanthus, ptosis, retrognathia, and in some cases eczema, mental retardation, poor fetal growth, short stature, poor postnatal growth.

Dwarfism and hypocalcemia.
0976   127000   759.8   AD
Persistent fontanelle, hyperopia, microphthalmos, dense bone with narrow marrow cavity, episodic hypocalcemia with hypophosphatemia, poor fetal growth, short stature, poor postnatal growth.

Ectrodactyly-ectodermal dysplasia-clefting syndrome. EEC syndrome.
0337   129900   759.8   AD
Blepharophimosis, lacrimal duct malformation, cleft lip or cleft lip and palate, retrognathia, microdontia, partial anodontia, hypoplastic nipples, thin skin, fine sparse hair, ectrodactyly, syndactyly.

Ectrodactyly-ectodermal dysplasia-macular dystrophy. EEM syndrome.
2793   225280   759.8   AR
Scant hair, hypodontia, microdontia, ectrodactyly, pigmentary macular dystrophy.

Ellis-Van Creveld syndrome. Chondroectodermal dysplasia.
0156   225500   756.55   AR
Short upper lip, accessory buccal frenulae, alveolar ridge defects, natal teeth, partial anodontia, atrial septal defect or other heart malformation, disproportionate irregularly short limbs, tibial hypoplasia, hamate-capitate fusion, polydactyly, hypoplastic nails, short stature.

Escobar syndrome. Pterygium syndrome.
2186   265000   759.8   AR
Ptosis, epicanthus, micrognathia, hypoplastic genitalia, pterygia of neck, axilla, elbow, knee, syndactyly, camptodactyly, equinovarus, rocker-bottom feet, short stature.

Exomphalos-macroglossia-gigantism syndrome.
EMG syndrome. Beckwith-Wiedemann syndrome.
0104   130650   759.8   AD

Macroglossia, linear creases in ear lobule, linear creases in posterior rim of helix, visceromegaly, gigantism, and in some cases, omphalocoele or other umbilical anomaly, neonatal hypoglycemia, mental retardation. Pathological studies show fetal adrenocortical cytomegaly.

Facioauriculoradial dysplasia.
0592   171480   759.8   AD
Midface hypoplasia, long philtrum, anomalies of external and internal ear, deafness, radial dysplasia, ectrodactyly most often of index finger, and, in some cases, vertebral anomalies and fibular hypoplasia.

Faciogenital dysplasia. Aarskog-Scott syndrome.
0001   305400   759.8   XD
Broad face, hypertelorism, short nose with anteverted nares, broad philtrum, hypodontia, hyperextensibility of fingers, genu recurvatum, hypermobility of cervical spine, umbilical protrusion, "saddle bag" scrotum, short stature, and in some cases, mental retardation.

Fanconi pancytopenia. Fanconi anemia.
2029   227650   284   AR
Small head, hypoplasia of thumb, patchy areas of hyperpigmentation, pancytopenia, short stature, and in some cases, mental retardation, aplasia of radius. Chromosome analysis shows enhanced chromosomal breakage.

Femoral-facial syndrome.
2027   134780   759.8   S
Upward eye slant, short nose, with hypoplastic alae nasi, long philtrum, thin upper lip, micrognathia, cleft palate, hypoplastic humerus, pelvic dysplasia, restricted elbow movement, hypoplastic or absent femur and fibula, short stature.

FG syndrome. Partial agenesis of corpus callosum.
0754   305450   759.8   XR
Large head, imperforate anus, seizures, hypotonia, mental retardation, short stature. Contrast studies show partial agenesis of corpus callosum.

Fibrodysplasia ossificans congenita. Myositis ossificans progressiva.
0700   135100   728.11   XR
Short monophalangeal hallux, painful swellings which ossify in fibrous tissues of neck, trunk, and proximal limbs, and in some cases, short thumbs.

Focal dermal hypoplasia. Goltz syndrome.
0281   305600   759.8   XD
Hypoplastic teeth, syndactyly, atrophy and linear hyperpigmentation of skin, herniation of fat through atrophic areas of skin, angiofibromatous nodules around lips and anus, and in some cases, coloboma, microphthalmia, polydactyly, mental retardation.

Fryns syndrome.
2265   229850   759.8   AR
Hypertelorism, macrostomia, brachytelephalangy, hypoplastic nails, diaphragmatic hernia, gastrointestinal anomalies, genitourinary anomalies.

Galactosialidosis. Gangliosidosis Gm1 type 4.
3110   256540   330.1   AR
Anasarca, cloudy cornea, cherry-red spot of retina, joint stiffness.

Gangliosidosis Gm1 type I.
0431   230500   330.1   AR
Prominent forehead, low nasal bridge, broad nose, flared alae nasi, long philtrum, prominent maxilla, gingival hypertrophy, thick wrists, short broad hands, edema, hypotonia. Hypertonia then develops, accompanied by claw hand, hyperacusis, joint stiffness, kyphoscoliosis, macrocephaly, mental retardation, poor fetal growth, short stature, poor postnatal growth, death in infancy. Some cases have cherry red spot of macula, hepatomegaly, excessive urinary keratan sulfate. Early bone x-rays of arms and legs show thin cortices and coarse trabeculations. Later, typical dysostosis multiplex is present. Pathological findings include vacuolated leukocytes and foam cells in marrow, visceral histiocytosis, neuronal lipidosis, and cytoplasmic vacuolization of renal glomerular cells. The basic defect is lack of beta-galactosidase A,B, and C.

Genital anomaly-cardiomyopathy. Najjar syndrome.
2246   212120   759.8   AR
Hypoplastic genitalia, hypergonadotrophic hypogonadism, progressive cardiomyopathy, mental retardation.

Geroderma osteodysplasticum. Walt Disney dwarfism.
2099   231700   759.8   AR
Lax wrinkled skin, joint hyperextensibility, prominent forehead, high-arched palate, kyphosis, scoliosis, dislocated hips, pes planus, vertebral compression, osteoporosis, poor postnatal growth, short stature.

Geleophysic dwarfism.

2020   231050   759.8   AR
Upward eye slant, anteverted nares, hypoplastic columella, smooth philtrum, upturned mouth commissures, cardiac valve defects, hepatomegaly, tight skin, short plump tubular bones, poor fetal growth, short stature, poor postnatal growth.

Goeminne syndrome.
2174   314300   759.8   XR
Congenital torticollis and cryptorchidism followed by keloids, progressive pyelonephritis, oligospermia, varicose veins.

Goldberg-Pashayan syndrome.
3042   186350   759.8   AD
Unusual complete cutaneous syndactyly of toes 1 and 2, ulnar polydactyly, earlobes with either a deep horizontal groove or a nodule, and, in some cases, a broad or bifid hallux or preaxial extra toe.

Gorlin syndrome.
0440   233500   759.8   AR
Brachycephaly, midface hypoplasia, small eyes, downslanting palpebral fissures, conductive hearing loss, high arched palate, oligodontia, microdontia, low hairline, hypertrichosis of scalp, hypoplasia of distal phalanges, short stature, poor postnatal growth.

Greig cephalopolysyndactyly syndrome.
2925   175700   759.8   AD
Megalencephaly with high forehead and bregma, syndactyly with pedunculated postminimi polydactyly of hands, preaxial polydactyl of feet, and in some cases, preaxial polydactyly of hands, syndactyly of feet, postaxial polydactyly of feet.

Hall-Pallister syndrome. Hypothalamic hamartoblastoma syndrome.
2285   146510   759.8   S
Neonatal hypothalamic hamartoblastoma, postaxial polydactyly, and imperforate anus, and in some cases, laryngeal cleft, abnormal lung lobulation, renal agenesis or dysplasia, short 4th metacarpals, nail dysplasia, multiple buccal frenula, hypoadrenalism, microphallus, congenital heart defect, and poor fetal growth. The anterior pituitary is replaced by a tumor composed mainly of cells resembling primitive, undifferentiated germinal cells. The gene at 3p25.3 is altered in some cases by a visible chromosome aberration; in others, the alteration is submicroscopic.

Hallerman-Streiff syndrome.

0738   234100   756   AR
Brachycephaly, frontal and parietal bossing, thin calvarium, delayed cranial suture closure, thin scalp skin, thin pointed hypoplastic nose with atrophic skin, microphthalmos, cataract, malar hypoplasia, micrognathia, microstomia, hypodontia, hypoplastic teeth, thin sparse light hair.

Hand-foot-genital syndrome.Hand-foot-uterus syndrome.
2570   140000   759.8   AD
Genital tract duplication in females, hypospadias, small hands, short thumb, mesobrachydactyly of fifth finger, short hallux. X-ray findings include short first metacarpal, trapezium-scaphoid fusion, short first metatarsal, cuneiform-navicular fusion.

Hays-Wells syndrome. Ankyloblepharon and cleft palate.
2590   106250   759.8   AD
Ankyloblepharon filiforme adnatum, oval face, broad nasal bridge, cleft lip/palate, hypodontia, conical teeth, palmar and plantar keratoderma, partial deficiency of sweat glands, anhidrosis, dysplastic nails, wiry sparse hair.

Heart hand syndrome-Spanish type.
3266   140450   759.8   AD
Brachydactyly, sinus conduction abnormality or intraventricular conduction defect. X-ray findings include short phalanges, especially the proximal and middle phalanges of the second and third fingers.

Herpes simplex syndrome.
2988   760.2   E
Hydrocephalus ex vacuuo, microcephaly, chorioretinitis, microphthalmia, natal vesicular rash, poor fetal growth.

Hirschsprung disease and brachydactyly.
306980   759.8   XR
Hypoplastic nails and distal phalanges of thumb and hallux, Hirschsprung disease.

Holt-Oram syndrome. Heart-hand syndrome.
0455   142900   759.8   AD
Thumb malformation, extra carpal bones, and heart malformation. A triphalangeal thumb and atrial septal defect are most characteristic, but there is a wide range of malformations.

Hydrolethalus syndrome.
2279   236680   759.8   AR

Hydramnios, poor fetal growth, hydrocephalus, microphthalmia, small nose, micrognathia, endocardial cushion defect, postaxial polydactyly of hands, preaxial polydactyly of feet. Contrast studies show external hydrocephalus, with ventricles open to subarachnoid space. X-ray shows key-hole shaped foramen magnum, tracheal stenosis, abnormal lobulation of lung.

Hypertelorism-microtia-facial clefting. HMC syndrome.

| 0506 | 239800 | 759.8 | AR |

Microcephaly, hypertelorism, cleft lip palate and nose, microtia, atresia of auditory canals, deafness, heart malformation, mental retardation. Pathological findings include ectopic kidneys.

Hypertension syndrome.

| | | 760.3 | E |

Microcephaly, patent ductus arteriosus, poor fetal growth.

Hyperthermia syndrome.

| 2385 | | 760.5 | E |

Neural tube defects, arthrogryposis, poor fetal growth.

Hypoglossia-hypodactyly. Aglossia-adactyly. . Charlie M syndrome.

| 0451 | 103300 | 759.8 | S |

Broad nose, telecanthus, lower eyelid coloboma, micrognathia, small mouth, small or absent tongue, cleft tongue, aberrant tongue attachment, hypodactyly or adactyly, syndactyly, peromelia, cranial nerve palsies, Moebius sequence.

Ichthyosiform erythroderma with hemidysplasia. CHILD syndrome.

| 2016 | 308050 | 759.8 | XD |

Rudimentary limbs and organs on one side, ichythyosiform erythroderma on same side, heart malformation, death in infancy.

Incontinentia pigmenti. Bloch-Sulzberger syndrome.

| 0526 | 308300 | 757.33 | xd |

Atrophic patchy alopecia, retinal dysplasia, blue sclerae, hypodontia, vertebral malformation, hemiatrophy, microcephaly, mental retardation, skin inflammation and vesiculation in whorl-like pattern followed by atrophy and pigmentation and in some cases, verrucous lichenoid lesions.

IVIC syndrome.

| 3043 | 147750 | 759.8 | AR |

Internal ophthalmoplegia, sensorineural deafness, hypoplastic thumb with short distal phalanx and slender metacarpal, radial carpal defects, thrombocytopenia, and in some cases, severe radial defect of arm, imperforate anus.

Jacobs syndrome.

| 2155 | 208250 | 759.8 | AR |

Flexion deformities of one or more fingers or thumb at birth, followed by synovitis of large joints, and restrictive pericarditis. Biopsy of synovium and pericardium shows hyperplasia , fibrosis and giant cells.

Johanson-Blizzard syndrome.

| 2026 | 243800 | 759.8 | AR |

Scalp defects, hypoplastic alae nasi, anodontia, deafness, hypothyroidism, pancreatic achylia, genital tract duplication in females, mental retardation.

Kabuki make-up sydrome. Niikawa-Kuroki syndrome.

| 2355 | 147920 | 759.8 | S |

Long palpebral fissures, eversion of lateral third of lower eyelid, high arch of lateral eyebrow, long thick eyelashes, large earlobes, depressed nasal tip, cleft or high-arched palate, fifth finger mesobrachydactyly, fetal finger pads, increased digital ulnar loop and hypothenar loop patterns, absence of the digital triradius c and/or d, heart malformation, scoliosis, vertebral anomalies, poor postnatal growth, mental retardation.

Kallman syndrome.

2301	147950	759.8	AD
	244200		AR
	308700		XR

Cryptorchidism, hypogonadism and hyposmia or anosmia, and, in some cases, unilateral renal agenesis, bimanual synkinesia, pes cavus, high-arched palate, and cerebellar ataxia. Olfactory bulbs are hypoplastic. The infertility is correctable with chorionic gonadotrophin. Prevalence among persons with hyposmia is 1:25 and, among males with hypogonadism, 1:30.

KBG syndrome.

| 0554 | 148050 | 759.8 | AD |

Brachycephaly, hypertelorism, broad eyebrows, macrodontia, poor postnatal growth, mental retardation, vertebral anomalies, short femoral neck, short metacarpals.

Kaufman oculocerebrofacial syndrome.

2179   244450   759.8   AR
Microcephaly, sparse broad eyebrows,
hypertelorism, epicanthus, microcornea, optic
atrophy, flat philtrum, narrow palate, micrognathia,
hypotonia, mental retardation, poor fetal growth,
short stature, poor postnatal growth.

Keutel syndrome.
0263   245150   759.8   AR
Midface hypoplasia, small alae nasi,
brachytelephalangy, multiple peripheral pulmonary
stenoses, calcification and/or ossification of the
cartilage in the external ears, nose, larynx, trachea
and ribs. X-ray shows stippled epiphyses in infants.

King syndrome.
2492   145600   759.8   AD
Mid-face hypoplasia, down slanted eyes, ptosis,
low-set ears, retrognathia, pectus carinatum, lumbar
lordosis, thoracic kyphosis, cryptorchidism, poor
postnatal growth, mild myopathy affecting mainly
the legs, elevated creatine phosphokinase, malignant
hyperthermia with muscle rigidity and lactic
acidosis upon exposure to depolarizing skeletal
muscle relaxants or volatile hydrocarbon
anesthetics. Other manifestations may be sudden
infant death syndrome (SIDS) or heat stroke in
adults. Dantrolene sodium may prevent the
hyperthermia. Survivors of the hyperthermia may
have neurological deficits and arthrogryposis.
Creatine phosphokinase may not identify all
hyperthermia-susceptible relatives. Other tests for
that purpose include caffeine contracture of biopsied
muscle fibers, and platelet ATP level after halothane
treatment of plasma. King syndrome is one of
several types of malignant hyperthermia.

Klippel-Fiel syndrome.
2032   148900   759.8   AD
Short neck, low posterior hair line, limitation of
head and neck movement, cervical vertebrae fusion
in variable associations with scoliosis, neural tube
defects, Sprengel deformity, deafness, rib anomalies,
eye anomalies, renal anomalies, genital anomalies.

Klippel-Trenaunay-Weber syndrome.
0055   149000   759.8   S
Hypertrophy of leg or arm, sometimes involving
head or genitalia, associated with hemangioma of
the same areas, as well as hemangioma of eye, brain,
viscera.

Kneist syndrome. Metatropic dwarfism type 2.
0557   156550   756.4   AD

Flat face, low nasal bridge, prominent eyes, myopia,
retinal detachment, deafness, cleft palate, enlarged
joints, limited joint mobility, arthritis, short
clavicles, short bowed limbs, kyphoscoliosis,
platyspondyly, vertically cleft vertebral bodies in
infancy.

Knuckle pads-leukonychia-deafness. Bart-Pumphrey
syndrome.
0558   149200   759.8   AD
Congenital sensorineural deafness followed later by
development of knuckle pads and leukonychia.
Older affected persons develop keratosis palmaris et
plantaris.

Kousseff syndrome.
2266   245210   759.8   AR
Sacral meningocele, conotruncal cardiac defects,
unilateral renal agenesis, low-set and posteriorly
angulated ears, retrognathia, and short neck with
low posterior hairline.

Lacrimoauriculodentodigital syndrome. LADD.
2180   149730   759.8   AD
Hypoplastic lacrimal puncta, cup-shaped ears,
sensorineural deafness, small peg-shaped lateral
maxillary incisors, triphalangeal thumb, finger 5
clinodactyly, and syndactyly.

Langer-Gideon syndrome. Trichorhinophalangeal
syndrome II.
2847   150230   759.8   AD
Microcephaly, bulbous nose, long prominent
philtrum, sparse thin hair, cone-shaped phalangeal
epiphyses, multiple exostoses, redundant skin,
mental retardation, and in some cases,
hyperextensible joints.

Laurence-Moon syndrome.
0578   245800   759.8   AR
Pigmentary retinopathy, hypogonadotrophic
hypogonadism, mental retardation, spastic
paraplegia.

Lead syndrome.
3194   760.79   E
Poor fetal growth, poor postnatal growth and
development.

Leg absence with congenital cataract.
            246000   759.8   AR
Congenital cataract, progressive scoliosis, unilateral
absence of leg.

Leopard syndrome. Multiple lentigines.
0586   151100   759.8   AD
Hypertelorism, sensorineural deafness, pulmonic stenosis, prolonged PR and QRS, abnormal P waves, winged scapula, hypogonadotrophic hypogonadism, short stature, generalized dark lentigines which are more numerous on neck and trunk.

Leprechaunism.
0587   246200   759.8   AR
Small face, prominent eyes, wide nares, thick lips, large ears, large breasts, large genitalia, hypoglycemia, hyperinsulinemia, mental retardation, frequent infections, poor fetal growth, short stature, poor postnatal growth, emaciation, death in infancy. Pathologic findings include pancreatic islet cell hyperplasia, Leydig cell hyperplasia, and cystic ovaries.

Limb and Mullerian anomalies.
2932   146160   759.8   AD
Limb anomalies varying from postaxial polydactyly to ectrodactyly to severe upper limb hypoplasia with split hand, associated with uterine anomalies varying from uterus didelphys to vertical vaginal septum.

Linear sebaceous nevus. Nevus Sebaceus of Jadassohn.
0593   163200   759.8   S
Linear sebaceous nevus of forehead, midface, and sometimes trunk and limbs, seizures, focal EEG abnormalities, mental retardation, and in some cases, eye malformation. The skin lesions develop basal cell epithelioma in adulthood.

Lowe oculocerebrorenal syndrome.
0736   309000   270.8   XR
Cortical cataract, glaucoma, renal tubular dysfunction, cryptorchidism, hypotonia, mental retardation, albuminuria, generalized aminoaciduria, phosphaturia, organic aciduria, poor postnatal growth, short stature.

Lymphedema with distichiasis.
2039   153400   759.8   AD
Distichiasis, generalized lymphedema which may appear localized and is of variable age onset, and in some cases, spinal epidural cyst, pterygium colli.

Mandibuloacral dysplasia. MAD.
2082   248370   759.8   AR
Wide cranial sutures, multiple Wormian bones, retrognathia, hypoplastic clavicles, acroosteolysis with progressive loss of bone from the distal

phalanges of the fingers and toes, stiff joints, atrophy of skin over hands and feet, alopecia, poor postnatal growth, short stature.

Mandibulofacial dysostosis. Treacher Collins syndrome.
0627   154500   756   AD
Downward eye slant, coloboma of lateral lower eyelid, hypoplastic zygomatic arch, macrostomia, micrognathia, microtia, malformed ear, and in some cases, deafness.

Marden-Walker syndrome.
0629   248700   759.8   AR
Blepharophimosis, micrognathia, immobile face, pectus carinatum, scoliosis, limb contractures, arachnodactyly, microcystic renal disease, cerebellar and brain stem hypoplasia, mental retardation, death in infancy.

Marinesco-Sjogren syndrome.
2031   248800   759.8   AR
Neonatal hypotonia, myopathy, and cerebellar hypoplasia, with later development of cataracts, microcephaly, cerebellar ataxia, mental retardation, poor postnatal growth, hypergonadotrophic hypogonadism, spasticity, contractures and neuromyopathic skeletal changes.

Marshall-Smith syndrome.
2193   759.8   S
Long head, prominent forehead, prominent eyes, anteverted nares, broad proximal and middle phalanges, tallness, mental retardation, accelerated linear growth, accelerated osseous maturation, poor weight gain, pneumonia, death in infancy.

McCune-Albright syndrome. Polyostotic fibrous dysplasia. Osteitis fibrosa cystica.
0391   174800   756.59   S
Irregular brown pigmentation over lower back and buttocks, fibrous dysplasia of long bones, pelvis and sometimes, face, with resulting deformity, sexual precocity, hyperthyroidism and other endocrinopathies.

McKusick-Kaufman syndrome.
0985   236700   759.8   AR
Heart malformation, polydactyly, hydrometrocolpos, glandular hypospadias, prominent scrotal raphe.

Meckel syndrome. Gruber syndrome. Dysencephalia splanchnocystica.
0634   249000   759.8   AR

Sloping forehead, encephalocoele, microcephaly, microphthalmia, cleft palate, retrognathia, polydactyly, polycystic kidneys, cryptorchidism, genital hypoplasia, brain malformation, death in infancy.

Megalocornea-mental retardation syndrome. MMR.
0638 249310 759.8 AR
Broad nasal bridge, antimongoloid eye slant, epicanthus, megalocornea, hypotonia, mental retardation, and in some cases, iris hypoplasia.

Menkes syndrome.
0643 309400 759.8 XR
Sparse stubby lightly pigmented hair, pili torti, Wormian bones, expressionless face, prominent cheeks, arterial elongation and tortuosity, deficient intestinal copper transport unresponsive to parenteral copper, excessive copper uptake by cultured amniocytes, metaphyseal widening with spurs similar to battered child syndrome, neurodegeneration, gliosis and atrophy of cerebral cortex, death in infancy.

Metaphyseal chondrodysplasia-McKusick type. Cartilage-hair hypoplasia.
0653 250250 759.9 AR
Short stature, rhizomelia, fine sparse hair, metaphyseal dysplasia, and in some cases, anemia, malabsorption, severe varicella.

Methimazole syndrome.
2926   760.79 E
Scalp defect, urachal defect.

Microcephaly-chorioretinitis.
2333 156590 759.8 AR
    251270   AR
Microcephaly, associated, in some cases, with encephalodysplasia; chorioretinitis, resembling, in some cases, toxoplasmosis; persistent primary vitreous remnants; varying degrees of mental and neurological deficiency.

Microcephaly-micromelia syndrome.
    251300 759.8 AR
Microcephaly, micromelia, fused elbow, short forearm with one bone, small hand with 2 to 4 malformed digits, poor fetal growth, death in infancy.

Microcephaly-hiatus hernia-nephrosis syndrome. Galloway syndrome.
2755 251300 759.8 AR

Microcephaly, large floppy ears, feeding difficulty, hiatus hernia, nephrosis, microcystic renal dysplasia, focal glomerulosclerosis, and in some cases, eye malformation.

Microphthalmia with multiple anomalies. Lenz dysplasia.
3171 309800 759.8 XR
Microcephaly, unilateral or bilateral microphthalmia or anophthalmos, agenesis of upper lateral incisors, irregular lower incisors, narrow shoulders, double thumb, scoliosis, heart malformation, hypospadias, cryptorchidism, renal dysgenesis, mental retardation.

Mietens syndrome.
2013 249600 759.8 AR
Corneal opacity, narrow nose with hypoplastic alae nasi, short forearm, dislocation of head of radius, flexion contracture of elbow, short stature, nystagmus, mental retardation.

Miller syndrome.
2126 154400 759.8 AR
Microtia, conductive deafness, downward eye slant, eyelid coloboma, ectropion, malar hypoplasia, cleft lip/palate, hypoplastic or absent radius and ulna, hypodactyly, syndactyly, digital arches excessive.

Miller-Dieker syndrome. Lissencephaly syndrome.
0603 247200 759.8 AR
Microcephaly, prominent forehead with vertical furrows, low-set ears, upward eye slant, small nose with anteverted nares, vertical furrow in upper lip, heart malformation, cryptorchidism, pachygyria or lissencephaly, heterotopia of gray matter, seizures, hypotonia followed by hypertonia, opisthotonus, hypsarrhytymia, poor postnatal growth, death in infancy. Many cases have visible or submicroscopic Chromosome 17p13.3 deletion.

Mohr syndrome. Oral-facial-digital syndrome II. OFD syndrome II.
0771 252100 759.8 AR
Telecanthus, lobate tongue, hypertrophied buccal frenula, flared alveolar ridge of mandible, cleft lip/palate, conductive deafness, Wormian bones in cranial sutures, brachydactyly, bifid hallux.

Mouth inability to open and short finger flexor tendons. Trismus-pseudocamptodactyly syndrome.
0882 158300 759.8 AD
Limitation of jaw excursion, short finger flexor tendons, short leg muscles.

Mucolipidosis II. I-cell disease.
0672   252500   272.7   AR
Prominent narrow forehead, low nasal bridge, puffy eyelids, short nose with anteverted nares, progressive gingival hypertrophy, stiff joints, thick tight skin, mental retardation, poor fetal growth, short stature, poor postnatal growth. Early x-rays may show periosteal new bone formation in limbs, while later x-rays show dysostosis multiplex. The basic defect is deficiency of N-acetylglucosamine-1-phosphotransferase.

Mulibrey nanism.
2081   253250   759.8   AR
Dolichocephaly, J-shaped sella turcica, triangular face, high pitched voice, yellow dots in ocular fundus, disproportionately large hands and feet, thick constrictive pericardium, hepatomegaly, nevus flammeus, fibrous dysplasia of tibia, hypotonia, gracility, poor fetal growth, poor postnatal growth, short stature.

MURCS association.
2406   759.8   S
Cervicothoracic vertebral defects, Klippel-Feil malformation, renal agenesis or ectopy, absent vagina, absent or hypoplastic uterus, short stature.

Muscle-eye-brain disease. MEB disease.
3047   253280   759.8   AR
Hydrocephalus, myopia, glaucoma, optic atrophy, retinal hypoplasia, congenital muscular dystrophy, mental retardation, myoclonic jerks, elevated serum creatine phosphokinase.

Myotonic myopathy-dwarfism-ocular-facial syndrome. Schwartz-Jampel syndrome. Chondrodystrophic myotonia.
0155   255800   756.89   AR
Blepharophimosis, myopia, long eyelashes, immobile face, low-set ears, retrognathia, high-pitched voice, myotonia, muscle wasting, limitation of joint movement, pectus carinatum, platyspondyly, fragmented femoral epiphyses, anesthetic hazard, poor postnatal growth, short stature.

Nager syndrome. Nager acrofacial dysostosis.
2167   154400   756   AR
Microtia, sensorineural deafness, preauricular tags, downward eye slant, malar hypoplasia, micrognathia, hypoplasia of radius, hypoplastic or absent thumb.

Nail-patella syndrome. Onychoosteodysplasia. Turner-Keiser syndrome. Fong disease.
0704   161200   756.89   AD
Onychodysplasia, absent or hypoplastic patella, iliac horn, hypoplastic capitellum, hypoplastic radial head, and in some cases, nephropathy with thickened glomerular basement membrane.

Nephrosialidosis.
          265150   759.8   AR
Coarse face, pericardial effusion, congenital ascites, hepatosplenomegaly, nephrosis, dysostosis multiplex, mental retardation, death in childhood. Cherry red spot of macula develops late. Foam cells are found in bone marrow, and leukocyte alpha-(2,6) neuraminidase is deficient.

Neu-Laxova syndrome.
2092   256520   759.8   AR
Microcephaly, arthromyodysplasia, edema, ectodermal dysplasia, genital malformation, abnormal placentation, poor fetal growth.

Neuraminidase deficiency I. Sialidosis I.
0671   256550   759.8   AR
Coarse facies, hepatosplenomegaly, followed by myoclonus, cherry red spot of macula, dysostosis multiplex. Urinary sialyloligosaccharides are elevated. Cultured fibroblasts are deficient in alpha-(2,6) neuraminidase.

Neurocutaneous melanosis.
2014   249400   759.8   S
Seizures, mental deterioration, thick pigmented pia arachnoid at base of brain, black thick hairy nevi which coalesce over lower trunk and upper thighs, malignant melanoma, death in childhood.

Neuroectodermal melanolysosomal disease.
2361   256710   759.8   AR
Hypopigmentation, silver colored hair, hypotonia, seizures, involuntary movements, mental retardation. Abnormal melanolysosomes in cells of skin and bone marrow.

Noonan syndrome. Pseudo-Turner syndrome.
0720   163950   759.8   AD
Epicanthus, ptosis, low-set ears, low posterior hairline, webbed neck, shield chest, pectus excavatum, pulmonic stenosis, septal defects, genital hypoplasia, cryptorchidism, cubitus valgus, vertebral malformation, mental retardation, poor postnatal growth, short stature.

Norrie disease.
0721   310600   759.8   XR
Microphthalmia, leukocoria, vitreoretinal dysplasia
which proceeds to phthisis bulbi, mental retardation,
sensorineural deafness.

Oculoauriculovertebral dysplasia. Goldenhar
syndrome.
0735   164210   756   P
Coloboma of eyelid, dermoid of conjunctiva,
microtia, accessory auricular appendages anterior to
ear, malar hypoplasia, macrostomia due to lateral
cleft-like extension of corner of mouth, hypoplastic
mandible, hemivertebrae, hypoplastic vertebrae.
Findings are variable and usually asymmetric.

Oculocerebral syndrome with hypopigmentation.
Cross syndrome.
0413   257800   759.8   AR
Ocular malformation, hypopigmentation, gingival
fibromatosis, athetosis, spasticity, mental
retardation.

Oculodentodigital dysplasia. Oculodentoosseous
dysplasia.
0737   164200   759.8   AD
Blepharophimosis, microphthalmos, microcornea,
glaucoma, hypoplastic alae nasi, enamelogenesis
imperfecta, fine sparse hair, finger 5 camptodactyly,
syndactyly of fingers 4 & 5, hypoplastic middle
phalanx toes.

Onychotrichodysplasia-neutropenia.
2331   258360   759.8   AR
Hypoplastic nails with koilonychia and
onychorrhexis; trichorrhexis; psychomotor
retardation; chronic neutropenia; recurrent
infections.

Ophthalmomandibulomelic dysplasia.
3259   164900   759.9   AD
Corneal clouding, temporomandibular fusion, absent
coronoid process, obtuse mandibular angle, aplasia
of lateral humeral condyle, aplasia of radial head,
aplasia of distal ulna.

Opitz syndrome. BBB syndrome.
0505   145410   759.8   AD
Widow's peak, hypertelorism, hypospadias,
cryptorchidism.

Opitz-Frias syndrome. G syndrome.
0401   145410   759.8   XR

Prominent occiput and parietum, broad flat nasal
bridge, low-set ears, hypertelorism, downward eye
slant, swallowing dysfunction, recurrent aspiration,
hypospadias.

Opitz trigonocephaly syndrome. C syndrome.
0121   211750   759.8   AR
Trigonocephaly, polydactyly, heart malformation,
cryptorchidism, death in infancy.

Oral-facial-digital syndrome type I.
0770   311200   759.8   XD
 Increased naso-sella-basion angle, hypoplastic alae
nasi, telecanthus, midline partial cleft lip, complex
cleft palate, lateral clefts of alveolar ridges and
tongue, renal microcysts, syndactyly, asymmetric
brachydactyly, coarse sparse hair, absence of corpus
callosum, heterotopia of gray matter, trembling,
mental retardation.

Oral-facial-digital syndrome III.
3058   258850   758.5   AR
Eyelid myoclonus, lobulated hamartomatous tongue,
dental malformation, bifid uvula, pectus excavatum,
short sternum, postaxial polydactyly, mental
retardation.

Osteoporosis-pseudoglioma syndrome.
0783   259770   759.9   AR
Pseudoglioma, hypotonia, ligamentous laxity,
osteoporosis, and in some cases, mental retardation.

Otodental dysplasia.
0784   166750   759.8   AD
High frequency sensorineural deafness, large
bulbous deciduous canines and deciduous and
permanent molars, absent premolars. X-ray shows 2
pulp chambers of deciduous molars, taurodontia,
and pulp stones.

Otopalatodigital syndrome I.
0786   311300   759.8   XD
Frontal and occipital prominence, increased naso-
sella-basion angle, thick frontal bone and skull base,
absent frontal and sphenoid sinuses, broad nasal
root, malar hypoplasia, partial anodontia, cleft soft
palate, conductive deafness, pectus excavatum, short
fingernails, broad thumb and hallux, finger 5
clinodactyly, secondary ossification center at base of
second metacarpal and metatarsal, short stature,
poor postnatal growth.

Otopalatodigital syndrome II.
2258   304120   759.8   XD

Wide cranial sutures in neonate, prominent forehead, downward eye slant, low nasal bridge, cleft palate, retrognathia, flexion deformity of fingers, overlapping fingers, conductive deafness.

Parietal foramina-hypoplastic clavicle.
2769   168550   759.8   AD
Megalencephaly, occipital dermoid with hair tuft, parietal foramina, hypoplastic clavicles.

Pena-Shokeir syndrome I. Arthrogryposis with pulmonary hypoplasia.
2080   208150   759.8   AR
Low-set ears, prominent eyes, hypertelorism, depressed tip of nose, small mouth, retrognathia, pulmonary hypoplasia, cryptorchidism, arthromyodysplasia, sparse dermal ridges, absent finger and palm creases, poor fetal growth, polymicrogyria, deficient anterior horn cells, polyhydramnios, poor postnatal growth, death in infancy.

Penchaszadeh syndrome.
3049   167730   759.8   AD
Nasopalpebral lipomas, colobomas of upper and lower eyelids, hypertelorism, maxillary hypoplasia.

Penicillamine syndrome.
2260   760.79   E
Skin hyperelastosis, joint hyperextensibility, contractures.

Pentalogy of Cantrell.
3121   313850   759.8   XD
Distal sternum cleft, midline supraumbilical abdominal wall defect with diastasis recti, anterior diaphragmatic hernia, pericardioperitoneal foramen, conotruncal heart malformation.

Perlman syndrome.
2241   267000   759.8   AR
Macrosomia, high anterior hairline, deep-set eyes, low nasal bridge, anteverted upper lip, bilateral renal hamartomas with or without nephroblastomatosis, hypertrophy of the islets of Langerhans, hypoglycemia, distended abdomen, cryptorchidism.

Perrault syndrome.
2350   233400   759.8   AR
Congenital sensorineural deafness, poor postnatal growth. Streak ovaries, elevated gonadotrophin and lack of sexual development in females.

Peters anomaly-short limb dwarfism. Peters-plus syndrome. Krause-Kivlin syndrome.
2812   261540   759.8   AR
Short-limb dwarfism, macrocephaly, corneal clouding, iridolenticulocorneal adhesions, lens opacity, glaucoma, anterior chamber cleavage anomalies, vision deficit, round face, blepharophimosis, low nasal bridge, anteverted nares, hypoplastic columella, smooth philtrum, retrognathia, small external auditory canals, deafness, cleft lip/palate, short hands, tapering brachydactyly, mesobrachydactyly of finger 5, hypogenitalism, hydrocephalus ex vacuuo, mental retardation.

Phenylketonuria-maternal.
2236   759.8   E
Microcephaly, round face, prominent glabella, heart malformation, poor fetal growth, hypertonia, mental retardation.

Piebald trait with neurologic defects.
            172850   759.8   AD
Dorsal and ventral areas of leukoderma, cerebellar ataxia, mental retardation, and in some cases, deafness.

Poland syndrome.
0813   173800   759.8   S
Unilateral symbrachydactyly and ipsilateral aplasia of the sternal head of the pectoralis major muscle. Severity is variable and so many patients have anomalies of nearby structures that this syndrome may be but one facet of a subclavian artery disruption sequence (SADS).

Polychlorinated biphenyl syndrome. PCB syndrome.
2733   760.79   E
Hyperpigmentation, onychodystrophy, natal teeth, natal acne, mental retardation, poor fetal growth.

Potter syndrome. Oligohydramnios sequence. Renal agenesis.
0856   191830   753   AD
Large low-set ears deficient in cartilage, flat nose, retrognathia, pulmonary hypoplasia, absent or hypoplastic kidneys, genital malformation, abnormal positioning of hands and feet, death in infancy.

Prader-Willi syndrome.
0823   176270   759.8   AR
Feeble fetal movements, poor fetal growth, hypotonia, narrow bifrontal diameter, small hands and feet, hypogonadotrophic hypogonadism, mental

retardation, obesity. Visible or submicroscopic deletions within the q11-q13 band of the paternally derived chromosome 15 causes some cases while others appear to be due to maternal uniparental isodisomy of chromosome 15.

Pre/postaxial polydactyly-absent corpus callosum. Acrocallosal syndrome-Schinzel type.

2263   200990   759.8   AR

Macrocephaly, prominent forehead, hypertelorism, low nasal bridge, epicanthus, partial duplication of hallux, postaxial polydactyly, toe 1-3 syndactyly, hypoplastic corpus callosum, hypotonia, mental retardation.

Progeroid syndrome. Wiedemann-Raustentrauch syndrome.

2593   264090   759.8   AR

Aged appearance, absent subcutaneous fat, mental retardation, poor fetal growth, poor postnatal growth, short stature.

Proteus syndrome.

2382   176920   759.8   AD

Deforming congenital extracranial or intracranial lipoma, macrocephaly, asymmetric partial gigantism of the limbs frequently accompanied by bizarre hypertrophy and angulation of digits, pigmented nevi, hemihypertrophy, subcutaneous hamartomatous tumors especially of the sole.

Pseudohermaphroditism with skeletal anomalies.

        264270   759.8   AR

Hypoplasia of mandibular condyles and maxilla, dislocated radial head, enlarged clitoris, labial fusion, primary amenorrhea.

Puretic syndrome.

0411   228600   759.8   AR

Malformation of head and face, poor postnatal growth, large calcified subcutaneous nodules, dermal atrophy, recurrent suppurative infections, osteolysis of terminal phalanges, painful flexion contractures of elbows, shoulders, and knees.

Radiation syndrome.

0383   760.5   E

Microcephaly, eye anomalies, genital hypoplasia, poor fetal growth.

Retinoic acid syndrome.

2261   760.79   E

Microtia, cleft lip/palate, hydrocephalus ex vacuuo, poor fetal growth.

Renal dysplasia and retinal aplasia.

2687   266900   759.8   AR

Congenital blindness due to retinal aplasia or hypoplasia, deterioration of renal function due to loss of glomeruli and tubules.

Rieger syndrome.

2139   180500   759.8   AD

Broad nasal root, telecanthus, microcornea with opacity, iris hypoplasia, anterior synechiae, maxillary hypoplasia, thin upper lip, protruding lower lip, hypodontia, protrusion of umbilical skin.

Roberts syndrome.

0875   268300   759.8   AR

Oxycephaly, prominent eyes, cleft lip/palate, genital enlargement, hypoplastic arm bones, aplastic leg bones.

Robinow syndrome.

0876   180700   759.8   AD

Macrocephaly, frontal prominence, hypertelorism, short nose, anteverted nares, long philtrum, crowded teeth, small chin, short limbs, small penis, hemivertebrae.

Rothmund-Thomson syndrome. Poikiloderma atrophicans and cataract.

2037   268400   757.33   AR

Low nasal bridge; sparse hair; dysplastic nails; hypogonadism; irregular erythema, telangiectasia, scarring, pigmentation, and atrophy of skin; poor postnatal growth, short stature. Juvenile zonular cataract occurs in the first few years of life. Some cases have radial anomalies, focal bone sclerosis, bone cysts.

Rubella syndrome.

0384   771   E

Microcephaly, deafness, cataract, glaucoma, chorioretinitis, microphthalmia, patent ductus arteriosus, peripheral pulmonic stenosis, septal defects, mental retardation, poor fetal growth, short stature, poor postnatal growth.

Rubinstein-Taybi syndrome.

0119   180849   759.8   AR

Small head, downward eye slant, strabismus, hypoplastic maxilla, beaked nose, low set ears, cryptorchidism, broad thumb with radial angulation, broad hallux, poor postnatal growth, short stature.

Russell-Silver syndrome.

0887   180860   759.8   S
Small triangular face, asymmetric limbs, finger 5 clinodactyly, delayed osseous maturation, weakness, cafe-au-lait spots, poor postnatal growth, short stature.

Rutledge syndrome. Smith-Lemli-Opitz syndrome type II.
2635   270400   759.8   AR
Oligohydramnios, feeble fetal movement, everted upper lip, microglossia, thick alveolar ridges, cleft palate, cataracts, postaxial polydactyly, hypoplastic genitalia, heart malformation, renal hypoplasia, islet cell hypoplasia, poor feeding, poor fetal growth, early death. Probably allelic to Smith-Lemli-Opitz syndrome. A defect in cholesterol biosynthesis causes elevated 7-dehydrocholesterol and low serum cholesterol.

Ruvalcaba syndrome.
2076   180870   759.8   AR
Microcephaly, hypoplastic alae nasi, small mouth, thin lips, narrow maxilla with crowded teeth, brachydactyly, short lateral metacarpals and metatarsals, finger 5 clinodactyly, cryptorchidism, delayed puberty, poor fetal growth, mental retardation, jovial personality, poor postnatal growth.

Ruvalcaba-Myhre syndrome.
2120   153480   759.8   S
Macrocephaly, ileal and colonic polyps, tan spots on penis, birth macrosomia, mental retardation.

SC phocomelia syndrome. Pseudothalidomide syndrome.
0875   269000   759.8   AR
Sparse silvery hair, capillary hemangioma of face, hypoplastic cartilage of nose and ear, cloudy cornea, retrognathia, hypoplastic bones of arms and legs, flexion contractures, poor fetal growth, short stature, poor postnatal growth.

Schinzel-Giedion syndrome.
2123   269150   759.8   AR
Bulging forehead and eyes and short upturned nose appear drawn in about the nasion; multiple skull anomalies including short and sclerotic base, Wormian bones, wide cranial sutures and fontanels;atrial septal defect; hydronephrosis; clubfeet; hypertrichosis. Increased density of tubular bones. Poor postnatal growth, apneic spells, death in infancy.

Seckel syndrome. Bird-headed dwarf. Nanocephalic dwarfism.
0881   210600   759.8   AR
Microcephaly, hypoplastic facies, prominent beaklike nose, retrognathia, joint dislocations, gap between toes 1 & 2, mental retardation, poor fetal growth, short stature, poor postnatal growth.

Senter syndrome.
2861   242150   759.8   AR
Alopecia, sensorineural deafness, corneal inflammation and vascularization, dental malformation, cryptorchidism, ichthyosiform erythroderma, keratosis palmaris and plantaris.

Shprintzen syndrome. Velocardiofacial syndrome.
2129   192430   749.8   AD
Microcephaly, ear malformation, deafness, blepharophimosis, square nasal root, prominent nose with small alae nasi, malar hypoplasia, long face, cleft palate, heart malformation, slender limbs, hyperextensible fingers, short stature, hypotonia, mental retardation.Most cases have microscopic or molecular deletions at chromosome 22q11.2. Deletions of other chromosome sites have been found in some cases instead. The DiGeorge syndrome may result from the similar deletions.

Shwachman syndrome.
0885   260400   759.8   AR
Short ribs, metaphyseal dysplasia, exocrine pancreatic insufficiency, variegate pancytopenia, poor development, poor postnatal growth, short stature.

Simpson dysmorphia syndrome.
2826   321700   759.8   XR
Large protruding jaw, wide nasal bridge, upturned nose, large tongue, broad short hands and fingers, prenatal and postnatal overgrowth.

Sirenomelia sequence.
3191   182940   759.8   S
Variable associations of imperforate anus, hypoplasia or absence of kidneys, bladder and genitalia except for gonads, fusion of legs.

Sjogren-Larsson syndrome.
2030   270200   757.1   AR
Congenital ichythyosiform erythroderma, spastic quadriplegia, mental retardation, and in some cases, pigmentary retinopathy, poor postnatal growth, short stature.

Smith-Lemli-Opitz syndrome.
0891   268670   759.8   AR
Microcephaly, prominent glabella, ptosis,
epicanthus, short nose with anteverted nares,
micrognathia, hypoplastic genitalia, cryptorchidism,
simian crease, excessive digital whorl patterns,
syndactyly of second and third toes, hypotonia,
seizures, mental retardation, poor fetal growth, short
stature, poor postnatal growth. Probably allelic to
Rutledge syndrome. A defect in cholesterol
biosynthesis causes elevated 7-dehydrocholesterol
and low serum cholesterol.

Sotos syndrome. Cerebral gigantism.
0137   117550   253   AD
Macrocephaly, prominent forehead, hypertelorism,
downward eye slant, prognathism, narrow anterior
mandible, large hands and feet, advanced osseous
maturation, mental retardation.

Spondyloepiphyseal dysplasia-congenital.
0897   183900   759.8   AD
Flat face, hypertelorism, myopia, retinal detachment,
short neck, short trunk, rhizomelia, weak abdominal
musculature, hypotonia, mental retardation. X-ray
findings include retarded ossification of pelvis and
legs, flattening of vertebral bodies, short wide
tubular bones, deformed fragmented juxta-truncal
epiphyses.

Steinert syndrome. Myotonic dystrophy.
0702   160900   359.2   AD
Premature frontal baldness, cataract, ptosis, expressionless face, dysarthria, cardiac arrhythmias,
hypogonadism, infantile hypotonia, myotonia
progressing to weakness, mental retardation,
hydramnios, swallowing dysfunction, poor postnatal
growth. 50-2000 copies of a CTG trinucleotide
repeat is found on Chromosome 19q in the 3'
untranslated region of mRNA for the myotonin-
protein kinase gene.

Stickler syndrome. Arthro-ophthalmopathy.
0090   108300   759.8   AD
Mixed deafness, epicanthus, iris hypoplasia, myopia,
cataract, retinal detachment, flat face, flat nasal
bridge, retrognathia, cleft palate, glossoptosis,
arthritis, hip dysplasia, spondyloepiphyseal
dysplasia, Marfanoid habitus, hypotonia.

Sturge-Weber syndrome.
0915   185300   759.6   S
Unilateral hemangioma of face, eye, meninges, and
brain, glaucoma, mental retardation, seizures.

Sulfocysteinuria. Sulfite oxidase deficiency.
0921   272300   759.8   AR
Congenital spastic paraplegia, blindness, ectopia
lentis, elevated urinary s-sulfo-1-cysteine, sulfite,
and thiosulfate. Sulfite oxidase is absent.

Summitt syndrome.
0013   272350   759.8   AR
Tower skull, craniosynostosis, syndactyly, obesity.

Symphalangism syndrome.
1001   185800   759.8   AR
Conductive deafness, narrow face, hypoplastic alae
nasi, hypoplastic nasal septum, fusions of
midphalangeal joints, elbows and carpal bones, talo-
navicular fusion, vertebral malformation.

Syphilis syndrome.
0385   760.2   E
Moist skin lesions, hepatosplenomegaly,
osteochondritis, meningitis, followed later in life by
interstitial keratitis, saddle nose, perennial rhinitis,
perioral rhagades, Clutton joints, saber shin,
Hutchinson teeth, mulberry molars, vestibular
dysfunction, sensorineural deafness, aortic
valvulitis, mental retardation, poor fetal growth.

Thalidomide syndrome.
0386   760.79   E
Microtia, eye malformation, dental malformation,
phocomelia.

Thrombocytopenia-absent radius syndrome. TAR
syndrome.
0941   274000   759.8   AR
Hypoplasia or aplasia of radius, thrombocytopenia
with inactive, decreased, or absent megakaryocytes.
Leukemoid granulocytosis and anemia occur during
bleeding episodes. Some cases have hypoplasia of
ulna and humerus, club hand, heart malformation.
Thumbs are present.

Thumb agenesis-dwarfism-immunodeficiency.
            274190   759.8   AR
Anosmia, delayed puberty, absent thumbs, unfused
olecranon, severe combined immunodeficiency,
poor postnatal growth, short stature.

Townes syndrome.
0072   107480   759.8   AD
Microtia or large ears, preauricular tags, hypoplastic,
double, or finger-like thumb and hallux,

imperforate, stenotic or anteriorly placed anus, renal hypoplasia, urinary malformation.

Toxoplasmosis syndrome.
0387   760.2   E
Microcephaly, hydrocephalus ex vacuuo, chorioretinitis, cerebral calcifications, poor fetal growth.

Tricho-dento-osseous syndrome.
0965   190320   759.8   AD
Kinky hair, dolichocephaly, square jaw, small widely spaced pitted teeth, taurodontism, brittle peeling nails, increased bone density.

Trichorhinophalangeal syndrome.
0966   190350   759.8   AD
Sparse thin hair, bulbous nose, prominent long philtrum, streblodactyly, cone-shaped phalangeal epiphyses, short metacarpals and metatarsals, winged scapula.

Trimethadione syndrome.
0388   760.79   E
Brachycephaly, prominent forehead, short upturned nose, broad low nasal bridge, long upslant of eyebrows, epicanthus, cleft lip/palate, folded upper helix, heart malformation, hypoplastic genitalia, mental retardation, speech defect, poor fetal growth, short stature, poor postnatal growth.

Twin syndrome.
2958   759.8   E
Variable associations of acephaly-acardia, anencephaly, holoprosencephaly, hydranencephaly, porencephaly, gastroschisis, intestinal atresia, exstrophy of cloaca, sacrococcygeal teratoma, sirenomelia, conjoining, aplasia cutis, poor fetal growth.

Ulnar-mammary syndrome.
0981   181450   759.8   AD
Congenital absence, hypoplasia or duplication of ulnar or its derivative carpals, metacarpals or phalanges; hypoplasia or absence of nipples, mammary glands and apocrine axillary glands.

Urethral obstruction sequence. Abdominal muscle absence. Prune belly syndrome.
2007   100100   756.7   S
Abdominal muscle deficiency, excess abdominal skin, colon malrotation, renal dysplasia, urinary malformation, persistent urachus, bladder wall

hypertrophy, genital malformation, absence defects of leg.

Urofacial syndrome.
2527   236730   759.8   AR
Congenital hydronephrosis and hydroureter due to neuropathic bladder, cryptorchidism, constipation, partial facial palsy causing a crying expression when laughing or smiling.

Valproic acid syndrome.
2496   760.74   E
Brachycephaly, microstomia, neural tube defects.

Van den Bosch syndrome.
0986   314500   759.8   XR
Nystagmus, choroideremia, myopia, acrokeratosis verruciformis, anhidrosis, winged scapula, mental retardation, short stature, poor postnatal growth.

Varicella syndrome.
2499   771.2   E
Chorioretinitis, limb hypoplasia, mental retardation, cutaneous scars, poor fetal growth, short stature, poor postnatal growth.

VATER association.
0987   192350   759.8   S
Tracheoesophageal fistula, heart malformation, renal malformation, imperforate anus, vertebral malformation, hypoplasia of radius and thumb, syndactyly, preaxial polydactyly.

Waardenberg syndrome.
0997   193500   759.8   AD
White forelock, wide nasal bridge, telecanthus, heterochromia irides, white eyelashes, cochlear deafness, isolated areas of leukoderma, and in some cases, cleft lip/palate, canites prematura.

Warfarin syndrome.
0389   760.79   E
Flat nasal bridge, small nose, deep groove between alae nasi and nasal tip, particulate mineralization of epiphyses, short fingers, hypoplastic nails, mental retardation, poor fetal growth.

Watson syndrome.
2776   193520   759.8   AD
Congenital pulmonic stenosis, macrocephaly, Lisch nodules, cafe-au-lait spots including axillary, and varying numbers of other features similar to Noonan syndrome including short stature, ptosis, midface hypoplasia, webbed neck, learning disabilities, and

muscle weakness, and, in some cases,
neurofibromas. The gene is an allele at the NF-1
locus 17q11.2.

Weaver syndrome.
2036   277590   759.8   S
Wide bifrontal diameter, flat occiput, hypertelorism,
large ears, long philtrum, retrognathia, hoarse low-
pitched cry, camptodactyly, broad thumb, prominent
fingertips, limited extension of elbow and knee,
macrosomia, hypertonia, mental retardation,
accelerated growth.

Weill-Marchesani syndrome.
0893   277600   759.8   AR
Brachycephaly, low nasal bridge, short stature,
limitation of extension of joints, brachydactyly,
microsperophakia, ectopia lentis.

Whistling face-windmill vane hand syndrome.
Freeman-Sheldon syndrome.
0223   193700   759.8   AD
Prominent forehead, expressionless face, epicanthus,
deep-set eyes, small nose, hypoplastic alae nasi,
long philtrum, small puckered mouth, small tongue,
limited palatal movement, H-shaped dimple of chin,
hernias, ulnar deviation and contracture of fingers at
metacarpophalangeal joint, adduction of thumb,
equinovarus with contracted toes, vertical talus,
hypertonia, short stature, poor postnatal growth, and
in some cases, scoliosis, hip dislocation.

Wildervanck syndrome. Cervicooculoacoustic
syndrome.
3180   314600   759.8   AD
Klippel-Fiel anomaly, retractio bulbi (Duane
anomaly), congenital sensorineural deafness.

Williams syndrome.
0999   194050   759.8   AD
Small head, low nasal bridge, malar hypoplasia,
stellate pattern in iris, short nose, anteverted nares,
long philtrum, prominent patulous lips, small chin,
open mouth, hypodontia, supravalvular aortic
stenosis, multiple peripheral pulmonary arterial
stenoses, aorta hypoplasia, renal artery stenosis,
bladder diverticula, mental retardation, poor fetal
growth, short stature, poor postnatal growth, and in
some cases, infantile hypercalcemia. Many cases
have submicroscopic Chromosome 17q11.23
deletion in the elastin gene.

Additional References:

Buyse ML (editor). *Birth Defects Encyclopedia.* Cambridge, MA: Blackwell Scientific, 1990.

DeGrouchy J, Turleau C. *Clinical Atlas of Human Chromosomes*, 2nd edition. New York: Wiley, 1984.

Jones KL. *Smith's Recognizable Patterns of Human Malformation.* Philadelphia: Saunders, 1988.

McKusick VA. *Mendelian Inheritance in Man. Catalogs of Autosomal Dominant, Autosomal Recessive, and X-linked phenotypes*, 10th Edition. Baltimore: The Johns Hopkins Press, 1992.

Schinzel A. The Human Cytogenetics Database. Oxford: Oxford University Press, 1994.

******

(01) Head

Aplasia cutis congenita-transverse limb defect:, 349
- ulceration
  - Chromosome 13 trisomy, 358
- scaphocephaly
  - Chromosome 11q23 to qter deletion, 357
- sella turcica J-shaped
  - Mulibrey nanism, 369
- sinuses
  - frontal & sphenoid
    - absent
      - Otopalatodigital syndrome I, 370
- skull base
  - short & sclerotic
    - Schinzel-Giedion syndrome, 373
  - thick
    - Otopalatodigital syndrome I, 370
- small
  - Bloom syndrome, 351
  - Borjeson-Forssman-Lehmann syndrome, 351
  - Carbamazepine syndrome, 351
  - Coffin-Siris syndrome, 361
  - Fanconi pancytopenia, 363
  - Rubenstein-Taybi syndrome, 372
  - Williams syndrome, 376
- tower skull
  - Summitt syndrome, 374
- trigonocephaly
  - Chromosome 09 ring, 356
  - Chromosome 09p to 22pter deletion, 356
  - Chromosome 11q23 to qter deletion, 357
  - Chromosome 13q31 to q32 deletion, 357
  - Chromosome 13q32 to q34 deletion., 358
  - Opitz trigonocephaly syndrome, 370
- turricephaly
  - Chromosome 12p12 to pter partial duplication, 357
- Wormian bones
  - multiple
    - Mandibuloacral dysplasia, 367
    - Menkes syndrome, 368
    - Mohr syndrome, 368
    - Schinzel-Giedion syndrome, 373

(02) Ear

- antihelix prominent
  - Chromosome 04p distal duplication, 354
  - Chromosome 11q23 to qter deletion, 357
  - Chromosome 18q21 to qter deletion, 359
- antitragus
  - prominent
    - Chromosome 18q21 to qter deletion, 359
- architecture
  - flattened
    - Chromosome 04q partial deletion, 354
- canal
  - atresia
    - Hypertelorism-microtia-facial clefting, 365
  - atretic
    - Chromosome 18q21 to qter deletion, 359
  - large
    - Chromosome 21q21 to pter deletion, 359
  - small
    - Peters anomaly-short limb dwarfism, 371
- cartilage
  - calcification/ossification

- Keutel syndrome, 366
- deficient
  - Potter syndrome, 371
- hypoplasia
  - SC phocomelia syndrome, 373
- cochlea apex hypoplastic
  - Branchiootorenal dysplasia, 351
- cup-shaped
  - Branchiootorenal dysplasia, 351
  - Lacrimoauriculodentodigital syndrome, 366
- faunesque
  - Chromosome 18 trisomy, 359
- helix
  - folded
    - Chromosome 04q distal duplication, 354
  - foldedf upper
    - Trimethadione syndrome, 375
  - linear creases in posterior rim
    - Exomphalos-macroglossia-gigantism syndrome, 363
  - pointed
    - Chromosome 04q partial deletion, 354
- hypoplasia
  - Alopecia-anosmia-deafness-hypogonadism, 350
- large
  - Borjeson-Forssman-Lehmann syndrome, 351
  - Cerebrooculofacioskeletal syndrome, 352
  - Chromosome 03p25 to p26 duplication, 353
  - Chromosome 04p distal duplication, 354
  - Chromosome 04q distal duplication, 354
  - Chromosome 04q partial deletion, 354
  - Chromosome 09p13 to pter duplication, 356
  - Chromosome 10p partial duplication, 356
  - Chromosome 13q14 to qter deletion, 357
  - Chromosome 13q32 to q34 deletion., 358
  - Chromosome 18p partial deletion, 359
  - Chromosome X monosomy, 360
  - Coffin-Lowry syndrome, 361
  - Leprechaunism, 367
  - Townes syndrome, 375
  - Weaver syndrome, 376
- large & floppy
  - Microcephaly-hiatus hernia-nephrosis syndrome, 368
- large and malformed
  - Chromosome 02p23 to pter duplication, 353
  - Chromosome 08 trisomy, 355
- lobes large
  - Kabuki make-up sydrome, 365
- lobule
  - horizontal crease
    - Goldberg-Pashayan syndrome, 364
  - linear creases
    - Exomphalos-macroglossia-gigantism syndrome, 363
  - nodule
    - Goldberg-Pashayan syndrome, 364
- long
  - Chromosome XYY syndrome, 360
- lop
  - Anus-hand-ear syndrome, 350
- low-set
  - Ablepharon-macrostomia, 349
  - Chromosome 01q25 to q32 duplication, 353
  - Chromosome 02q23 to q32 deletion, 353
  - Chromosome 02q34 to qter duplication, 353
  - Chromosome 04q distal duplication, 354
  - Chromosome 05p partial duplication, 354
  - Chromosome 05q31 to qter duplication, 354
  - Chromosome 07p22 deletion, 355

Chromosome 08p partial duplication, 355
Chromosome 09q12 to q21 deletion, 356
Chromosome 10q24 to qter duplication, 356
Chromosome 11q23 to qter deletion, 357
Chromosome 11q23 to qter duplication, 357
Chromosome 12p12 to pter partial duplication, 357
Chromosome 13q31 to q32 deletion, 357
Chromosome 15pter to q21 duplication, 358
Chromosome triploidy, 360
King syndrome, 366
Miller-Dieker syndrome, 368
Myotonic myopathy-dwarfism-ocular-facial syndrome, 369
Noonan syndrome, 369
Opitz-Frias syndrome, 370
Pena-Shokeir syndrome I, 371
Rubenstein-Taybi syndrome, 372
low-set large
Chromosome 12p11 to p13 partial deletion, 357
Potter syndrome, 371
low-set malformed
Chromosome 01q25 to qter duplication, 353
Chromosome 03p25 to pter deletion, 353
Chromosome 03q21 to qter duplication, 353
Chromosome 06 ring, 355
Chromosome 06p distal duplication, 355
Chromosome 07q partial deletion, 355
Chromosome 07q32 to qter duplication, 355
Chromosome 09 trisomy, 356
Chromosome 09p to 22pter deletion, 356
Chromosome 09q partial duplication, 356
Chromosome 10p partial duplication, 356
Chromosome 10p13 to pter deletion, 356
Chromosome 13 trisomy, 358
Chromosome 13q13 to qter duplication, 358
Chromosome 18p partial deletion, 359
Chromosome 21q21 to pter deletion, 359
Chromosome 22 trisomy, 360
low-set posterior angulated
Kousseff syndrome, 366
malformation
Charge association, 352
Chromosome 05q31 to qter duplication, 354
Chromosome 06q partial duplication, 355
Chromosome 09 ring, 356
Chromosome 22q proximal duplication, 360
Cryptophthalmos syndrome, 361
DiGeorge syndrome, 362
Facioauriculoradial dysplasia, 363
internal
Facioauriculoradial dysplasia, 363
Mandibulofacial dysostosis, 367
Shprintzen syndrome, 373
unusual
Amniotic band syndrome, 350
microtia
Anus-hand-ear syndrome, 350
Hypertelorism-microtia-facial clefting, 365
Mandibulofacial dysostosis, 367
Miller syndrome, 368
Nager syndrome, 369
Oculoauriculovertebral dysplasia, 370
Retinoic acid syndrome, 372
Thalidomide syndrome, 374
Townes syndrome, 375
pinna
anteverted
Branchiootorenal dysplasia, 351

anteverted prominent
Cataract-dental syndrome, 351
pit prehelical
Branchiootorenal dysplasia, 351
preauricular tags
Chromosome 22 trisomy, 360
Chromosome 22q proximal duplication, 360
Nager syndrome, 369
Oculoauriculovertebral dysplasia, 370
Townes syndrome, 375
satyr
Anus-hand-ear syndrome, 350
simple
Chromosome 04p16 to pter deletion, 354
small
Chromosome 21 trisomy, 360

(03) Eye

albinism
Albinism with hemorrhagic diathesis, 349
almond-shaped
Chromosome 15pter to q21 duplication, 358
Chromosome 22 ring, 360
aniridia
Chromosome 11p13 partial deletion, 357
ankyloblepharon
Curly hair-ankyloblepharon-nail dysplasia syndrome, 361
ankyloblepharon filiforme adnatum
Cleft lip-palate and popliteal pterygium, 361
anophthalmos
Microphthalmia with multiple anomalies, 368
anterior chamber cleavage malformation
Peters anomaly-short limb dwarfism, 371
anterior synechiae
Rieger syndrome, 372
blepharophimosis
Alcohol syndrome, 350
Blepharophimosis-ptosis-epicanthus inversus, 351
Borjeson-Forssman-Lehmann syndrome, 351
Chromosome 04p distal duplication, 354
Chromosome 04q distal duplication, 354
Chromosome 06p distal duplication, 355
Chromosome 07q32 to qter duplication, 355
Chromosome 09 trisomy, 356
Chromosome 10q24 to qter duplication, 356
Chromosome 15pter to q21 duplication, 358
Chromosome 21q21 to pter deletion, 359
Cleft palate-contractures-Dandy-Walker malformation, 349
Ectrodactyly-ectrodermal dysplasia-clefting syndrome, 362
Marden-Walker syndrome, 367
Myotonic myopathy-dwarfism-ocular-facial syndrome, 369
Oculodentodigital dysplasia, 370
Peters anomaly-short limb dwarfism, 371
Shprintzen syndrome, 373
blepharophimosis lateral telecanthus
Dubowitz syndrome, 362
blindness
congenital
Renal dysplasia and retinal aplasia, 372
Sulfocysteinuria, 374
Brushfield spots
Cerebro-hepato-renal syndrome, 352
Chromosome 21 trisomy, 360
bulging

(04) Face

(05) Mouth

Angelman syndrome, 350
    Chromosome 03p25 to p26 duplication, 353
    Fryns syndrome, 363
    Mandibulofacial dysostosis, 367
    Oculoauriculovertebral dysplasia, 370
mandibular alveolar ridge flared
    Mohr syndrome, 368
microstomia
    Chromosome 13q14 to pter duplication, 358
    Hallerman-Streiff syndrome, 364
    Valproic acid syndrome, 375
open
    Williams syndrome, 376
open with protruding tongue
    Chromosome 21 trisomy, 360
palate
    high arch
        Kabuki make-up sydrome, 365
        Kallman syndrome, 365
    high arched
        Gorlin syndrome, 364
    movement limited
        Whistling face-windmill vane hand syndrome, 376
    narrow
        Kaufman oculocerebrofacial syndrome, 366
palate high arched
    Geroderma osteodysplasticum, 363
pursed, 354
rhagades
    perioral
        Syphilis syndrome, 374
small
    Chromosome 01q25 to q32 duplication, 353
    Chromosome 01q25 to qter duplication, 353
    Chromosome 06p distal duplication, 355
    Chromosome 09q partial duplication, 356
    Chromosome 21 monosomy, 359
    Pena-Shokeir syndrome I, 371
    Ruvalcaba syndrome, 373
small & puckered
    Whistling face-windmill vane hand syndrome, 376
smile asymmetric
    Chromosome 09p13 to pter duplication, 356
teeth
    anodontia
        Johanson-Blizzard syndrome, 365
        partial
            Deafness-congenital with onychodystrophy, 362
            Ellis-Van Creveld syndrome, 362
            Otopalatodigital syndrome I, 370
    anodontia partial
        Ectrodactyly-ectrodermal dysplasia-clefting syndrome, 362
    anomalies
        Chromosome 02q23 to q32 deletion, 353
        Chromosome 04p distal duplication, 354
    canines,molars
        large & bulbous
            Otodental dysplasia, 370
    conical
        Hays-Wells syndrome, 364
    coniform
        Deafness-congenital with onychodystrophy, 362
    crowded
        Robinow syndrome, 372
        Ruvalcaba syndrome, 373
    diastema
        Cataract-dental syndrome, 351

enamelogenesis imperfecta
    Oculodentodigital dysplasia, 370
Hutchinson
    Syphilis syndrome, 374
hypodontia
    Ectrodactyly-ectodermal dysplasia-macular dystrophy, 362
    Gorlin syndrome, 364
    Hallerman-Streiff syndrome, 364
    Hays-Wells syndrome, 364
    Incontinentia pigmenti, 365
    Williams syndrome, 376
hypoplasia
    Ablepharon-macrostomia, 349
    Focal dermal hypoplasia, 363
    Hallerman-Streiff syndrome, 364
incisors
    cone-shaped
        Cataract-dental syndrome, 351
    Hutchinsonian
        Cataract-dental syndrome, 351
incisors lower
    irregular
        Microphthalmia with multiple anomalies, 368
incisors upper lateral
    agenesis
        Microphthalmia with multiple anomalies, 368
large
    Chromosome XYY syndrome, 360
macrodontia
    KBG syndrome, 365
malformation
    Chromosome 20p11 to pter duplication, 359
    Cranioectodermal dysplasia, 361
    Oral-facial-digital syndrome III, 370
    Senter syndrome, 373
    Thalidomide syndrome, 374
maxillary incisors lateral
    peg-shaped & small
        Lacrimoauriculodentodigital syndrome, 366
microdontia
    Ectrodactyly-ectodermal dysplasia-macular dystrophy, 362
    Ectrodactyly-ectrodermal dysplasia-clefting syndrome, 362
molars
    mulberry
        Syphilis syndrome, 374
natal
    Ellis-Van Creveld syndrome, 362
    Polychlorinated biphenyl syndrome, 371
oligodontia
    Gorlin syndrome, 364
periodontal disease
    Alopecia-seizures-mental retardation, 350
premolar
    absence
        Otodental dysplasia, 370
pulp stones
    Otodental dysplasia, 370
small
    Tricho-dento-osseous syndrome, 375
supernumerary
    Cataract-dental syndrome, 351
taurodontia
    Otodental dysplasia, 370
taurodontism
    Tricho-dento-osseous syndrome, 375
wide-spaced & pitted
    Tricho-dento-osseous syndrome, 375

tongue
  absent
    Hypoglossia-hypodactyly, 365
  attachment aberrant
    Hypoglossia-hypodactyly, 365
  cleft
    Hypoglossia-hypodactyly, 365
  hamartoma
    Oral-facial-digital syndrome III, 370
  large
    Simpson dysmorphia syndrome, 373
  lateral clefts
    Oral-facial-digital syndrome type I, 370
  lobate
    Mohr syndrome, 368
  lobulated
    Oral-facial-digital syndrome III, 370
  macroglossia
    Chromosome 05p partial duplication, 354
    Chromosome 07q32 to qter duplication, 355
    Exomphalos-macroglossia-gigantism syndrome, 363
  microglossia
    Rutledge syndrome, 373
  small
    Hypoglossia-hypodactyly, 365
    Whistling face-windmill vane hand syndrome, 376
tongue thrusting
  Angelman syndrome, 350
uvula
  bifid
    Oral-facial-digital syndrome III, 370
wide
  Chromosome 14 trisomy, 358

(06) Neck

branchial cleft fistula
  Branchiootorenal dysplasia, 351
broad
  Chromosome 09p to 22pter deletion, 356
cervical spine hypermobility
  Faciogenital dysplasia, 363
Klippel-Fiel malformation
  MURCS association, 369
  Wildervanck syndrome, 376
movement limited
  Klippel-Fiel syndrome, 366
pterygium colli
  Chromosome 03q21 to qter duplication, 353
  Chromosome 18 trisomy, 359
  Chromosome 18 ring, 359
  Chromosome 18p partial deletion, 359
  Chromosome X monosomy, 360
  Lymphedema with distichiasis, 367
  Noonan syndrome, 369
  Watson syndrome, 376
short
  Chromosome 04p distal duplication, 354
  Chromosome 04q distal duplication, 354
  Chromosome 05q12 to q22 deletion, 354
  Chromosome 06 ring, 355
  Chromosome 07q32 to qter duplication, 355
  Chromosome 08p21 to pter deletion, 355
  Chromosome 09p13 to pter duplication, 356
  Chromosome 10q24 to qter duplication, 356

Chromosome 11q23 to qter duplication, 357
Chromosome 12p12 to pter partial duplication, 357
Chromosome 14pter to q23 duplication, 358
Chromosome 18 trisomy, 359
Chromosome 18 ring, 359
Chromosome 18p partial deletion, 359
Chromosome 19q13 to qter duplication, 359
Chromosome 21 trisomy, 360
Klippel-Fiel syndrome, 366
Kousseff syndrome, 366
Spondyloepiphyseal dysplasia-congenital, 374
skin
  redundant
    Cerebro-hepato-renal syndrome, 352
    Chromosome 01q32 to qter duplication, 353
    Chromosome 19q13 to qter duplication, 359

(07) Chest

breasts
  large
    Leprechaunism, 367
  broad
    Chromosome X monosomy, 360
    Noonan syndrome, 369
gynecomastia
  Chromosome XXY syndrome, 360
mammary glands
  absent
    Ulnar-mammary syndrome, 375
nipple
  absence
    Ulnar-mammary syndrome, 375
  hypoplasia
    Ablepharon-macrostomia, 349
    Ectrodactyly-ectrodermal dysplasia-clefting syndrome, 362
    Ulnar-mammary syndrome, 375
  wide-spaced
    Cerebrooculofacioskeletal syndrome, 352
    Chromosome 01q32 to qter duplication, 353
    Chromosome 03q21 to qter duplication, 353
    Chromosome 04p distal duplication, 354
    Chromosome 04q distal duplication, 354
    Chromosome 08p21 to pter deletion, 355
    Chromosome 09p to 22pter deletion, 356
    Chromosome 09p13 to pter duplication, 356
    Chromosome 10p13 to pter deletion, 356
    Chromosome 11q23 to qter duplication, 357
    Chromosome 18p partial deletion, 359
    Chromosome 18q21 to qter deletion, 359
    Chromosome 19q13 to qter duplication, 359
    Chromosome 20p11 to pter duplication, 359
    Chromosome X monosomy, 360
pectoralis major sternal head aplasia
  Poland syndrome, 371
pectus carinatum
  Coffin-Lowry syndrome, 361
  King syndrome, 366
  Marden-Walker syndrome, 367
  Myotonic myopathy-dwarfism-ocular-facial syndrome, 369
pectus excavatum
  Chromosome 03p25 to pter deletion, 353
  Noonan syndrome, 369
  Oral-facial-digital syndrome III, 370
  Otopalatodigital syndrome I, 370

shield
 Chromosome X monosomy, 360
 Noonan syndrome, 369
sternum
 distal cleft
  Pentalogy of Cantrell, 371
 malformation
  Chromosome 08 trisomy, 355
  Chromosome 08q2 to qter duplication, 355
 short
  Chromosome 12p12 to pter partial duplication, 357
  Chromosome 18 trisomy, 359
  Oral-facial-digital syndrome III, 370
 upper
  narrow
   Chromosome 09p13 to pter duplication, 356
   Chromosome 18 ring, 359
 wall defect
  Amniotic band syndrome, 350

(08) Respiratory

aspiration
 recurrent
  Opitz-Frias syndrome, 370
bronchi
 epiarterial
  Asplenia with cardiovascular anomalies, 350
 hyparterial
  Asplenia with cardiovascular anomalies, 350
choanal atresia
 Amniotic band syndrome, 350
 Charge association, 352
cry
 see voice, 352
diaphragmatic hernia
 anterior
  Pentalogy of Cantrell, 371
 Chromosome 19q13 to qter duplication, 359
 Fryns syndrome, 363
dysarthria
 Steinert syndrome, 374
larynx
 cartilage
  calcification/ossification
   Keutel syndrome, 366
 cleft
  Hall-Pallister syndrome, 364
lung
 bi-lobed bilaterally
  Asplenia with cardiovascular anomalies, 350
 lobulation abnormal
  Hall-Pallister syndrome, 364
  Hydrolethalus syndrome, 365
 tri-lobed bilaterally
  Asplenia with cardiovascular anomalies, 350
pulmonary fibrosis
 Albinism with hemorrhagic diathesis, 349
pulmonary hypoplasia
 Cloacal dysgenesis with female virilization, 361
 Pena-Shokeir syndrome I, 371
 Potter syndrome, 371
rhinitis
 perennial
  Syphilis syndrome, 374

trachea
 cartilage
  calcification/ossification
   Keutel syndrome, 366
 stenosis
  Hydrolethalus syndrome, 365
tracheoesophageal fistula
 VATER association, 375
voice
 dysphonic
  Chromosome 11p partial duplication, 357
 high-pitched
  Chromosome 01q partial deletion, 352
  Mulibrey nanism, 369
  Myotonic myopathy-dwarfism-ocular-facial syndrome, 369
 high-pitched and mewing
  Chromosome 05p15 deletion, 354
 hoarse & low-pitched
  Weaver syndrome, 376
 low and growling
  Cornelia de Lange syndrome, 361

(09) Cardiovascular

acrocyanosis
 Bullous dystrophy with macules, 351
arteries
 elongation and tortuosity
  Menkes syndrome, 368
asplenia
 Asplenia with cardiovascular anomalies, 350
cadiomyopathy
 progressive
  Genital anomaly-cardiomyopathy, 363
heart
 acardia
  Twin syndrome, 375
 aorta
  coarctation
   Chromosome X monosomy, 360
  hypoplasia
   Williams syndrome, 376
  supravalvular stenosis
   Williams syndrome, 376
 aortic arch anomalies
  DiGeorge syndrome, 362
 aortic valvulitis
  Syphilis syndrome, 374
 arrhythmia
  intervertricular conduction
   Heart hand syndrome-Spanish type, 364
  sinus conduction
   Heart hand syndrome-Spanish type, 364
  Steinert syndrome, 374
 atrial septal defect
  Alcohol syndrome, 350
  Ellis-Van Creveld syndrome, 362
  Holt-Oram syndrome, 364
  Schinzel-Giedion syndrome, 373
 conotruncal malformation
  Diabetes syndrome, 362
  Kousseff syndrome, 366
  Pentalogy of Cantrell, 371
 endocardial cushion defect
  Hydrolethalus syndrome, 365

left atria bilaterally
    Asplenia with cardiovascular anomalies, 350
malformation
    Catel-Manzke syndrome, 351
    Cerebro-hepato-renal syndrome, 352
    Charge association, 352
    Chromosome 01q25 to q32 duplication, 353
    Chromosome 02q23 to q32 deletion, 353
    Chromosome 02q34 to qter duplication, 353
    Chromosome 03p25 to p26 duplication, 353
    Chromosome 03q21 to qter duplication, 353
    Chromosome 04p16 to pter deletion, 354
    Chromosome 04q distal duplication, 354
    Chromosome 04q partial deletion, 354
    Chromosome 05p partial duplication, 354
    Chromosome 05p15 deletion, 354
    Chromosome 05q31 to qter duplication, 354
    Chromosome 06p distal duplication, 355
    Chromosome 07p22 deletion, 355
    Chromosome 08p partial duplication, 355
    Chromosome 08p21 to pter deletion, 355
    Chromosome 08q2 to qter duplication, 355
    Chromosome 09 trisomy, 356
    Chromosome 09 ring, 356
    Chromosome 09p to 22pter deletion, 356
    Chromosome 10p partial duplication, 356
    Chromosome 10p13 to pter deletion, 356
    Chromosome 10q24 to qter duplication, 356
    Chromosome 11q23 to qter deletion, 357
    Chromosome 11q23 to qter duplication, 357
    Chromosome 12p11 to p13 partial deletion, 357
    Chromosome 13 trisomy, 358
    Chromosome 13q14 to qter deletion, 357
    Chromosome 14 trisomy, 358
    Chromosome 14pter to q23 duplication, 358
    Chromosome 16q partial duplication, 358
    Chromosome 18 trisomy, 359
    Chromosome 18p partial deletion, 359
    Chromosome 18q21 to qter deletion, 359
    Chromosome 19q13 to qter duplication, 359
    Chromosome 20p11 to pter duplication, 359
    Chromosome 21 monosomy, 359
    Chromosome 21 trisomy, 360
    Chromosome 21q21 to pter deletion, 359
    Chromosome 22q proximal duplication, 360
    Chromosome triploidy, 360
    Chromosome X polysomy, 360
    Cocaine syndrome, 361
    complex
        Asplenia with cardiovascular anomalies, 350
    conotruncal
        Chromosome 01q25 to qter duplication, 353
        Chromosome 01q32 to qter duplication, 353
    Ellis-Van Creveld syndrome, 362
    Hall-Pallister syndrome, 364
    Holt-Oram syndrome, 364
    Hypertelorism-microtia-facial clefting, 365
    Ichthyosiform erythroderma with hemidysplasia, 365
    Kabuki make-up sydrome, 365
    McKusick-Kaufman syndrome, 367
    Microphthalmia with multiple anomalies, 368
    Miller-Dieker syndrome, 368
    Opitz trigonocephaly syndrome, 370
    Phenylketonuria-maternal, 371
    Rutledge syndrome, 373
    Shprintzen syndrome, 373
    Thrombocytopenia-absent radius syndrome, 374

    Trimethadione syndrome, 375
    VATER association, 375
P waves abnormal
    Leopard syndrome, 367
patent ductus arteriosus
    Hypertension syndrome, 365
    Rubella syndrome, 372
pericardial effusion
    Nephrosialidosis, 369
pericardioperitoneal foramen
    Pentalogy of Cantrell, 371
pericarditis
    restrictive
        Jacobs syndrome, 365
pericardium
    hyperplasia, fibrosis, giant cells
        Jacobs syndrome, 365
    thick & constrictive
        Mulibrey nanism, 369
peripheral pulmonic stenosis
    Cholestasis with peripheral pulmonary stenosis, 352
    Keutel syndrome, 366
    Rubella syndrome, 372
    Williams syndrome, 376
PR & QRS prolonged
    Leopard syndrome, 367
pulmonary vein anomalies
    Asplenia with cardiovascular anomalies, 350
pulmonic stenosis
    Cholestasis with peripheral pulmonary stenosis, 352
    Leopard syndrome, 367
    Noonan syndrome, 369
    Watson syndrome, 376
right atria bilaterally
    Asplenia with cardiovascular anomalies, 350
septal defect
    Noonan syndrome, 369
    Rubella syndrome, 372
tetralogy of Fallot
    DiGeorge syndrome, 362
valve defects
    Geleophysic dwarfism, 364
ventricular septal defect
    Alcohol syndrome, 350
    Asymmetric crying face syndrome, 350
    DiGeorge syndrome, 362
hypertension
    Brachydactyly and hypertension, 351
polysplenia
    Asplenia with cardiovascular anomalies, 350
systemic vein anomalies
    Asplenia with cardiovascular anomalies, 350
varicose veins
    Goeminne syndrome, 364

(10) Hematologic

agammaglobulinemia
    Metaphyseal chondrodysplasia-thymolymphopenia, 349
anemia
    hypoplastic congenital
        Anemia and triphalangeal thumb, 350
    Metaphyseal chondrodysplasia-McKusick type, 368
    Thrombocytopenia-absent radius syndrome, 374
bleeding diathesis

(11) Enteric

(12) Abdomen

(13) Renal

(14) Urinary

(15) Genital

(16) Skeletal

(17) Arm

transverse
  Aplasia cutis congenita-transverse limb defect, 349
humerus
  hypoplasia
    Femoral-facial syndrome, 363
    Thrombocytopenia-absent radius syndrome, 374
  lateral condyle aplasia
    Ophthalmomandibulomelic dysplasia, 370
  hypoplasia
    Amniotic band syndrome, 350
    Limb and Mullerian anomalies, 367
  long
    Chromosome 08 trisomy, 355
  malformation
    radial
      Chromosome 04q partial deletion, 354
  mesomelia
    Aminopterin syndrome, 350
  phocomelia
    Amniotic band syndrome, 350
  radioulnar synostosis
    Chromosome X polysomy, 360
radius
  aplasia
    Craniosynostosis with radial defects, 361
    Fanconi pancytopenia, 363
    Miller syndrome, 368
    Nager syndrome, 369
    Thrombocytopenia-absent radius syndrome, 374
  defect
    IVIC syndrome, 365
  dislocation
    Coffin-Siris syndrome, 361
  dysplasia
    Facioauriculoradial dysplasia, 363
  head
    dislocation
      Mietens syndrome, 368
      Pseudohermaphroditism with skeletal anomalies, 372
    hypoplastic
      Nail-patella syndrome, 369
  hypoplasia
    Anemia and triphalangeal thumb, 350
    Miller syndrome, 368
    Nager syndrome, 369
    Thrombocytopenia-absent radius syndrome, 374
    VATER association, 375
  malformation
    Rothmund-Thomson syndrome, 372
ulna
  aplasia
    Miller syndrome, 368
    Ulnar-mammary syndrome, 375
  distal aplasia
    Ophthalmomandibulomelic dysplasia, 370
  duplication
    Ulnar-mammary syndrome, 375
  hypoplasia
    Miller syndrome, 368
    Thrombocytopenia-absent radius syndrome, 374
    Ulnar-mammary syndrome, 375
  short and curved
    Craniosynostosis with radial defects, 361

(18) Hand

acheiria
  Aplasia cutis congenita-transverse limb defect:, 349
adactylia
  Aplasia cutis congenita-transverse limb defect, 349
broad
  Chromosome 12p12 to pter partial duplication, 357
clinodactyly
  Chromosome 02q34 to qter duplication, 353
  Chromosome 05q31 to qter duplication, 354
  Chromosome 06q partial duplication, 355
deformity
  positional
    Chromosome 04p distal duplication, 354
dermatoglyphics
  axial palmar triradius
    distal
      Chromosome 08p21 to pter deletion, 355
  axial triradius distal
    Chromosome 04p distal duplication, 354
  dermal ridge hypoplasia
    Chromosome 04p16 to pter deletion, 354
  dermal ridges sparse
    Pena-Shokeir syndrome I, 371
  digital arches excessive
    Chromosome 02p23 to pter duplication, 353
    Chromosome 04p16 to pter deletion, 354
    Chromosome 06q partial duplication, 355
    Chromosome 09p13 to pter duplication, 356
    Chromosome 18 trisomy, 359
    Deafness-congenital with onychodystrophy, 362
    Miller syndrome, 368
  digital large composite paterns excessive
    Chromosome 18q21 to qter deletion, 359
  digital low arches excessive
    Dilantin syndrome, 362
  digital radial loops excessive
    Chromosome 13 trisomy, 358
  digital ridge count low
    Chromosome 02q34 to qter duplication, 353
  digital triradius c and/or d absent
    Kabuki make-up sydrome, 365
  digital ulnar loops excessive
    Chromosome 05p partial duplication, 354
    Chromosome 21 trisomy, 360
    Kabuki make-up sydrome, 365
  digital whorls excessive
    Chromosome 03p25 to p26 duplication, 353
    Chromosome 04p distal duplication, 354
    Chromosome 09 ring, 356
    Chromosome 09p to 22pter deletion, 356
    Chromosome 18 ring, 359
    Smith-Lemli-Opitz syndrome, 374
  finger and palm creases absent
    Pena-Shokeir syndrome I, 371
  finger flexion creases
    absent
      Chromosome 08p partial duplication, 355
      Cleft palate-contractures-Dandy-Walker malformation, 349
    supernumerary
      Chromosome 09p to 22pter deletion, 356
  hypothenar loop
    Kabuki make-up sydrome, 365
  palmar axial triradius distal
    Chromosome 02q34 to qter duplication, 353

Chromosome 19q13 to qter duplication, 359
broad
  Anus-hand-ear syndrome, 350
  Chromosome 03q21 to qter duplication, 353
  Otopalatodigital syndrome I, 370
  Weaver syndrome, 376
broad & radial angulation
  Rubenstein-Taybi syndrome, 372
distal phalanx
  short
    IVIC syndrome, 365
distal phalanx hypoplastic
  Hirschsprung disease and brachydactyly, 364
double
  Microphthalmia with multiple anomalies, 368
  Townes syndrome, 375
finger-like
  Chromosome 22 trisomy, 360
  Dilantin syndrome, 362
  Townes syndrome, 375
flexion deformity
  Jacobs syndrome, 365
hypoplasia
  Chromosome 13q14 to qter deletion, 357
  Chromosome 13q21 deletion, 357
  Craniosynostosis with radial defects, 361
  Fanconi pancytopenia, 363
  IVIC syndrome, 365
  Nager syndrome, 369
  Townes syndrome, 375
  VATER association, 375
malformation
  Chromosome 04q distal duplication, 354
  Holt-Oram syndrome, 364
malposition
  Chromosome 09p13 to pter duplication, 356
  Chromosome 20p11 to pter duplication, 359
posterior placement
  Cornelia de Lange syndrome, 361
short
  Fibrodysplasia ossificans congenita, 363
  Hand-foot-genital syndrome, 364
supernumerary
  Anus-hand-ear syndrome, 350
triphalangeal
  Anemia and triphalangeal thumb, 350
  Anus-hand-ear syndrome, 350
  Deafness-congenital with onychodystrophy, 362
  Holt-Oram syndrome, 364
  Lacrimoauriculodentodigital syndrome, 366
wrinkled dorsal skin
  Acrodysostosis syndrome, 349
wrist
  bony anomalies
    Anus-hand-ear syndrome, 350
  carpal
    ulnar malformation
      Ulnar-mammary syndrome, 375
  carpal bone fusion
    Symphalangism syndrome, 374
  carpal bones accessory
    Holt-Oram syndrome, 364
  carpal defect
    radial
      IVIC syndrome, 365
  carpal malformation
    Craniosynostosis with radial defects, 361

contracture
  Cleft palate-contractures-Dandy-Walker malformation, 349
trapezoid-scaphoid fusion
  Hand-foot-genital syndrome, 364
wrist thick
  Gangliosidosis Gm1 type I, 363

(19) Leg

absence
  unilateral
    Leg absence with congenital cataract, 366
absence defect
  Urethral obstruction sequence, 375
amputation
  Amniotic band syndrome, 350
bones
  aplastic
    Roberts syndrome, 372
  hypoplasia
    SC phocomelia syndrome, 373
constriction bands
  Amniotic band syndrome, 350
femoral epiphysis
  fragmented
    Myotonic myopathy-dwarfism-ocular-facial syndrome, 369
femoral neck
  short
    KBG syndrome, 365
femur
  hypoplasia
    Femoral-facial syndrome, 363
fibula
  hypoplasia
    Facioauriculoradial dysplasia, 363
    Femoral-facial syndrome, 363
fusion
  Sirenomelia sequence, 373
genu recurvatum
  Faciogenital dysplasia, 363
hemangioma hypertrophy
  Klippel-Trenaunay-Weber syndrome, 366
hemimelia
  transverse
    Aplasia cutis congenita-transverse limb defect, 349
hip
  dislocation
    Cleidocranial dysplasia, 361
    Dilantin syndrome, 362
    Geroderma osteodysplasticum, 363
    Whistling face-windmill vane hand syndrome, 376
  dysplasia
    Caudal regression syndrome, 351
    Chromosome 05q12 to q22 deletion, 354
    Stickler syndrome, 374
  malformation
    Chromosome 11q23 to qter duplication, 357
    Chromosome 20p11 to pter duplication, 359
    Chromosome 22 trisomy, 360
  narrow
    Chromosome 08 trisomy, 355
    Chromosome 08q2 to qter duplication, 355
    Chromosome 09q partial duplication, 356
  narrow malformed
    Chromosome 18 trisomy, 359

hypoplasia
  Amniotic band syndrome, 350
knee
  extension limited
    Weaver syndrome, 376
long
  Chromosome 08 trisomy, 355
muscles short
  Mouth inability to open and short finger flexor tendons, 368
ossification delayed
  Spondyloepiphyseal dysplasia-congenital, 374
patella
  absent
    Nail-patella syndrome, 369
  hypoplasia
    Nail-patella syndrome, 369
phocomelia
  Amniotic band syndrome, 350
popliteal pterygium
  Cleft lip-palate and popliteal pterygium, 361
shin
  saber
    Syphilis syndrome, 374
sirenomelia
  Sirenomelia sequence, 373
  Twin syndrome, 375
tibia
  fibrous dysplasia
    Mulibrey nanism, 369
  hypoplasia
    Ellis-Van Creveld syndrome, 362

(20) Foot

ankle
  bony anomalies
    Anus-hand-ear syndrome, 350
apodia
  Aplasia cutis congenita-transverse limb defect, 349
club
  Catel-Manzke syndrome, 351
  Chromosome 04p16 to pter deletion, 354
  Chromosome 05q12 to q22 deletion, 354
  Chromosome 10p partial duplication, 356
  Cleft palate-contractures-Dandy-Walker malformation, 349
  Schinzel-Giedion syndrome, 373
cuneiform-navicular fusion
  Hand-foot-genital syndrome, 364
deformity
  positional
    Chromosome 04p distal duplication, 354
dermatoglyphics
  hallucal arch fibular or S
    Chromosome 13 trisomy, 358
  hallucal loop tibial
    Chromosome 13 trisomy, 358
equinovarus
  Escobar syndrome, 362
equinovarus with contracted toes
  Whistling face-windmill vane hand syndrome, 376
hallux
  bifid
    Goldberg-Pashayan syndrome, 364
    Mohr syndrome, 368
  broad

Goldberg-Pashayan syndrome, 364
    Otopalatodigital syndrome I, 370
    Rubenstein-Taybi syndrome, 372
  distal phalanx absence
    Cleidocranial dysplasia, 361
  distal phalanx hypoplastic
    Hirschsprung disease and brachydactyly, 364
  double
    Townes syndrome, 375
  duplication partial
    Pre/postaxial polydactyly-absent corpus callosum, 372
  finger-like
    Townes syndrome, 375
  hammer toe
    Chromosome 10q24 to qter duplication, 356
  hypoplasia
    Townes syndrome, 375
  proximal phalanx hypoplasia
    Cleidocranial dysplasia, 361
  short
    Hand-foot-genital syndrome, 364
  short dorsiflexed
    Chromosome 18 trisomy, 359
  short monophalangeal
    Fibrodysplasia ossificans congenita, 363
hamartoma
  subcutaneous
    Proteus syndrome, 372
ketatosis plantaris
  Knuckle pads-leukonychia-deafness, 366
large
  Mulibrey nanism, 369
  Sotos syndrome, 374
long
  Chromosome 09p to 22pter deletion, 356
malformation
  Chromosome 03q21 to qter duplication, 353
metatarsal
  lateral short
    Ruvalcaba syndrome, 373
metatarsal 1 short
  Hand-foot-genital syndrome, 364
metatarsal fusion
  Anus-hand-ear syndrome, 350
metatarsals
  short
    Trichorhinophalangeal syndrome, 375
pes cavus
  Kallman syndrome, 365
pes planus
  Chromosome 12p12 to pter partial duplication, 357
  Geroderma osteodysplasticum, 363
polydactyly
  Amniotic band syndrome, 350
  postaxial
    Pre/postaxial polydactyly-absent corpus callosum, 372
position abnormal
  Potter syndrome, 371
positional deformity
  Chromosome 01q partial deletion, 352
rocker-bottom
  Bowen Hutterite syndrome, 351
  Chromosome 13 trisomy, 358
  Escobar syndrome, 362
short broad
  Chromosome 21 trisomy, 360
small

(21) Integument

newborn
    Herpes simplex syndrome, 364
vesiculation
    whorl-like
        Incontinentia pigmenti, 365
vitiligo
    Deafness-congenital-vitiligo-achalasia, 362

(22) Neurologic

anencephaly
    Amniotic band syndrome, 350
    Twin syndrome, 375
anosmia
    Kallman syndrome, 365
    Thumb agenesis-dwarfism-immunodeficiency, 374
anterior horn cells deficient
    Pena-Shokeir syndrome I, 371
apnea
    Chromosome 19q13 to qter duplication, 359
apneic spells
    Schinzel-Giedion syndrome, 373
areflexia
    Cerebro-hepato-renal syndrome, 352
    Cholestasis with peripheral pulmonary stenosis, 352
arrhinencephaly
    Chromosome 13 trisomy, 358
    Chromosome 18 ring, 359
    Chromosome 18p partial deletion, 359
arthrogryposis
    Cerebrooculofacioskeletal syndrome, 352
    King syndrome, 366
ataxic gait
    Angelman syndrome, 350
athetosis
    Oculocerebral syndrome with hypopigmentation, 370
behavior
    aberrant
        Chromosome 20 ring, 359
    abrupt
        Chromosome XYY syndrome, 360
    antisocial
        Chromosome XXY syndrome, 360
        Chromosome XYY syndrome, 360
brain
    hemangioma
        Klippel-Trenaunay-Weber syndrome, 366
        Sturge-Weber syndrome, 374
    malformation
        Meckel syndrome, 368
brain stem
    hypoplasia
        Marden-Walker syndrome, 367
cebocephaly
    Chromosome 18 ring, 359
cerebellar ataxia
    Kallman syndrome, 365
    Marinesco-Sjogren syndrome, 367
    Piebald trait with neurologic defects, 371
cerebellum
    hypoplasia
        Bowen Hutterite syndrome, 351
        Marden-Walker syndrome, 367
        Marinesco-Sjogren syndrome, 367
cerebral calcifications

Cytomegalovirus syndrome, 361
    Toxoplasmosis syndrome, 375
cerebral cortex
    gliosis and atrophy
        Menkes syndrome, 368
cerebral malformation
    Chromosome 21q21 to pter deletion, 359
claw hand
    Gangliosidosis Gm1 type I, 363
contractures
    Chromosome 12p tetrasomy mosaicism, 357
    Marinesco-Sjogren syndrome, 367
coordination
    poor
        Chromosome 08 trisomy, 355
        Chromosome 09p13 to pter duplication, 356
        Chromosome XYY syndrome, 360
corpus callosum
    absence
        Chromosome 08p partial duplication, 355
        Oral-facial-digital syndrome type I, 370
    absent or hypoplastic
        Pre/postaxial polydactyly-absent corpus callosum, 372
    agenesis partial
        FG syndrome, 363
    hypoplasia
        Cerebro-hepato-renal syndrome, 352
cranial nerve palsies
    Hypoglossia-hypodactyly, 365
Dandy-Walker malformation
    Cleft palate-contractures-Dandy-Walker malformation, 349
deafness
    Chromosome 13 trisomy, 358
    Chromosome 21 trisomy, 360
    cochlear
        Waardenberg syndrome, 375
    Cockayne syndrome II, 361
    conductive
        Alopecia-anosmia-deafness-hypogonadism, 350
        Craniosynostosis with radial defects, 361
        Gorlin syndrome, 364
        Miller syndrome, 368
        Mohr syndrome, 368
        Otopalatodigital syndrome I, 370
        Otopalatodigital syndrome II, 371
        Symphalangism syndrome, 374
    congenital
        sensorineural
            Deafness-congenital with onychodystrophy, 362
    Cytomegalovirus syndrome, 361
    Facioauriculoradial dysplasia, 363
    Hypertelorism-microtia-facial clefting, 365
    Johanson-Blizzard syndrome, 365
    Klippel-Fiel syndrome, 366
    Kneist syndrome, 366
    Mandibulofacial dysostosis, 367
    neural
        Albinism-deafness syndrome, 349
    Peters anomaly-short limb dwarfism, 371
    Piebald trait with neurologic defects, 371
    Rubella syndrome, 372
    sensorineural
        Anus-hand-ear syndrome, 350
        Branchiootorenal dysplasia, 351
        Charge association, 352
        congenital
            Knuckle pads-leukonychia-deafness, 366

(23) Endocrine

(24) Dimension

(25) Course

elevated in urine
    Sulfocysteinuria, 374
sulfite oxidase absent
    Sulfocysteinuria, 374
sweat electrolytes elevated
    Deafness-congenital with onychodystrophy, 362
thiosulfate
    elevated in urine
        Sulfocysteinuria, 374
toxoplasmosis
    Microcephaly-chorioretinitis, 368
urinary keratan sulfate excessive
    Gangliosidosis Gm1 type I, 363
varicella severe
    Metaphyseal chondrodysplasia-McKusick type, 368
weight gain
    poor
        Marshall-Smith syndrome, 367
Wilms tumor
    Chromosome 11p13 partial deletion, 357

(26) Disorder

Ablepharon-macrostomia, 349
Acrodysostosis syndrome, 349
Albinism with hemorrhagic diathesis, 349
Albinism-deafness syndrome, 349
Alcohol syndrome, 349
Alopecia-anosmia-deafness-hypogonadism, 350
Alopecia-mental retardation, 350
Alopecia-seizures-mental retardation, 350
Alopecia-skeletal anomalies-mental retardation, 350
Aminopterin syndrome, 350
Amniotic band syndrome, 350
Anemia and triphalangeal thumb, 350
Angelman syndrome, 350
Anus-hand-ear syndrome, 350
Aplasia cutis congenita-transverse limb defect, 349
Asplenia-polysplenia syndrome, 350
Asymmetric crying face syndrome, 350
Bardet-Biedl syndrome, 350
Biemond II syndrome, 351
Blepharochalasis and double lip, 351
Blepharophimosis-ptosis-epicanthus inversus, 351
Bloom syndrome, 351
Borjeson-Forssman-Lehmann syndrome, 351
Bowen Hutterite syndrome, 351
Brachydactyly and hypertension, 351
Branchiootorenal dysplasia, 351
Bullous dystrophy with macules, 351
Carbamazepine syndrome, 351
Cataract-dental syndrome, 351
Cataract-ichthyosis syndrome, 351
Catel-Manzke syndrome, 351
Caudal regression syndrome, 351
Cerebrocostomandibular syndrome, 351
Cerebro-hepato-renal syndrome, 352
Cerebrooculofacioskeletal syndrome, 352
Charge association, 352
Chediak-Higashi syndrome, 352
Cholestasis with peripheral pulmonary stenosis, 352
Chondrodysplasia punctata-asymmetric, 352
Chondrodysplasia punctata-mild, 352
Chondrodysplasia punctata-rhizomelic, 352
Chromosome 01 ring, 353

Chromosome 01q25 to q32 duplication, 353
Chromosome 01q25 to qter duplication, 352
Chromosome 01q32 to qter duplication, 353
Chromosome 01q42 to qter deletion, 352
Chromosome 02p23 to pter duplication, 353
Chromosome 02q23 to q32 deletion, 353
Chromosome 02q34 to qter duplication, 353
Chromosome 03p25 to p26 duplication, 353
Chromosome 03p25 to pter deletion, 353
Chromosome 03q21 to qter duplication, 353
Chromosome 04 ring
    see Chromosome 04q partial deletion, 354
Chromosome 04p distal duplication, 354
Chromosome 04p16 to pter deletion, 353
Chromosome 04q distal duplication, 354
Chromosome 04q partial deletion, 354
Chromosome 05p partial duplication, 354
Chromosome 05p15 deletion, 354
Chromosome 05q12 to q22 deletion, 354
Chromosome 05q31 to qter duplication, 354
Chromosome 06 ring, 355
Chromosome 06p distal duplication, 354
Chromosome 06q partial duplication, 355
Chromosome 07p22 deletion, 355
Chromosome 07q partial deletion, 355
Chromosome 07q32 to qter duplication, 355
Chromosome 08 trisomy, 355
Chromosome 08p partial duplication, 355
Chromosome 08p21 to pter deletion, 355
Chromosome 08q2 to qter duplication, 355
Chromosome 09 ring, 356
Chromosome 09 trisomy, 356
Chromosome 09q partial duplication, 356
Chromosome 10p partial duplication, 356
Chromosome 10p13 to pter deletion, 356
Chromosome 10q24 to qter duplication, 356
Chromosome 11p partial duplication, 357
Chromosome 11p13 partial deletion, 357
Chromosome 11q23 to qter deletion, 357
Chromosome 11q23 to qter duplication, 357
Chromosome 12p tetrasomy mosaicism, 357
Chromosome 12p11 to p13 partial deletion, 357
Chromosome 12p12 to pter partial duplication, 357
Chromosome 13 ring
    see Chromosome 13q31 to q32 deletion, 357
    see Chromosome 13q32 to q34 deletion, 358
Chromosome 13 trisomy, 358
Chromosome 13q13 to pter duplication, 358
Chromosome 13q14 to pter duplication, 358
Chromosome 13q14 to qter deletion, 357
Chromosome 13q21 deletion, 357
Chromosome 13q31 to q32 deletion, 357
Chromosome 13q32 to q34 deletion, 358
Chromosome 14 trisomy, 358
Chromosome 14pter to q23 duplication, 358
Chromosome 15 distal duplication, 358
Chromosome 15 maternal uniparental disomy
    Prader-Willi syndrome, 372
Chromosome 15 paternal uniparental disomy
    Angelman syndrome, 350
Chromosome 15 ring, 358
Chromosome 15pter to q21 duplication, 358
Chromosome 15q11-q13 deletion
    Angelman syndrome, 350
    Prader-Willi syndrome, 372
Chromosome 16q partial duplication, 358
Chromosome 17p13.3 deletion, 368

organic gas chromatography, 125
organism
    invading, 141
organomegaly, 214
Oriental, 152
Orkin SH (1987), 256
ornithine, 128
ornithine amino transferase, 128
ornithine carbamyl transcarbamyl, 133
Ornithine transcarbamalase deficiency
    DNA diagnosis, 104
ornithine transcarbamylase, 128
ornithine transcarbamylase deficiency
    treatment, 267, 268
ornithinemia with gyrate atrophy, 128
oro-facio-digital 1 syndrome
    corpus callosum anomaly, 55
orofaciodigital syndrome I, 171
oropharynx
    small, 109
orotate, 125
orotic, 128
orotic aciduria, 138
    treatment, 267
ossified ear cartilage, 335
osteodysplasia
    corpus callosum anomaly, 55
osteogenesis imperfecta, 238
osteogenesis imperfecta II, 190
osteogenesis imperfectas, 138
osteogensis imperfecta phenotype variability, 245
osteogensis imperfecta types, 245
osteoma, 214
osteomas, 57
osteoporosis, 239
OTC deficiency, 128, 131, 133
otopalatodigital syndrome I, 171
otosclerosis, 204
ototoxicity
    drug induced, 263
outbreak of deformed children, 88
outbred population, 48
outer canthal norms, 318
Outhit MC (1933), 56, 196
ovarian cancer, 214
ovarian carcinoma, 119
ovarian cystadenocarcinoma, 207
ovaries
    hypoplastic, 119
    primordial, 119
ovary
    polycystic, 216
ovulation, 25, 26, 28
    multiple, 146
ovulation induction, 147
ovum, 16, 27
    mitochondria, 16
oxaluria, 138
oxidative phosphorylation defect, 253
oxydative phosphorylation enzyme, 16

P arm, 14

P site, 18
p53, 208, 214
pachytene, 25
pain in toes, 52

palatal anomaly, 273
palatal shelf, 170
palate
    cleft, 170
    high-arched, 170
    primary, 170
    submucous cleft, 170
palate formation, 170
palindromic, 28
palm dermatoglyphic pattern, 334
palm dermatoglyphic symmetry, 334
palm length norms, 328
palmar pits, 214
palpebral fissure
    down-slanting, 171
palpebral fissure norms, 318
palpitation, 218
pamaquine
    adverse effect, 263
pancreas
    cancer, 214
    tumor, 187
pancreatic enzymopathies, 138
pancreatic lipase deficiency, 138
pancytopenia, 191
pancytopenia, 112
papilloma, 114
paracentric inversion, 40
parallelism, 201
paralysis, 253
    anesthesia, 259
    drug induced, 264
paranoia, 84
paraplegia, 55
parasitic twin, 147, 148
parathyroid
    tumor, 187
parent, 153, 285
    infertile, 289
    surrogate, 289
parent counseling, 291
parent of origin, 59
parentage, 146
    exclusion, 146
    likelihood of, 154
    local population data, 146
    proof, 146
    proof of, 154
parentage exclusion, 152
parentage testing, 96, 143, 144, 152
    DNA, 144
parental age, 84
parental consanguinity, 54
parental exclusion, 144, 153
parental genotype, 67
parent-child mating, 60
parenthood norms, 286
parents
    consanguineous, 60
parietal foramina, 335
Parker LS (1994), 296
parkinsonian movements, 54
Parkinsonism
    Charcot-Marie-Tooth disease, 53
paroxysmal hypertension, 218
paroxysmal noctournal hemoglobinuria, 114
Parrish ML, Roessmann U, Levinsohn MW (1979), 65